AF342558

KIN, GENE, COMMUNITY

Fertility, Reproduction and Sexuality

Volume 1
Managing Reproductive Life: Cross-Cultural Themes in Fertility & Sexuality
Edited by Soraya Tremayne

Volume 2
Modern Babylon? Prostituting Children in Thailand
Heather Montgomery

Volume 3
Reproductive Agency, Medicine & the State: Cultural Transformations in Childbearing
Edited by Maya Unnithan-Kumar

Volume 4
A New Look at Thai AIDS: Perspectives from the Margin
Graham Fordham

Volume 5
Breast Feeding & Sexuality: Behaviour, Beliefs & Taboos among the Gogo Mothers in Tanzania
Mara Mabilia

Volume 6
Ageing without Children: European & Asian Perspectives on Elderly Access to Support Networks
Philip Kreager & Elisabeth Schröder-Butterfill

Volume 7
Nameless Relations: Anonymity, Melanesia and Reproductive Gift Exchange between British Ova Donors and Recipients
Monica Konrad

Volume 8
Population, Reproduction & Fertility in Melanesia
Edited by Stanley J. Ulijaszek

Volume 9
Conceiving Kinship: Assisted Conception, Procreation & Family in Southern Europe
Monica M. E. Bonaccorso

Volume 10
Where There is No Midwife: Birth & Loss in Rural India
Sarah Pinto

Volume 11
Reproductive Disruptions: Gender, Technology, & Biopolitics in the New Millennium
Edited by Marcia C. Inhorn

Volume 12
Reconceiving the Second Sex: Men, Masculinity, and Reproduction
Edited by Marcia C. Inhorn, Tine Tjørnhøj- Thomsen, Helene Goldberg & Maruska la Cour Mosegaard

Volume 13
Transgressive Sex: Subversion & Control in Erotic Encounters
Edited by Hastings Donnan & Fiona Magowan

Volume 14
European Kinship in the Age of Biotechnology
Edited by Jeanette Edwards & Carles Salazar

Volume 15
Kinship and Beyond: The Genealogical Model Reconsidered
Edited by Sandra Bamford & James Leach

Volume 16
Islam and New Kinship: Reproductive Technology & the Shariah in Lebanon
Morgan Clarke

Volume 17
Childbirth: Midwifery & Concepts of Time
Edited by Chris McCourt

Volume 18
Assisting Reproduction, Testing Genes: Global Encounters with the New Biotechnologies
Edited by Daphna Birenbaum-Carmeli & Marcia C. Inhorn

Volume 19
Kin, Gene, Community: Reproductive Technologies among Jewish Israelis
Edited by Daphna Birenbaum-Carmeli & Yoram S. Carmeli

KIN, GENE, COMMUNITY
REPRODUCTIVE TECHNOLOGIES AMONG JEWISH ISRAELIS

Edited by

Daphna Birenbaum-Carmeli
and Yoram S. Carmeli

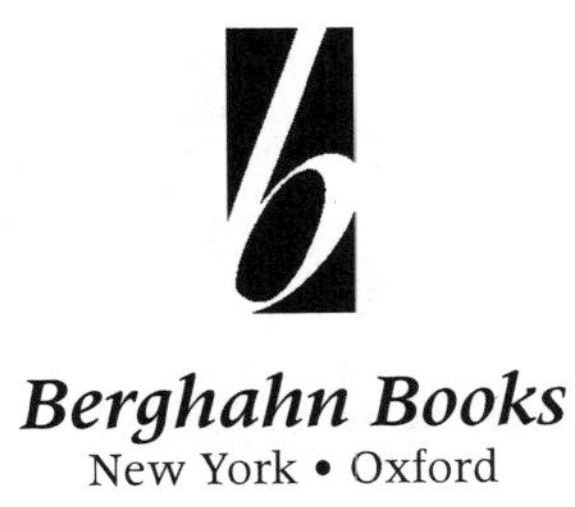

Berghahn Books
New York • Oxford

Library of Congress Cataloging-in-Publication Data

Kin, gene, community : reproductive technologies among Jewish
    Israelis / edited by Daphna Birenbaum-Carmeli and Yoram S.
    Carmeli.
        p. cm. — (Fertility, reproduction, and sexuality ; v. 19)
    Includes bibliographical references and index.
    ISBN 978-1-84545-688-7 (hardback : alk. paper)
    1. Human reproductive technology—Israel.   I. Birenbaum-
Carmeli, Daphna.   II. Carmeli, Yoram S.
    RG133.5.K56 2010
    362.198'1780095694—dc22   2010007980

British Library Cataloguing in Publication Data

A catalogue record for this book is available
from the British Library.
Printed in the United States on acid-free paper

ISBN 978-1-84545-688-7 (hardback)

CONTENTS

List of Tables and Figures   vii

Introduction: Reproductive Technologies among Jewish Israelis:
Setting the Ground   1
Daphna Birenbaum-Carmeli and Yoram S. Carmeli

PART I
Kin: Reproductive Technologies and
The Quest For Biogenetic Parenthood

1. The Contribution of Israeli Researchers to Reproductive
Medicine: Fertility Experts' Perspectives   51
*Shlomo Mashiach, Daphna Birenbaum-Carmeli, Roy Mashiach
and Martha Dirnfeld*

2. The Regulation of Preimplantation Genetic Diagnosis
for Sibling Donors in Israel, Germany, and England:
A Comparative Look at Balancing Risks and Benefits   61
Yael Hashiloni-Dolev and Shiri Shkedi

3. The Man in the Sperm: Kinship and Fatherhood in Light
of Male Infertility in Israel   84
Helene Goldberg

4. The Last Outpost of the Nuclear Family: A Cultural
Critique of Israeli Surrogacy Policy   107
Elly Teman

5. Adoption and Assisted Reproduction Technologies:
A Comparative Reading of Israeli Policies   127
Daphna Birenbaum-Carmeli and Yoram S. Carmeli

PART II
Gene: Reproductive Technologies and
The Quest For The Perfect Child

6. Genetic Testing and Screening in Religious Groups:
Perspectives of Jewish *Haredi* Communities   153
Barbara Prainsack and Gil Sigal

7. Ultrasonic Challenges to Pro-Natalism   174
Tsipy Ivry

8. Abortion Committees as Agents of Eugenics: Medical
and Public Views on Selective Abortion Following
Mild or Likely Fetal Pathology   202
Nitzan Rimon-Zarfaty and Aviad Raz

9. Cultural Values in Action: The Israeli Approach to
Human Cloning   226
Gali Ben-Or and Vardit Ravitsky

PART III
Community: A Self-Portrait With Technology

10. ART, Community, and Beyond: Human Embryonic Stem Cell
Research in Israel—Interviews with Prof. Nissim Benvenisty
and Prof. Karl Skorecki   255
Interview and Introduction: *Daphna Birenbaum-Carmeli*

11. Medicine and the State: The Medicalization of Reproduction
in Israel   271
Yali Hashash

12. The Mirth of the Clinic: Fieldnotes from an Israeli
Fertility Center   296
Susan Martha. Kahn

13. Between Reproductive Citizenship and Consumerism:
Attitudes towards Assisted Reproductive Technologies
among Jewish and Arab Israeli Women   318
Larissa Remennick

14. Ethnography, Exegesis, and Jewish Ethical Reflection:
The New Reproductive Technologies in Israel   340
Don Seeman

Notes on Contributors   363

Index   369

Tables and Figures

Tables

Introduction

1. Israel – General and Family Characteristics   5

2. Fertility rates by year and religion   9

3. TFR in the Orthodox community vs. all other Jewish Israelis   11

4. Child allowance in various countries (in USD)   14

5. Maternity Leave regulations in selected industrialized countries   15

6. Uptake of prenatal screening tests: Jewish Israeli women by religiosity and age (as percentage)   26

Chapter 2

7. Appendix: The main differences between Israel, England and Germany   79

Chapter 5

8. Selected adoption guidelines: International profiles   130

9. Intercountry adoptions per 1,000 live births   131

Chapter 6

10. Demographic parameters (in %)   162

11. Knowledge and Practices (in %)   164

12. Attitudes towards genetic testing in general and DY in
particular (in %)   165

Chapter 13

13. Socio-demographic characteristics of focus group participants   322

Figures

Introduction

1. TFR by religious groups, 1996, 2000, 2006   9

2. Number of IVF cycles per year in Israel   17

3. Number of IVF cycles per million per annum   18

Introduction

Reproductive Technologies among Jewish Israelis: Setting the Ground

---

Daphna Birenbaum-Carmeli and Yoram S. Carmeli

The tremendous expansion of medical technologies involved in various aspects of human reproduction has been described and analyzed extensively over more than two decades now. Generally speaking, technologies in this domain can be divided into three subcategories. The first includes procreative, namely conception-enabling technologies, currently centered around in vitro fertilization (IVF) and its varied derivatives: intracytoplasmic sperm injection (ICSI) to overcome male infertility; testicular biopsy and aspiration; electro-ejaculation for spinal-cord-injured males; ooplasmic transfer from a younger woman's to an older woman's ova to improve ova quality; third-party donation (and sale) of sperm, ova, and embryos; removal and freezing of human ovaries for later use in cancer survivors and postmenopausal women; cryopreservation, or long-term freezing of sperm, embryos, and, most recently, ova; and surrogacy. It is estimated that since 1978, over three million children have been born using these technologies (ESHRE 2006). We refer to this assortment of technologies as assisted reproduction technologies (ARTs).

The second category of technologies is applied in order to obtain information regarding a future or existing fetus. Central, though not exclusive, to this category are genetic tests, such as premarital genetic profiling of potential spouses, preimplantation genetic diagnoses to screen IVF embryos for genetic defects or to select embryos of a certain sex (PGD); microsorting of sperm for the purposes of sex selection; multifetal pregnancy reduction (so-called "selective abortion") in high-order IVF pregnancies; as well as older technologies like obstetrical ultrasound, alpha fetoprotein screening, chorionic villus sampling (CVS) and amniocentesis. Aiming at an existing child rather than a fetus is the technology of DNA-based paternity testing of children. To distinguish this group of technologies from the former, we call them reproductive technologies (RTs).

A third group of technologies uses reproductive medicine as a platform for the development of new domains of medical research and therapy. Most prominent in this category is the burgeoning field of human embryonic stem cell (hESC) research, and the disputed cloning of genetic material for the production of animals (e.g., Dolly the sheep) or, potentially, humans.[1]

The impact of these technologies has been observed through the private and the public, the biological and the social, the local and the global, and they have influenced major contemporary processes like the conceptual deconstruction of the human body, the commodification of human gametes and body parts, and the biopolitics of individual and communal identities (Strathern 1992a, 1992b, 2005; Franklin 1997, 2007; Franklin and McKinnon 2001, Franklin and Roberts 2006; Nelkin and Lindee 2004). So much so that reproductive technologies may themselves be considered a prominent emblem of the era.

Our general theoretical perspective in this volume is that reproductive technologies, like all technologies, are a socio-technical product shaped by their economic, political, and cultural environment, finding social acceptance and application when compatible with and as part of existing perceptions, interests, and power relations (Wyatt 2007). Technology, identity, and power, in the wide societal sense, are therefore viewed as mutually constitutive, each being a source and a consequence of the others. Through probing the application of a variety of reproductive technologies, ranging from donor insemination to surrogacy, adoption, abortion, pre-implantation genetic diagnosis, and human embryonic stem cell research, and through applying a variety of methodological approaches—ethnography, interviews, focus groups, policy analysis, and textual analysis—the chapters here add up to offer a composite portrait of a social reproductive landscape. Political, economic, historical, and cultural processes comprise a vehicle through which technologies and social contexts are examined as forming and reforming one another. Thus, on a still more general level, the issues addressed in this volume illuminate how nature is being construed as a technology of dominance; how genetics is weaved into the production and reproduction of politicized identities; and how the endorsement of reproductive technologies can be used to govern populations as well as scientific work and to enhance internal and external collective boundaries.

This volume juxtaposes "bottom up" with "top down" perspectives. A few chapters focus on the personal encounters of women and men with reproductive technologies in Israel, describing and analyzing individual adaptation to, modification of, and resistance to these technologies. Other chapters take a more macrosociological perspective when tracing Israel's political economy of fertility, showing the embeddedness of community institutions in cultural, political, economic, and professional structures and processes that operate at the local and global levels. The activity of human subjects is thus located within structured contexts that are themselves the products of past activity, but which currently exert power influence on individuals, enabling yet also limiting their actions and agency (Bates 2006; Roseberry 1989; Greenhalgh 1990: 87). We therefore look at both internalized social conventions and aspirations alongside external limitations as factors shaping and constraining individual decisions and behavior.

The context of our study is Israel, a country of moderate "Western" characteristics according to parameters like GDP, life expectancy, and infant mortality (see Table 1). Contemporary Israel is a thoroughly unequal country, ranking first in the Western world on the Gini Index of inequality (Israel—39; OECD average—31; Prime Minister's Office 2007, No. 43). Israel's population consists of over seven million citizens. Roughly eighty percent of the citizenry is Jewish while the remaining twenty percent consists of Palestinian (Muslim—16.5 percent; Christian—1.65 percent) and Druze (1.66 percent) minorities (Central Bureau of Statistics 2007f).

In this volume our focus is on the country's Jewish population. The choice of this axis stems from the view of inter-group differences as substantive. Dissimilar religions, histories, socio-demographic structures, sense of collective identity, and position within the local politics have resulted in distinct fertility and infertility patterns in each community (Kanaaneh 2002). The specific patterns of each subpopulation are, however, molded in reference to those of the others, thereby weaving and reproducing a complex system of power relations. Concentrating on the Jewish sector thus does not mean ignoring the others. Nor does it imply that Israel's reproductive policy, formed predominantly by the Jewish majority, is shaped exclusively or even primarily vis-à-vis "the Arab Other" or by the so-called "demographic struggle." Rather, as shown in this book's chapters, a wider array of factors appears to influence Israel's reproductive policy. The diverse cultural backgrounds within the Jewish sector and inter-ethnic relations, religious vs. non-religious Jewish camps, internal state politics, professional interests, consumer culture, state vs. citizens, and general Jewish tradition—each seems to have its contribution, and none would be independent of the Israeli-Palestinian conflict. In fact, the opposite is true. It is our hope that the emerging analysis of Israel's Jewish population, which ties together global processes with an array of local particularities, will reveal interrelations between seemingly remote issues, thereby turning the study of reproduction into a more seminal perspective for the understanding of broader complexities of the Israeli reality.

A.   Family and Natality among Jewish Israelis

Characteristics and possible origins

Jewish Israelis generally subscribe to a familial mode of living. A comparative reference to North America and West Europe shows that despite some erosion of the traditional family, Jewish Israelis still exhibit more familial social patterns along several major parameters like cohabitation, births out of wedlock, single parenthood, and divorce rate. The difference is especially visible in comparison to Europe (see Table 1).

Also in terms of total fertility rates (TFR) Jewish Israelis are more family-oriented, having more children than their West European and North American counterparts. Whereas the US and EU averages are 2.09 and 1.47[2] respectively, Jewish Israelis' TFR is 2.75 (Central Bureau of Statistics 2007i), i.e., roughly one child more per family. Children are therefore relatively prominent in Israel, comprising 33 percent of the local population (vs. 25 percent in the USA and 17 percent in Italy) (Central Bureau of Statistics 2007e). The difference is significant especially given the roughly similar levels of women's education and labor-market participation (50.4 percent in Israel in 2006 vs. 60 percent in the EU) (Central Bureau of Statistics 2006b, and Nimwegen et al. 2006, respectively). A vivid indication of the significance of children for Jewish Israelis was provided in a survey reporting that the majority of respondents stated that the lives of

Table 1   Israel – General and Family Characteristics

	ISRAEL	EUROPE	USA
Life expectancy			
-Men	78.5 years[a]	76.0[c]	75.2[e]
-Women	82.2 years[b]	81.2[d]	80.4[f]
GDP per capita (USD)	26,884[g]	30,121[h] (EU-25)	43,883[i]
Infant mortality rate	4.0[j]	Finland, Sweden – 2.8[k] (min) UK – 5.1 Romania – 13.9 (max)	6.8[l]
Crude marriage rate	5.9[m] (down from 11.2 in 1950-54)	EU – 4.82[n] (2005)	7.4[o]
Mean age at first marriage[p]		Sweden Spain	
-Men	27.6 years	34.1 31.2	27.1
-Women	25.2 years	31.5 29.3	25.3
Percentage of cohabitation	3%[q]	EU – 9%[r] Sweden – 23%[s] UK – 14%[t]	7.4%[u]
Age at first birth	26.8 years[v]	Sweden, Germany – 29[w] Ireland, Finland[x]- 28	25.1[y] (2002)
Births out of wedlock	5.64%[z]	33% in the EU[aa] 55% in Sweden,[bb] 95% in Norway[cc]	36.9[dd]
Single parented families with young children	5.7%	9%[ee]	16%[ff]
Crude divorce rate	1.9[gg]	Belgium – 3.01[hh] Germany – 2.45 Switzerland – 2.86	3.7[ii]

Sources: Central Bureau of Statistics (2005b), (2006a), (2007a), (2007b), (2007c), (2007d), Europa (N.D), National Center for Health Statistics (2007 [2006]), (2006c), (2007a), (2007b), US Department of State (2006), EconStats (N.D), Eurostat (N.Da) and (N.Db), Institute for the Study of Civil Society (2006), BBC News (2007), Eurofound (N.Da), (N.Db), Center for Disease Control and Prevention (2003), University of Helsinki (N.D), United Nations Statistics Division (2005)

a. Central Bureau of Statistics (2007a); b. Central Bureau of Statistics (2007a); c. Europa (N.D); d. Europa (N.D); e. National Center for Health Statistics (2007 [2006]); f. National Center for Health Statistics (2007 [2006]); g. Central Bureau of Statistics (2007a); h. US Department of State (2006); i. EconStats (N.D).; j. Central Bureau of Statistics (2007a); k. Eurostat (N.Da); l. National Center for Health Statistics (2007a); m. Central Bureau of Statistics (2007b); n. Eurostat (N.Db); o. National Center for Health Statistics (2007b); p. Central Bureau of Statistics (2007c); q. Central Bureau of Statistics (2007d); r. Central Bureau of Statistics (2007d); s. Institute for the Study of Civil Society (2006); t. BBC News (2007); u. Central Bureau of Statistics (2007d); v. Central Bureau of Statistics (2006a); w. Eurofound (N.Da); x. Eurofound (N.Da); y. Center for Disease Control and Prevention (2003); z. Central Bureau of Statistics (2006a); aa. Eurofound (N.Db); bb. The Institute for the Study of Civil Society (2006); cc. University of Helsinki (N.D).; dd. National Center for Health Statistics (2007c); ee. Central Bureau of Statistics (2007d); ff. Central Bureau of Statistics (2007d); gg. Central Bureau of Statistics (2005b); hh. United Nations Statistics Division (2005); ii. National Center for Health Statistics (2007b).

childless people were virtually empty and that raising one's children was life's greatest joy (Glickman 2003).

Jewish Israeli familism has commonly been traced by researchers to three major sources: Biblical prescription, the trauma of the Holocaust, and present day demographic politics.

The Jewish *Halachah* (the body of literature interpreting Biblical laws) establishes the significance of biological maternity and paternity in allocating each a distinct role in forming a person's belonging to the Jewish people. Jewish identity is passed matrilineally, i.e., the child of a Jewish woman is Jewish. The technology-induced disintegration of motherhood into genetic, gestational and social components has destabilized this formerly straightforward definition: Is it the egg, the womb, or the raising mother that defines a child's Jewish identity? While most rabbis focus on pregnancy and birth as the source of Jewish identity, others prefer a genetic, ova-based definition (Kahn 2000: 129; 2002). More progressive streams (Reform) in Judaism invoke early Judaic practices in an attempt to pursue paternal transferring of Jewishness (see Goldberg, this volume). The State of Israel has endorsed the traditional definition, viewing any offspring of a Jewish woman as Jewish. (This definition has clear political implications as it entitles any bearer to Israeli citizenship.) Biological paternity has its own identity forming aspects. In biblical texts and prayers, a child is referred to as "the son of his father." When the mother is Jewish, the father transfers to his son the "tribal" status as Cohen, Levi, or "ordinary Israel."[3]

Natality itself can be traced to the Bible. Emerging from the deepest historical reaches is the biblical commandment "Be fruitful and multiply," which may be viewed as construing procreation as a key constituent of a Jewish person's moral integrity. The centrality that this commandment has been charged with over the years can most likely be attributed to the function it fulfilled in the communal quest for survival. Establishing procreation as transcending one's own family and as crucial to the collectivity's regeneration, the commandment acquired a moral significance as a main goal in one's life (Gold 1988: 23). At the same time, collective strategies of survival were rooted in the familial body, rendering reproduction a collective mission (e.g., Gold 1988: 27; Safir 1991). Reproduction thus became a sphere of convergence between the private and the political, in which individual survival was virtually equated with the survival of the collectivity (Swirski 1976: 129–30).

The emphasis on familial procreation as the primary vehicle for collective regeneration needs to be explored within changing historical contexts. Going back to biblical times and into the second century BCE through late antiquity and the early Middle Ages, the Jewish collectivity seemed rather amenable to exogamy and conversion. This has changed in later periods (see Birenbaum-Carmeli and Carmeli, this volume).

In more recent history, the Holocaust has enhanced a local view of childbearing as a response to the Nazi devastation and threat of extermination. Holocaust survivors wished, and were actively encouraged, to establish families in order to heal from their traumatic past. This pronatalist approach to Holocaust survivors fit smoothly with the Zionist ideology that declared the enlargement of the Jewish population in the land of Israel an important component of the nation-building effort. Mothers were expected to follow medical advice aimed to nurture the "new Jew," who would serve the national cause, even at the price of risking her/ his life (Stoler-Liss 2003). State policies reproduced and echoed the values and interests that the emerging state and other influential bodies brought to bear during the "manufacturing process" (Drake 1999: 37). The state installed paid maternity leave before any other social benefit (Barkai 1998: 44); it allocated child allowances to particular families; workers in the public sector were remunerated in proportion to the number of their children (during the 1940s and 1950s); employed mothers were eligible for special tax reductions; national awards were granted to "Heroine Mothers" who delivered their tenth child, and to "families blessed with many children," as they were called (Portugese 1998). Though they were most likely geared at the Jewish population, these policy measures applied to the country's entire citizenry.

Several years later, in 1968, The Demographic Centre was established by the government, defining its goal in its founding document as "Carry[ing] out a reproductive policy intended to create a psychologically favorable climate that will encourage and stimulate natality; an increase in natality in Israel being crucial for the future of the whole Jewish people (1968: 2).

The following decades saw a further expansion of publicly funded pronatalist measures like obstetric follow-up, maternity care, and child allowances as well as fertility treatments (on the last, see below.) In the labor market, "mother-friendly" taxation was applied. Laws protected pregnant workers and women in fertility treatment from redundancy and granted the latter up to 80 days of annual paid leave. Currently, men, too, are entitled to twelve days of paid leave on account of fertility treatments (Ministry of Industry, Commerce and Employment).

In some predominantly female employment areas (e.g., teaching), a mother's position entitled her to full-time payment and benefits for fewer hours.

On the other hand, researchers pointed to the insufficiency of sex education and contraceptives (Doron and Kramer 1991: 119–40; Portugese 1998: 91–149) and to the humiliation that accompanied abortion committees' approval of the procedure (Amir and Benjamin 1992).

The enhancement of family and pronatalism amongst Jewish–Israelis also manifests in practical and everyday discourse. Establishing a family and raising children is construed as the "normal" accomplishment of mature adulthood, and parenthood as a morally obliging status. This family that one is expected to establish is both patterned and further legitimated by a broader collective narrative which it reproduces. Even the fiercely disputed claim on the land is legitimized through the tribal/familial/biblical myth of ancestry (Birenbaum-Carmeli and Carmeli, this volume), as are the politics of immigration[4] and the "demographic struggle" discourse. With its diffused religious, collective, and individual significance, the familial conviction has been profoundly internalized by Israeli Jews, rendering individual agency a crucial factor in the regulation and regeneration of the Jewish population in Israel (Prainsack 2006).

Complementary and countervailing evidence

Significant as pronatalism is in official state rhetoric, a closer scrutiny suggests that it is not a straightforward coherent policy of the Jewish-dominated State of Israel. Rather, more complex and varied dynamics appear to be at work, some of which are more likely to discourage natality, among both Jewish and non-Jewish Israelis. These countervailing measures problematize the accepted monolithic picture of Israeli pronatalism.

We start out with a historical look at group-specific total fertility rates (TFR). As shown in Table 2, over the last four and a half decades, all Israeli religion-defined population sectors have lowered their fertility rates. The decrease has been especially pronounced in the non-Jewish sectors: Among Muslim citizens of Israel, TFR dropped to less than half, from 9.23 to just under four. Israeli Druze's TFR plummeted from 7.49 to 2.64, and Israel's Christian citizens' fertility levels fell from 4.68 to 2.14. The change in the Jewish sector has been smaller but still in the same direction, decreasing from 3.39 to 2.75. On the whole, the country's TFR has declined from 3.85 in the early 1960s to 2.88 in 2006.

Table 2   Fertility rates by year and religion

TFR	1960–1964	1965–1969	1970–1974	1975–1979	1980–1984	1985–1989	1990–1994	1995–1999	2000–2004	2005	2006
Israel	3.85	3.83	3.80	3.47	3.13	3.07	2.93	2.93	2.92	2.84	2.88
Jews	3.39	3.36	3.28	3.00	2.80	2.79	2.62	2.62	2.67	2.69	2.75
Muslims	9.23	9.22	8.47	7.25	5.54	4.70	4.67	4.67	4.57	4.03	3.97
Druze	7.49	7.30	7.25	6.93	5.40	4.19	3.77	3.24	2.87	2.59	2.64
Christians	4.68	4.26	3.65	3.12	2.41	2.49	2.18	2.56	2.35	2.15	2.14

Source: Adapted from Central Bureau of Statistics 2007[i]

A few scholars (e.g., Portugese 1998) have claimed that the reduction of fertility among non-Jewish women is in fact congruent with the state's pronatalism that targets the Jewish population alone. The modest decrease in Jewish fertility, which further coincides with an observable increase in TFR in the last few years, may support this theory (see Figure 1).

While generally accepting this perspective, we will now take a closer look at different processes within Israel's Jewish population. The broader framework is that of a consistent decline in Jewish TFR in Israel over four decades, resulting in roughly 20 percent fewer children in Jewish families today as compared to the 1960s. Several concurrent processes seem to have taken place among four Jewish subpopulations in Israel: Orthodox Jews, non-religious Oriental

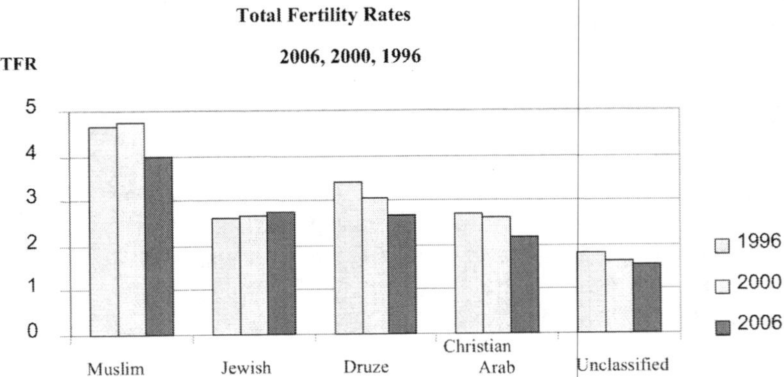

Figure 1   TFR by religious groups, 1996, 2000, 2006
Source: Angel 2007

Jews, non-religious Ashkenazi Jews, and immigrants from the Former Soviet Union (FSU).

Orthodox Jews in Israel exhibit very distinct fertility patterns from those of all other local sectors. Having always presented high TFR, orthodox women had 6.5 children on average in 1980, 7.6 in 1995 (Rebibo 2002) and 7.7 in 2004 (Gurovich and Cohen-Castro 2004: 25). In some young Orthodox communities present figures have exceeded even this number, reaching 9 children per woman (ibid.). Though pertaining to a relatively small sector (7 percent of the country's population) (Central Bureau of Statistics 2007g), this rise still contributes to the recent increase in Jewish TFR and has moderated the decrease in previous years.

The main and most prevalent explanation to this exceptional reproductive pattern is an interpretation of the biblical command to "Be fruitful and multiply" as demanding the birth of numerous children and forbidding contraception and abortion. Some practical support that helped maintain this interpretation was provided by the state's relatively generous child allowances that were allocated to large families during the 1990s. These allowances rose proportionately with the number of the child (i.e., the allowance for the fifth child was higher than that for the second child), thus adding up to a substantial sum, allowing Orthodox families to survive if only at poverty level. Fifty-eight percent of Orthodox families are below the poverty line (Prime Minister's Office 2007).[5]

The role of state funding seems especially crucial given the community's low participation in the labor market. Among women, the primary bearers of the immense household burden, 45 percent are gainfully employed. Among men, however, the majority are engaged in full-time religious learning, with only 30 percent earning any money (Fogel and Friedman 2006). In these families, in the mid 1990s child allowances comprised over 30 percent of the family's income (Berman 2000). Though it is difficult to assess the influence of policy on fertility (Nimwegen et al. 2006; Ophir and Eliav 2005), the rarity of full-time learning among Jewish Orthodox men abroad (e.g., in London, Montreal, and New York) seems to underscore the contribution of Israel's child allowance policy to the shaping, or at least the enabling, of the exceptional TFR among Orthodox Israelis (Berman 2000; Gonen 2005).

A different outlook could, however, view the high fertility rate as a form of resistance undertaken by a marginal population. From this perspective, the Orthodox sector, largely alienated from the state (on grounds of religious disapproval of a Jewish state before the arrival of the Messiah), prioritizes its own interpretation of the biblical commandment above surrounding reproductive expectations. A current reform that gradually reduces and levels allowances for every child which has been completed in 2009 (see below), will provide an opportunity to probe these two explanations and to decipher the role of state allowances in Orthodox fertility patterns: A reduction in fecundity will support the more pragmatic economic explanation; stability will enhance the resistance line. As this chapter is being written, preliminary figures have been published suggesting a decrease in TFR since 2001 among Orthodox Jewish women in Israel (Schtrassler 2008). More years of research are still required to affirm these new findings.

In contrast to the Orthodox community, TFRs of all other Jewish sectors have been on a decline, as shown in Table 3. This trend somewhat problematizes the monolithic pronatalist image commonly conferred on Israeli policy.

Zooming in on non-religious Ashkenazi Jews (Jews of European descent), we observe a decrease in TFR from 2.8 in 1970 to 2.2 in the late 1990s. The decline, which in this group was the mildest of all Jewish Israeli populations, has in fact been moderated by rising fecundity among FSU immigrants who are included under the same rubric. From 1993 to 1994, Jewish women in the FSU had 0.8 children on average (Jewish Agency for Israel 2007). Israeli figures of the early 1990s estimated TFR in this sector at 1.3. However, having assimilated the surrounding Israeli patterns and having improved their financial situation, the immigrants or their children started expanding their families (Nahmias 2004), reaching 1.7 in 1994 (Gurovich and Cohen-Castro 2005; Central Bureau of Statistics 2005a).

A more significant reduction in fertility took place among non-religious Jews of Oriental origin (i.e., Asian and African), nearly halving from 5.7 in 1955, to just over 3 in the 1970s. Towards the end of the 1990s, this group, too, started to approach replacement level (Goldscheider 1996; Friedlander). It is this steep decline that may pose the main challenge to the sweeping theorem regarding Jewish Israeli pronatalism.

Table 3   TFR in the Orthodox community vs. all other Jewish Israelis

	Orthodox Jews	Other Jewish Israelis
1980/1982	6.49	2.61
1995/1996	7.61	2.27

Extrapolated from Berman 2000: 936

"Traditionally," researchers attributed the drastic reduction in family size to the "Oriental" immigrants' encounter with modern norms, the increase in age limit on marriage, greater access to higher education for women, and the lower rates of infant mortality, as compared to the newcomers' countries of origin (Goldscheider 1996; Okun 1997). However, other researchers have viewed the process more critically, arguing for the existence of more active state input in this sphere. According to these scholars, in the 1950s and 1960s an association was created between Oriental Jews and economic deprivation and high fertility, the latter of which was construed as a symbol of backwardness and "Arabness," to be presumably "rectified" by (Ashkenazi) Zionism and child allowances that were allocated only to large families (Shohat 1998: 5). The geographical spread of the few family planning clinics that operated in the country in those years in Oriental immigrant areas may be taken as additional evidence in support of this argument. At the same time, small, mostly Ashkenazi families were granted financial support under different titles. Tax exemptions, for instance, privileged this more affluent sector, whose women were employed in the formal sector and earned the qualifying sum (Barkai 1998: 22, 160; Hashash 2004). State assistance in child education and accommodation improvement further helped those families who could afford initial funding for these purposes. The combined effect of these policy measures, so the argument goes, was a stigmatization of high fertility and reduction of natality among Oriental Jews alongside encouragement of natality in small Ashkenazi families. An explicit declaration of this policy was provided in The Demographic Center campaign of 1968 that overtly aimed to encourage "families with two children to increase their families to 3–4 children, and advise large families on family planning" (Hashash 2004).

Thus, in some disparity from its image of nearly unbounded pronatalism, Israel's early reproductive discourse emerges from these descriptions as more dual: overtly pronatalist, presumably encouraging Jewish natality per se for the sake of national regeneration, but with a more clandestine anti-natalist undercurrent that equates large families with backwardness and deprivation (Ducker 2006). A succinct representation of this approach was given by Joseph Meir, former head of Israel's largest Health Fund and the general director of the Ministry of Health in the mid 1940s: "We have no interest in the tenth or even the seventh child of the poor Mizrahi families. . .we must pray for the second child of the families of the intelligentsia" (Ducker 2006: 43). Notably, just as large families were stigmatized, so having a single child was condemned as a mode of spoiling one's child, a severe charge in mid twentieth-century Israel.

Subsequent policy measures appear to further support this line of argument and illuminate the above mentioned changes in TFR. Once again we take child allowance as our illustration. Israel's first child allowance scheme was ratified in 1959, eleven years after independence, as a response to the *Wadi Salib* riots, in which Jewish Israelis of Oriental origin protested against ethnic discrimination. The modest benefits that were allocated after the riots to families with four children or more (Doron and Kramer 1991: 82) might have somewhat alleviated poverty but at the same time reinvigorated the large family stigma, now further highlighted in the context of poverty (Shenhav and Melamed 2006). The next significant change in child allowances—universalization and increase—took place in 1975, when widening ethnic-economic gaps in the increasingly capitalistic state coincided with the post-1973 war unrest, which threatened the historical hegemony of the Labor party. These changes were largely reversed between 1983 and 1994, when child allowances were generally eroded, with the exception of large families with four or more children whose allowances were raised (Portuguese 1998: 104). At this point in time, large families were primarily Ultra-Orthodox, and the higher allowances reflected the growing power of Ultra-Orthodox parties in coalition formation negotiations (Birenbaum-Carmeli 2003). In 2002, a scheme to reduce and level all child allowances was ratified, reflecting once again local processes—namely, the increasing domination of market economy governed by neo-liberal advocates. The shifts seem to disclose great responsiveness of child allowances to ongoing political dynamics. Starting out from tax reductions that primarily benefited the then hegemonic Ashkenazi middle class, child allowances were raised in the 1960s and 1970s as part of an attempt to calm social unrest. In the following two decades it was primarily the empowered Orthodox sector that benefited from allowances to very large families, and the situation was reversed yet again in favor of smaller families in 2002 with the strengthening of the market economy.

The proposed correspondence between child allowance policy and internal politics may suggest that rather than a mere goal in its own right, pronatalism, represented here via child allowance policy, is also a means to internal political ends. Some researchers have further politicized the link. Underscoring the persistence of economic and social gaps between Israeli Jews of Oriental vs. Ashkenazi origin, Ducker (2006) views Israel's reproductive discourse as a means to enhance the local ethnic class hierarchy while concealing the establishment's role in its creation (Hashash 2004). Even more broadly, critics have analyzed the state's reproductive discourse as reflecting and serving the leaders' Neo-Malthusian conviction to generate a class, ethnicity and gender system that would be conducive to Western- and market-oriented schemes of development (Shenhav and Melamed 2006; Hashash 2004).

In the light of these understandings, which complicate and problematize Israel's reproductive policy, we will now turn to a brief international comparison in order to locate Israel's investment in and encouragement of natality vis-à-vis other industrialized countries.

Starting with child allowance, the comparison shows (Table 4) that in contrast to popular notions that prevail among Israelis, state contribution towards childrearing is lower in Israel than in West European countries.

A broader survey that compared child allowances on the basis of national GDP also ranked Israel at the low end of the European spectrum (Ophir and Eliav 2005), and a more extensive historical perspective showed a steep decline in Israel's relative investment in child support starting in 2001 and ending in 2009. Notably, one-third of Israel's children live below the poverty line, even after redistributive transfers. This percentage is expected to rise even higher after 2009 when the child allowance reform will have been fully applied (ibid. 32, 33, 35).

A similar picture emerges from an international comparison of maternity leave. Often hailed in its early legalization as a local social accomplishment, Israel's 12-week maternity leave also ranks low when compared to most West European countries (Table 5), which provide from 15 to 16 weeks of paid leave, up to a whole year (Norway) or even longer (Estonia, Sweden).

Table 4   Child allowance in various countries (in USD)

No. of Children	1	2	3	4	Cost of Living Index[6]
Belgium[7]	107	307	600	900	86.5
Germany[8]	224	448	672	932	87.5
Sweden[9]	165	346	566	866	93.1
Israel[10]	**40**	**80**	**127**	**215**	**97.7**
Ireland[11]	233	466	750	1,033	99.6
France[12]	—	173	394	616	101.4
UK[13]	169	284	369	511	126.3
Norway[14]	181	362	543	724	105.8

Table 5 Maternity Leave regulations in selected industrialized countries

Country	Maternity Leave Regulations
Australia	None
USA	None
Germany, New Zealand	14 weeks at 100%. In Germany a further 12 months at 67%. Must have private health insurance for part of paid leave
Israel	**14 weeks at 75% of average last 3 months (to be extended to 16 weeks)**
Belgium, Canada, Finland	15 weeks
Austria, France, Greece, Luxembourg, Netherlands, Poland, Spain, Switzerland	16 weeks, 100% pay
Portugal	120 days at 100% pay
Denmark	18 weeks at 90%. Can be extended to 28 weeks. A further 32 weeks is paid by the State at DKK 3,335.00.
Italy	5 months at 100% of pay plus an optional 6 months at 30% of pay.
Hungary	24 weeks at 100% pay
Ireland	26 weeks at 75% pay
UK	39 weeks, first 6 weeks at 90%; thereafter—£112.75 per week
Norway	54 weeks at 80% or 44 weeks at 100% of pay; *paternity leave*—45 weeks at 80% or 35 weeks at 100% shared with mother.
Estonia	15 months (455 days) at 100%; up to 3 years unpaid leave.
Sweden	16 months at 80% ; flat rate for last 3 months

Source: British Employment Law (2007)

Considered within a still broader framework of a whole array of child-related benefits—income tax, income and non-income related benefits, net rent, net local tax, school costs benefits, health costs, and other benefits—Israel offers lower state support than the twenty-one industrialized countries included in Bradshaw and Finch's comparison (2002).

Israeli pronatalism is also problematized from a different perspective. The state offers generous state funding and subsidies to prenatal screening and applies a liberal abortion policy, especially in cases of potential fetal anomalies. We will elaborate on this aspect in section B. below.

Taken together, these measures complicate the notion of Israel's pronatalism, which is often associated with sweeping generalizations about "Jewish tradition and interests." Even when focusing on the Jewish population, as we do in the present volume, we must acknowledge internal divisions and address each sector's distinct position and interests that may be competing and occasionally antagonistic to one another. The preceding data suggests that Israel's reproductive policy was applied to serve a variety of state interests in such domains as inter-ethnic relations, economics, or coalition politics. Thus, Ashkenazis competed with Oriental Jews, religious parties with their non-religious rivals, rich vs. poor, and, beyond the national-religious divide, Israeli Jews competed with the local non-Jewish minorities. The overview has also suggested that alongside pronatalist policies, other policy measures seemed to have been implemented in order to discourage certain types of natality. On the basis of this depiction we understand Israel's reproductive policy as a compound social product reflecting an ideological commitment to, as well as state interest in, (Jewish) natality for a diversity of political, economic, and cultural purposes. This multifaceted approach will furnish the backdrop for our exploration of the government and usage of reproductive technologies in Israel, which stand at the center of the present collection.

B.   Reproductive Technologies in Israel

Both tradition and contemporary discourses of reproduction and parenthood reverberate in the pain and shame that infertility entails in Israel. Comprising the archetypal image of women's suffering and man's failure to fulfill his prime duty to procreate (which is, in Judaism, a man's duty only), infertility is constituted in Judaism as a major personal tragedy (Kahn 2000; Jakobovits 1967). The anguish is further amplified by the role given to "natural" relatedness in the construction and reproduction of the Jewish collectivity. Both outsiders, who had imposed collective definitions on Jews during centuries of exile, and Jewish communities themselves have traditionally privileged "natural" over "social" forms of relatedness, thus marginalizing options like third-party procreation or adoption as solutions to infertility (see Birenbaum-Carmeli and Carmeli, this volume). In this section we look at various technologies of procreation and prenatal screening, as applied and embedded in the Israeli reality, which is thereby transformed.

Technologies of procreation

The particularity of Israel's RT scene has by now been well documented. Israel is the only country that fully funds nearly universal procreative medicine services. Treatment is offered to couples as well as single women of all sexual orientations until the age of 45. If using a donor egg, funded treatment is extended to the age of 51 and/or until the woman has two children with her present partner, where applicable (see Yogev et al. 2003). Women aged 45 to 51 are entitled to unlimited state-subsidized egg donation within Israel (Rabinerson et al. 2002). Any treatment combination—e.g., gamete donation with IVF—is allowed. Surrogacy is also permitted in compliance with the 1996 Embryo Carrying Agreement Law, the world's first law to regulate surrogacy.

It therefore comes as no surprise that Israel has one of the world's highest ratios of IVF centers per capita (22 units per 7 million people) (Collins 2002). The volume of treatment in these centers is particularly high, showing a five-fold increase over a course of 15 years, from 1990 to 2005 (see Figure 2). The increase is attributable to the introduction of ICSI as a routine treatment of male infertility, the influx of immigrants from the Former Soviet Union who were keen to

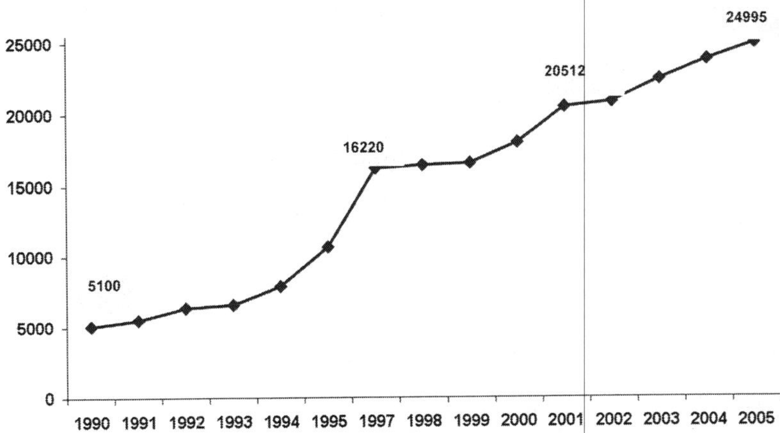

Figure 2   Number of IVF cycles per year in Israel
Source: Ministry of Health Periodical Database 2007

resolve untreated infertility, as well as a rise in the average number of cycles per woman.

These figures render Israeli women the world's heaviest consumers of the technology. For the sake of comparison, we can look at the year 2003, when 22,449 IVF cycles were conducted in Israel, for a population of 6.7484 million (Central Bureau of Statistics 2007h). The resulting figure of 3,327 cycles per million placed Israel at the top of the world's list (see Figure 3); in 2005, the figure rose to 3,575, with IVF being used three times more frequently there than in the average EU country (EU average = 1022) (Nyboe Andersen et al. 2007). Three percent of all births in Israel follow IVF and related technological interventions (ESHRE [European Society for Human Reproduction and Embryology] 2006). Treatment is available to Israeli citizens of all religious and national affiliations (Birenbaum-Carmeli and Inhorn 2009).

Despite, or perhaps because of the high level of consumption, treatment-related risks have always been marginalized in Israel's IVF discourse (Landau 2003). Though the treatment may entail substantial complications to the mother and the baby, including menopause symptoms, pregnancy induced hypertension, birth complications, and multiple births, as well as potentially life threatening ovarian

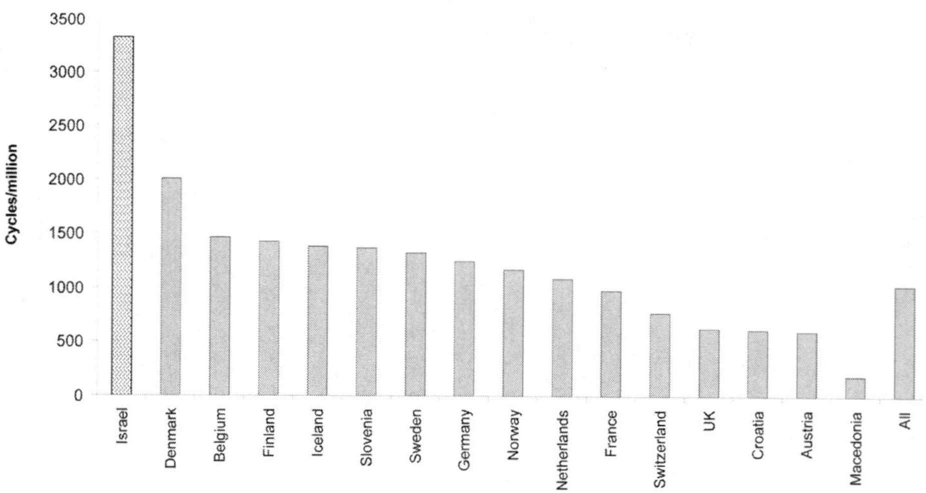

Figure 3   Number of IVF cycles per million per annum

Source: Adapted from Nyboe Andersen et al. (2007)

** Israeli figures: 22,449 cycles in 2003 (Ministry of Health); 6.7484 million citizens (Central Bureau of Statistics 2007h)*

hyperstimulation and possible increased risk of gynecological cancers (Lerner-Geva 2003), these risks are rarely mentioned in the local discourse of IVF. Since the early 1980s, when Israeli physicians introduced the technology to the country and delivered the world's fifth "IVF baby," and throughout its proliferation and routinization into standard treatment (for male as well as female infertility), IVF has been consistently presented as a source of hope, while its riskier aspects have been sidelined and silenced (Birenbaum-Carmeli 1997; Birenbaum-Carmeli and Dirnfeld 2007). The silence becomes especially significant when considering that IVF is an elective treatment, one that is often performed on a healthy woman in order to address her partner's impairment. In the rare instances that the risks have been raised publically (e.g., in parliamentary discussions on rationing IVF), such claims were swiftly rejected as unfounded and manipulative, aiming to cut state expenditure at the expense of citizens' basic human right to parenthood (Birenbaum-Carmeli 2004a). Interestingly enough, as this chapter is going to press, the headline on the front page of Israel's widest read newspaper declared, "The Heavy Price of Fertility Treatment" (Rosenblum 2008). The article, which covered the whole two subsequent pages, thereby making IVF the subject of the newspaper's three front pages, reported increased prevalence of breast cancer among women who had undergone IVF and defined them as being at a high risk for the disease. Whether this finding will prompt a public debate or change consumption patterns remains to be seen in the following weeks, months and years.

Another marginalized aspect of RT provision in Israel is economic. Though Israel indeed funds fertility treatments more comprehensively than any other country, consumer contribution—roughly $150 (U.S.) per cycle—is still an obstacle for some potential patients, who cannot afford this and concomitant expenses like traveling and work absence. Consequently, though accessible to a much larger clientele, IVF is still beyond the reach of the lower social strata.

In contrast to the silencing of these potentially problematic aspects of reproductive technologies, much publicity and support has been conferred on potentially controversial cases. Israeli courts have approved transplanting cryopreserved embryos in a surrogate woman after the intended parents divorced and despite strong objection of the male partner (Birenbaum-Carmeli 2007), post-mortem sperm aspiration at a widow's request, which has become standard practice in Israel since 2003 (see Siegel-Itzkovich 2003 and Landau 2004), and even at the parents' request (Hasson 2007). These and similar cases were broadly and emphatically reported in all major Israeli newspapers.

The high scope of treatment translates into a substantial state expense. Available figures are dated but can provide a rough indication: In 1995, the cost of one IVF cycle in Israel was estimated at $3,000 (U.S.) (Schenker and Shushan 1996) and that of a "take home (IVF) baby" at $19,267 (U.S.) (Stern et al. 1995). Translated into more recent figures (Collins 2002), the cost was raised to $3,817 (U.S.) per IVF cycle in Israel. On the basis of this estimate, Israel's 2005 IVF expenditure is over $95 million,(U.S.) roughly equaling 400 million NIS at the time. Calculated as percentage of the 22 billion NIS cost of the health basket in 2005 (Government decision no. 3551 2005), the country's 2005 IVF budget accounted for 1.8 percent of the annual health basket cost.

To this sum, one should add the cost of ICSI and other related technologies as well as the increased neonatal expenses associated with IVF. Recent calculations estimated prenatal and neonatal costs as 2.7–3.2-fold for twins compared to singletons, and pediatric health care as 1.3-fold for IVF singletons and 1.1-fold for IVF twins, compared to respective controls (Koivurova et al. 2004).

These figures are especially relevant to Israel, where embryo transfer practices are also more "liberal" than in many West European and North American settings, resulting in a higher frequency of multiple births. Whereas in Finland, Sweden, and Belgium, only one embryo is transferred back to the woman (Nyboe-Andersen et al. 2004), in Israel, gynecologists still transfer two or three embryos, and even four to five in older women. Consequently, 23.6 percent of IVF deliveries in Israel are multiple births, and 28.6 percent are pre-term (Israel Women's Network). Nearly half (47 percent) of IVF-assisted births are by Caesarean section, and the share of babies born in multiple births has increased by 12 percent during the last decade, reaching 4.4 percent of Israeli babies and 4.8 percent of Jewish babies (Central Bureau of Statistics 2007b).

A more concrete sense of the significance of IVF and related costs may be provided by the recent negotiation, not to say struggle, over the inclusion of new medications including life prolonging ones in the publicly funded "medication basket." The missing sum was $75 million (U.S.) (Azoulay 2007; Swirski 2007).

The burden on the public budget has indeed been the primary motivation for the recurring attempts to ration ARTs. However, to date, all such proposals, even when made in harder times of recession, have been rejected with severe condemnation (Birenbaum-Carmeli 2004a). At the popular level, too, no serious challenge to the local RT policy has been put forward.

The emerging picture of ART in Israel then is one of virtually unbounded acceptance. The general public endorses the technology without any significant questioning, together with politicians, women activists, professionals and journalists, who all seem to marginalize potential health risks. Even the exceptional public investment in funding has never raised serious concerns. This wholehearted endorsement of a technology that results in failure more often than in a live birth is not self explanatory, especially if we accept that Israel's reproductive policy is actually more ambivalent, as suggested in the preceding section. In the following we outline several possible explanations. Rather than suggesting a fully fledged solution to the question, we attempt to chart out a web of concerns, interests, and agencies that we consider influential in forming and sustaining the present situation. These will set the groundwork for the ensuing chapters in the collection.

We may start from the discursive power that the biblical commandment "Be fruitful and multiply" has been charged with over decades—maybe centuries—of pronatalist rhetoric. The supreme significance that has been conferred on childbearing at both the individual and collective levels has rendered the subject formative of foundational self-perceptions like gender, life cycle, citizenship, and social participation. This meaning has enabled the construction of parenthood as a human right and state obligation, which then translated into the right to fertility treatment. Various stakeholders each have their distinct interests in maintaining the existing status quo.

Consumer interest seems self-evident at first: being faced by infertility, women and couples would obviously prefer to have their treatment publicly funded rather than pay out of pocket (see Remmenick, this volume). However, on a closer look, it is less clear what it is that drives Israeli women, especially those who have undergone numerous ineffective cycles, to subordinate their bodies once and again over years, sometimes decades, to intrusive treatments whose likelihood of success diminishes, and which jeopardize their health and career prospects along the way. Why would Israelis choose to undergo so many treatment cycles before opting for simpler and more efficient—if less "biogenetic"—alternatives like donor insemination or adoption?

One line of interpretation could focus on women's internalization of the hegemonic significance allocated to motherhood in Jewish tradition and Zionist discourse. Since its early days and then for decades following, Zionist ideology and the State of Israel constituted motherhood as a woman's primary obligation and privilege that granted her place in society and accomplished her female normalcy

(Berkowitch 1997, 2000). Within this framework, the quest for motherhood—biogenetic motherhood, to be precise—has been perceived as justifying, indeed requiring, any investment of energy, time and, if inevitable, also money for its fulfillment. (The expanding practice of overseas ova donation, owing to local restrictions on donation, amply illustrates the need for money.) This line of interpretation would also help in understanding women's tendency to overestimate the likelihood of treatment success while downplaying its complications, risks, and toll on their lives (Birenbaum-Carmeli and Dirnfeld 2007) (for a somewhat higher emphasis on treatment implications for treated women, see Remennick, this volume). This "rosy" perception of the technology, which probably underpins Israeli women's willingness to undergo "as many IVF cycles as needed" as the vast majority have declared (Birenbaum-Carmeli and Dirnfeld 2007) thus nurtures both the need for the technology as well as one's right to demand its provision.

For Israeli men, too, IVF is a scene for negotiating male images. As noted, it is the man who is religiously obliged to fulfill the biblical commandment. It is also the man's name that will be carried on to the future by his children and it is his "manhood," with its "macho" elements that imbue Jewish Israeli culture (Shadmi 2000), that needs to be "rescued" through genetic fatherhood. Social family formations would at best provide a partial solution for these concerns, by putting on a thin external appearance. They will, however, leave unresolved the subjective sense of impairment and even the continuity of the "tribal status" (Cohen, Levy, or Israelite). That so many Israeli couples choose to undergo numerous IVF cycles in order to resolve a man's infertility problem suggests that at least to some extent, women share this perception.

Another source of influence that might have contributed to the favorable attitude of Israeli consumers towards ART is physicians' encouragement, which some researchers consider crucial. In their major domain of power, the hospital clinic, doctors praise not only the treatment but the patients' perseverance as a moral virtue (Carmeli and Birenbaum-Carmeli 2000a). Also, in their public appearances, e.g., as experts in Knesset discussions on the subject, practitioners have consistently commended the local policy of universal access to treatment as superior to any known alternative (Birenbaum-Carmeli 2004a). The doctors have centered their arguments exclusively on the capacity to allay an infertile person's agony, which, in turn, will supposedly contribute to the country's prosperity.

Though doctors are indeed most likely absorbed in the powerful local discourse of pronatalism, they also have a professional stake in the continuation of the current policy.[15] One could assume that beyond their earnings, experts would have a scientific interest in sustaining an extensive IVF practice. Israeli researchers have been prominent in IVF research since its early days and seem to have managed to retain this exceptional visibility to the present (Mashiach et al., this volume).[16] The origins of this emphasis can be traced back to the 1940s, when the eminent Jewish German gynecologist Prof. Bernhard Zondek arrived in Jerusalem, bringing cutting-edge science to the barely existing local bioresearch.[17] In subsequent years, especially following the Holocaust, this early head start developed into international acclaim, turning reproductive medicine into a symbol of Jewish regeneration and ingenuity. In recent years, the evolving domain of human embryonic stem cell research has possibly acquired a somewhat similar significance, though probably not to the same extent (see Chapters 9 and 10, this volume). To the best of our knowledge, the scientific or lucrative interests that doctors might have in sustaining a massive IVF practice have never been mentioned in any public discussion of the subject. Rather, doctors' opinions have been construed as disinterested professional assessments, humanized and enriched by personal acquaintance with infertile women and couples (Birenbaum-Carmeli 2004a).[18]

However, neither professionals' nor consumers' interests can fully account for the state's extensive funding of ARTs. If the state's actual interest in natality is more contingent and limited, as suggested in previous sections, why would it invest so exceptionally in fertility treatments? Moreover, even when acting pronatalistically, the state could apply other policy measures (e.g., anti-abortion or pro-adoption policies), none of which are implemented (Birenbaum-Carmeli and Carmeli, this volume). Here again, rather than a fully coherent answer we would like to point in several directions that we consider central to the explanation.

We start with a plain logistical factor that seems to have contributed to the emergence of the local policy. From its introduction to Israel in 1981, through to 1995, IVF was provided and funded by the four local Health Maintenance Organizations (HMOs). Three HMOs limited service to seven IVF cycles and to woman younger than 47 (limits somewhat varied among HMOs), offering additional cycles through a basic private supplementary insurance (Shalev and Lev 1999). The forth and largest HMO, *Clalit*, was limited by its computer infrastructure which could not trace a woman's treatment history and therefore placed no restrictions on usage. However, in 1995, when the National Health Law came into effect, services in all HMOs were leveled so as to match *Clalit*'s services, now deemed

Israel's "service basket." Although all local HMOs, including *Clalit*, wanted to ration IVF at that point, the law applied the most liberal policy possible, with practically unlimited access (Birenbaum-Carmeli 2004a). While this historical origin may account for the mid 1990s policy it does not explain its continued persistence. To gain a deeper insight into Israel's ART policy we now turn to look at what we identify as the state's preference for biogenetic relatedness.

Together with physicians and consumers, Israel's policy makers have consistently prioritized treatments that aim to generate biogenetically related offspring: ovulation induction precedes the use of a donor egg; ICSI—despite its toll on women's health and its lower success rates—is pursued prior to donor insemination; and all treatments, including donor gametes and surrogacy are seen as better than adoption. This hierarchy is almost explicit in the Ministry of Health's recommendation to mix the male partner's sperm with that of the donor (Carmeli and Birenbaum-Carmeli 2000b), and to encourage adoption applicants to continue fertility treatment while waiting for an adopted baby (Birenbaum-Carmeli and Carmeli, this volume). The same spirit underpins the secrecy policy in gamete donation and the intention of many parents to conceal genetic origin details from the resulting children (Birenbaum-Carmeli, Carmeli and Yavetz 2000; Nachman 2005; Goldberg, this volume). All these measures convey a clear message regarding the superiority of "natural" relatedness vs. alternatives, thereby establishing the great public investment in IVF as proportional to the magnitude of its symbolic significance. Within this framework, Israel's generous ART funding can be viewed as a "tribute" to its pronatalist discourse. This line of exploration leads us to probing the power and legitimacy of this ritual discourse (Bell 1992).

As described, for years Israeli officials have endorsed a pronatalist language, locating procreation at the momentous intersection of Jewish tradition, the Holocaust, and national renewal. These "weighty" meanings, alongside the notion of self accomplishment through family founding and child rearing, are construed as vital elements in the formative core symbolism of the Jewish-Israeli political body. Anchoring reproduction within this "sacred" ritualized realm practically delegitimizes any limiting discourse regarding fertility treatment. If having children is a paramount goal in one's life, and if it justifies, maybe requires, any effort in the name of personal and national accomplishment, then consumers, who willingly subject their bodies to prolonged treatment, can readily claim funding from the state, and the state—across all coalition formations—can hardly defend rationing of the service. Pursuing this line of thought one could further suggest that Israel's ART policy serves governments in garnering substantial symbolic profit. State-funded treatment in the presumably optional domain of infertility becomes a ritual manifestation of the State caring for personal anguish, the relief of which also helps heal national traumas and serves presumed collective needs. Pushed a step further, it may be viewed as indirectly—maybe also unintentionally—nurturing public demographic fears.[18]

Indeed, within and beyond these ideological and symbolic politics, Israeli politicians may well have a pragmatic interest in the resulting babies. IVF consumers, though more socially heterogeneous in Israel than elsewhere, are still largely within the broad confines of the middle class. Patients must have the time, some money, and the rational disposition required in order to pursue the complicated treatment. The public funding of RT thus coheres with the state's policy of encouraging natality in natural, mid-sized, self-reliant families. That treatment is provided as generously to non-Jewish Israelis is apparently a fortunate consequence of the state's democratic claim, which in this matter, lives up to its promise (Inhorn and Birenbaum-Carmeli 2008).

To sum up, Israel's exceptional funding of ART emerges as thoroughly context dependent. A discourse of biogenetic procreation as of paramount import has enhanced Israelis' resolve to seek and expect funded treatment; it has rendered doctors' pro-funding views readily acceptable, and has delegitimized any limitation on fertility treatment. From the State's point of view, it has symbolically enhanced the legitimacy of its broader reproductive policy that appears to encourage fairly specific modes of reproduction rather than others. The following section will look at another aspect of reproductive policy and practice, that of prenatal screening.

Prenatal screening tests

In our preceding discussion of ART we have mentioned Jewish Israelis' silence regarding IVF-related risks. In striking contrast, we find heightened awareness and concern regarding the "normalcy" of a newborn child. Jewish Israelis are avid consumers of pre-marital, pre-pregnancy, and prenatal screening tests, many of which are also state funded. First in the sequence are *Dor Yeshorim* tests that screen applicants for several common "Jewish" genetic mutations (e.g., Tay-Sachs). These tests originated in the Ultra-Orthodox sector to serve the particular needs of a community that fully rejects abortion. Today, *Dor Yeshorim* tests have become integral to marriage arrangement procedures in these communities (Vizner 2007;

Table 6 Uptake of prenatal screening tests: Jewish Israeli women by religiosity and age (as percentage)

	Secular	Traditional	Religious	Ultra-Orthodox	All women < 35y
Triple test	88.9	87.5	59.2	5.7	65.6
Fragile X	39.7	27.0	26.7	3.4	25.0
Amniocentesis (Women>35y)	94.4	62.5	36.4	0.0	50.8 (women>35y)
Tay-Zachs (via *Dor Yeshorim*)	79.9	73.2	44.9	47.7	88.9
Nuchal translucency					21.7

Source: Based on Romano-Zelicha et al. (2002)

Prainsack and Siegal, this volume), and have been swiftly endorsed by non-Orthodox women (see Table 6), albeit the latter commonly undertake testing in later stages of their marital life.

In less observant sectors, testing continues well beyond *Dor Yeshorim* tests. Prior to pregnancy, Jewish Israeli women and couples generally embark on a series of screening tests, proactively encouraged by the local HMOs. *Clalit*, for instance, declares on its pregnancy website that "modern pregnancy lasts 12 months, the first three being devoted to preparations and consultations." The pre-conception appointment is defined as "the most crucial of all pregnancy-related consultations" (Riskin-Mashiach 2007). All prospective parents are advised to be tested and even warned that "not knowing of a genetic disease in the family is not a reason to exempt oneself from pre-conception testing" (Shohat and Levy 2007). Women are further advised that even a condition as seemingly trivial as influenza may increase the fetus' risk for schizophrenia, and therefore warrants immunization. Seventeen genetic conditions are listed as pre-conception screening options.

Many of the tests are state funded (e.g., weekly monitoring of blood pressure, urine culture and edema; various blood tests; Rh typification; VDRL, rubella, glucose challenge test, the first trimester ultrasound, and the triple test). Others are subsidized for holders of basic supplementary insurance: nuchal translucency, 17 genetic diseases, CVS, amniocentesis, and second and third trimester ultrasound would each cost some $30 to $150 (U.S.), adding up to $800 to $1,000 (U.S.) if undertaken in their entirety, based on *Clalit* and

Meuhedet HMO prices. Though a significant amount, and for some women and couples a serious obstacle, these prices are affordable for most Israelis, as reflected in the high uptake levels. Yet, while nearly all (99.2 percent) pregnant Israelis were under obstetrical monitoring, prenatal testing increases with the woman's income (Romano-Zelicha et al 2002: 14), as well as age and education (Mishori-Dery, Carmi and Shoham Vardi 2007).

This intensive testing is reflected at the ideological level. Recent studies have shown that Jewish Israelis increasingly equate "good mothering" with assuming "genetic responsibility." This perception adds to the fear of coping with the burden of caring for a disabled child and of the encounter with a stigmatizing excluding environment, to account for Israelis' effort to diagnose congenital anomalies prenatally (Remennick 2006). A recent survey reaffirmed the prevalence of this view, with 82 percent of the respondents approving prenatal testing aimed at preventing the birth of affected children, and over a third (36 percent) unsure whether a neurologically impaired baby should be actively helped to survive. Among Former Soviet Union immigrants, 58 percent expressed such hesitation (Sinai 2007a). Notably, Israeli geneticists and even people with disabilities seem to subscribe to similar views (Mishori-Dery, Carmi and Shoham Vardi 2007; Raz 2004; Hashiloni-Dolev 2007).

The local openness to genetic screening is also evident when looking at newly developed testing options. Similar to the unquestioning welcome of IVF in the early 1980s (Birenbaum-Carmeli 1997), so in the early 2000s preimplantation genetic diagnosis (PGD), which raised profound ethical dilemmas elsewhere (e.g., in Germany and England [see Hashiloni-Dolev and Shkedi, and Ben-Or and Ravitzki, this volume]), was accepted in Israel with practically no public or professional debate. Moreover, using the technology in order to generate a bone marrow sibling donor—again, a heavy concern in other countries—has served in Israeli policy discussions as a self-evident example of the technology's benefits (Science and Technology Knesset Committee 2005). At present, the range of PGD applications has expanded to screening for predisposing mutations for late-onset diseases (e.g., breast and ovarian cancer in later life), and for particular cases of non-medical sex selection.

If a test does reveal an anomaly, the vast majority of Israelis choose to terminate the pregnancy. It is very difficult to provide international comparative figures regarding the termination of pregnancies of affected fetuses.[19] We can however note that in the year 2003, of 148 "Jewish fetuses" diagnosed prenatally with Down Syndrome, all but three were aborted (Ministry of Health 2005; see also Rimon-Zarfati and Raz, this volume, on genetic counselors' support of pregnancy termination).

Researchers generally agree on the main factors that have shaped the keen endorsement of genetic screening by Jewish Israelis. Prominent in the list is the perception of the embryo as acquiring its human status only gradually in the course of pregnancy, which is claimed to prevail in Jewish *Halachic* thought. Thus, embryos outside the uterus are not regarded as human life, and even developing fetuses do not have full human rights until birth (Prainsack 2006; Weiss 2002; Kahn 2000; Ben-Or and Ravitzki, this volume). As such, they are not as keenly protected in Israel as they are for instance in the Catholic world, rendering abortion more acceptable.

The Jewish tradition is also assumed to underpin a more diffused approval of human intervention in the reproductive process. In fact, some researchers even claim that such intervention is part of an obligation to fight imperfections, including diseases presumably implied in the Biblical dictate, "Conquer the land and subdue it." A similar understanding has been suggested by Douglas (1966) who claimed to have identified in Judaic scriptures an emphasized quest for perfection and clarity (e.g., in the *kosher* rules). This concern is especially relevant for our discussion given the body's centrality as a symbol and expression of the collectivity in Judaic thought (Douglas 1975). Using technology to prevent the affliction of affected newborns is thus perceived as a dignified human quest (Wahrman 2002; Heyd 1992) that accords with foundational Jewish values (Prainsack 2006; Prainsack and Siegal 2006: 26; Hashash, this volume; Ben-Or and Ravitzky, this volume).[20]

The coincidence of this religious approach with a centuries-long history of endogamy inserts additional layers of sensitivity to prenatal screening. In the last two decades, with the advent of genetics, the increased prevalence of recessive mutations in the Jewish population has been highlighted and quantified, inducing a sense of susceptibility in some Jewish communities (Birenbaum-Carmeli 2004b). Awareness of the risk of congenital anomalies has increased, often translating into a personal concern. According to Ivry (this volume), a fear of imminent catastrophe imbues the pregnancy experience of local Jewish women, which may reflect a more diffused, typically Jewish-Israeli anxiety. The concern regarding fetal pathology is apparently so intense it renders abortion reasonable even on grounds of what may objectively appear as a mild risk or impairment and even in late stages of pregnancy (for a comparative foreign reference, see Gammeltoft 2007). These concerns are all couched in a broader outlook that seems to lack the Western "suspicion" regarding science and technology (Beck 1992), but rather views these spheres as positive developments, especially in the reproductive context, where they help secure the continuity of the Jewish people (Prainsack and Firestine 2006).

Plausible and convincing as these religion- and history-based explanations appear to be, we would somewhat challenge them by revisiting Table 6, in which Orthodox Jews are shown to be visibly more reluctant towards prenatal screening than non-Orthodox Jews. Among the Orthodox, the absence of any attempt to predict or prevent the birth of an affected baby, and the readiness to acquiesce with any newborn, stand in striking opposition to the norms that prevail among non-religious Jewish Israelis. Nevertheless, the Orthodox view is obviously claimed to be as deeply rooted in Jewish tradition. Accounting for the coexistence of these incongruent approaches is beyond the scope of this introduction. However, we consider it important to highlight the incongruence as it challenges a simple straightforward attribution of the prevalence of prenatal screening and abortion among Jewish Israelis to the Jewish tradition.

Beyond Jewish tradition, Zionism and related politics seem to have added to Jewish Israelis' quest to ensure fetal normalcy. Alongside the emphasis on procreation as a means for national regeneration, Zionist writing has glorified a specific body form, that of the healthy strong "New Jew" (Weiss 2002; Gluzman 2007). This ideology was translated into practice when the medical establishment in the pre-state and early years of independence created an association between one's Zionist conviction and the height, strength, and health of babies (Stoler-Liss 2003; Khazoom 2003; Weiss 2002). These early beginnings perhaps underlay the contemporary acceptance of directivity in counseling (Shuval and Anson 2000), and even eugenic practices (Wertz 1998), which Israeli health professionals have supported in some situations. They may also underpin the relatively generous support that the state currently offers to prenatal screening (Remennick 2006), which appears to be embedded in the same ideological conviction.

Beyond the religious, historical, and ideological commitment to Jewish tradition and continuity, and to helping its citizens in securing healthy offspring, the state also operates here as a "meta" service provider whose policy needs to be weighed in economic terms. At one level, state-funded tests may be financially cost effective. At another level, the developing professional industry, alongside a burgeoning market of supplementary (private) health insurance, has its own interest in expanding prenatal testing. The women who get tested, on their part, are not just pregnant women, "Jewish women," or citizens (in a Jewish state). They are consumers as well. Though reproductive choice cannot be reduced to financial considerations (Birenbaum-Carmeli and Carmeli 2002a, 2002b), aspects of class and market seem to acquire increasing significance also in this sphere. Prenatal and fetal bodies are fragmented into systems and genes, competed over by clinics offering comparable prices, and become the objects of consumer decisions. In this increasingly commodified and privatized reality, the resulting baby is probably less of a state "possession" than it has been in the past and more clearly her or his parents'. Further, the parents are left alone, dismantled of their historic collective belonging (Remennick, this volume).

To sum up, a complex picture is evolving. Jewish Israelis emerge as proactively attempting to diagnose and prevent congenital anomalies. To some extent this is true even in the Orthodox sector where premarital testing aims to reduce the likelihood of impairment. This attitude can be traced, at least partly, to Jewish leniency regarding the humanity of the fetus, to its pronounced quest for categorical clarity and perfection as well as to increased genetic risk following centuries of endogamy. However, the fatalistic rejection of any prenatal testing or abortion that prevails among Orthodox Jews in Israel stems from a similar background, thus challenging this explanation. To this religious historical backdrop, one should add Zionism's praising of the New Jew's bodily stature and the involvement of the medical establishment in the effort to materialize this ideal, which seem to have further enhanced the local significance of able-bodiedness. Market economy drives furnish the last, though not least, component in the list of the contributing factors that we see as formative of Jewish Israelis' reproductive practices.

Bodies and identities

Reproduction and the application of new reproductive technologies, cuts across a variety of collective and private spaces. Traditional Jewish texts (religious, secular, ideological), corridors and chambers of governing bodies, medical conventions and publications, doctors' careers, hospitals' laboratories and clinics, committees deliberations, the particular biographies of women and men, single individuals and couples—all these take part in the shaping of new family experiences and structures. As they are processed through government and practice, reproductive technologies are not only a site of demographic, national, and political negotiation. They also demarcate, maybe primarily, a realm of pain, stress, shame, exposure, hope and despair, all mixing with tubes, with objectified living materials, bureaucratic forms to fill, and lines to queue. While these life processes are ongoing, and partly as a consequence, society changes, cosmology changes, gender and sex, parenthood, couplehood, all become "deconstructed," and turn liquid, to use Sigmund Bauman's concept. Perhaps more than in other spheres, the process of individuation, as manifested in the choices that must be made without clear parameters, is especially evident here. Jewish Israeli bodies—public and private—represent myths, collective memory, trauma, and the particular embeddedness of individuals in families and collective bodies. And yet, beyond and within the collectivity, cleavages are growing and tension becomes immanent in the rifts between religious and secular Jewish Israelis, different "cohorts" of immigrants, rich and poor, making the Jewish-Israeli reality an intriguing intersection between the local and the global. The following and final section will outline these aspects of Israel's reproductive landscape, which are tackled in the volume's chapters.

C.   Volume Themes and Chapters

Kin: Reproductive Technologies and the Quest for Biogenetic Parenthood

The first part of this book probes the social/biological interface of ARTs. Tracing the hardships that Jewish Israeli consumers of ARTs are ready to endure while undergoing gamete donation, surrogacy, genetic tests or adoption, the authors probe the significance conferred on biogenetic parenthood by Jewish Israelis. These chapters look at prospective parents, health professionals, and policies to reveal tacit assumptions and practices that underlie the production and reproduction of the privileging of "natural" biogenetic relatedness, which emerges as a main motivation for embarking on fertility treatment in the first place. In line with this notion, the chapters illustrate the extensive effort—on the part of policy makers, professionals, and individuals—to avert the destabilizing potential of ARTs, while sustaining traditional significances of biological kinship, some of which are expanded so they can encompass even problematic technology-generated cases.

Part I opens with an overview of the contribution of Israeli researchers to reproductive medicine. Often stated as a matter of course, local accomplishments in this field are traced in this chapter in some detail by Mashiach et al. from their historical roots in the 1940s to the present.

In chapter 2, Hashiloni-Dolev and Shkedi analyze the welcoming ethical discourse and regulation of Preimplantation Genetic Diagnosis (PGD) for sibling donors in Israel. A comparison to the U.K. and Germany, where the technology was a source of concern and tightly restricted, underscores the Jewish Israeli particularity. The latter is explained by the prioritization of the welfare of the biogenetic family over that of the individual. Generalized into a more encompassing reading, this understanding would suggest that Jewish Israelis tend to assume and expect an especially enhanced bond and mutual liability among family members.

Jewish Israeli notions of relatedness are also examined in Helene Goldberg's study of men in fertility treatments. Though largely marginalized in the treatment setting, the male partner still has to provide the sperm, a task that may pose serious religious and psychological difficulties for some men. Interviewees' accounts regarding these difficulties illustrate the embeddedness of ARTs in culture-specific ideas about kinship, gender, and sexuality, as well as the distance that Jewish Israelis will go to achieve biogenetic parenthood. They also show how traditional ideas, though challenged through ART practices, are ultimately reinforced rather than destabilized.

In chapter 4, Elly Teman takes a critical look at another obstacle riddled route to biogenetic parenthood, that of surrogacy. An analysis of the making of Israel's Surrogacy Law highlights the law's restrictive aspects that subject all applicants to close state control, which eventually enhances conservative biogenetic notions of kinship. The tight monitoring of this specific technology is interpreted as the state's response to the symbolic challenges that surrogacy presents to traditional definitions of "mother" and "family," to biogenetic parenthood, and to the national collective boundaries that are constructed and maintained through the bodies and families of its citizens.

Going beyond ART, Birenbaum-Carmeli and Carmeli compare Israel's ART policy to the state regulation of adoption. Their chapter points at the striking difference between the inclusive state funding of ARTs and the tight conservative requirements presented to applicants of domestic adoption. Inter-country adoption sets more accessible eligibility criteria but entails very high costs which render it unattainable for most Israelis. The differences are accounted for in terms of the symbolic significance bestowed on biogenetic relatedness in contemporary Jewish Israel, particularly as a constitutive element of the Jewish collectivity. It is this definition, which is currently challenged by various historical processes, that the state seems to be trying to protect by privileging biogenetic over social forms of relatedness.

Gene: Reproductive Technologies and the Quest for the Perfect Child

Part II of the collection probes the social ramifications of applying various prenatal screening technologies in Israel, analyzing the opportunities they open up for active decision making on issues traditionally considered a matter of destiny. Local attitudes towards the expanding ability to assess and predict the health of a fetus are explored at various stages along the reproductive process, from premarital genetic screening of potential spouses, to obstetrical ultrasound and abortion decisions on grounds of potential embryopathy. The final chapter in this part includes a contribution by legal experts on the IVF-based research domain of human embryonic stem cells. This account expands its perspective beyond the social sciences.

Part II begins with Prainsack and Siegal's study of *Dor Yeshorim* premarital genetic screening, which defines the "genetic compatibility" of prospective spouses in Orthodox communities. The study offers an insight into the paramount significance bestowed on the health of the unborn in a community that rejects abortion. A comparison to the Cypriot premarital screening program for Thalassemia highlights Dor Yeshorim's notion of "genetic couplehood" that associates an existing risk to the bond of two individuals rather than to one person. By so doing, *Dor Yeshorim* avoids some of the pressing issues that occupy "secular" genetic screening, like the perils of "knowing too much." A preliminary survey of Orthodox students reveals how screening has come to be perceived as a social rather than a medical procedure.

Moving further along the reproductive process, Ivry takes a critical look at obstetrical ultrasound. On the basis of an analysis of public presentations by experts, Ivry contends that the technology is routinely used in Israel to present ultrasound detectable fetal anomalies to pregnant women and their partners, thereby infusing terror into the social imagery of gestation. The unreserved embrace of prenatal diagnostic technologies and selective abortions and the absence of a meaningful public debate about the eugenic implications of these "selective" technologies are associated with a diffused Jewish-Israeli sense of threat that renders prenatal screening most attractive to local professionals and prospective parents. In this respect, obstetric ultrasound is applied in Israel in a way that (also) nurtures parents' fears of anomalies to counter the prevailing image of pronatalism.

A complementary perspective on the importance of fetal "normalcy" and the limits of Israeli pronatalism is provided in Rimon-Zarfaty's and Raz's analysis of professional and lay views on selective abortion following mild or likely fetal pathology. In the absence of clear definitions and guidelines, responses to mild embryopathy are left to abortion committees, genetic counselors, and prospective parents. Interviews and media analysis reveal that unlike their foreign counterparts, Israelis are pleased with the existing legal ambiguity and the greater flexibility it grants them in decision making, and are generally supportive of abortion even in relatively mild or less probable cases, and in late-stage pregnancies.

The last chapter in Part II looks at human embryonic stem cell research from a judicial point of view. In this field, products of the reproductive technology of IVF comprise a platform for the investigation of foundational scientific questions, assumed to be of unparalleled therapeutic potential. Israel was one of the first countries to regulate this research field via law. From their participants' standpoint, Ben-Or and Ravitsky offer a jurist's and a bioethicist's perspective on the making of Israel's cloning law. The legislative processes leading to the formulation of the law in 1999 and its extension in 2004 are analyzed as reflecting a unique Israeli approach to key ethical issues such as the moral status of the human embryo, the importance of actively seeking therapeutic potentials, and scientific progress as key to Jewish Israel's prosperity and survival. To the desire to help humankind by developing new therapies that is at the center of the chapter, we would add the likely contribution to researchers' professional development and a broader Israeli ambition to take part in the international scientific community, for which reproductive medicine has long been an established vehicle.

Community: A Self-Portrait with Technology

The application and governing of technologies are local cultural products, ones that are congruent with the past and further reproduce it. In the case of RT, the technological similarity across international contexts renders the surrounding field of practice an intriguing lens for community self-reflection, for the exploration of local particularities, and for collective positioning vs. globalization processes. The positions of various categories of citizens/patients/consumers vis-à-vis the state can be explored through their entitlement to, perception of, and utilization of RT services. Social critics can use RT as a platform to question the role of professionals' scientific and career interests in the development of the domain. Culture analysts can examine seemingly revolutionary technological-legal developments that may be understood, on a deeper reading, as coherent with or even succeeding ancient practices. This significance of RT as a vantage point has been invoked in the descriptions of Israeli fertility practitioners of their research as part of the international RT endeavor (chapter 1), as well as in the practitioners' reflections on local legislation in the field of hESC (chapter 9). In this last part of the book, the chapters aim to project a broader picture of Israel as emerging from RT-related issues. No less than ends in themselves, RTs serve here as a vantage point for the scrutiny of the social system within which they take place. The studies take a reflexive look, listening to lay Israelis, health professionals and policy makers as they reason and enact local and broader international contexts. An analysis of the religious underpinning of Israel's ART policy concludes this composite portrait.

The first three chapters in this part look at the actual "craft" of IVF from the professionals' perspective. In chapter 10, two senior Israeli researchers, Nissim Benvenisty and Karl Skorecki, present their views on the principles and concerns that guide their daily research. Assuming, as we do, that genetics and society are mutually intertwined, we present their views on what is "Jewish" in Israel's policy and practice and how they locate Israel's hESC research and regulation within international laws, norms, and networks in this thoroughly globalized scientific domain.

In chapter 11, Yali Hashash looks at professionals' work through a more politicized lens. Unlike the accepted view of doctors' practice and recommendations as professionally neutral and as a tribute to the Zionist nation building project, Hashash analyzes the medicalization of reproduction as a process of power accumulation. Three moments in the politics of reproduction are explored to illustrate how the interests of medical experts, cloaked or aided by national rhetoric and enacted through state apparatuses, have served professionals' interests and research agendas by expanding their jurisdiction into wider aspects of the reproductive process.

For the doctors, nurses, technicians, *mashgichot* and secretaries in IVF clinics, operating theaters and laboratories, the hospital is one's workplace. Susan Kahn's ethnography conveys a rare glance at the daily life of the clinic as operated and experienced by its employees. On the basis of her fieldwork, Kahn describes, in detail, the health professionals' work, integrating craftwork, surgical skills, emotional labor, teamwork, and administrative aspects in a way that resonates with broader, culture-specific perceptions and modes of work. A somewhat chaotic blend of irony, irreverence, and impatience, alongside profound compassion, heartfelt identification, and intense joy is depicted in defining the clinic as intensely Israeli, forming a setting that mirrors and dramatizes the world outside its walls.

The subsequent chapter moves beyond the monolithic focus on Jewish Israelis to venture into wider citizens' circles, and their respective positions and agencies. Remennick's comparison of attitudes toward ARTs looks at three local sectors of Israeli women: native Jewish Israelis, native Palestinian Israelis, and Jewish immigrants from the Former Soviet Union. The observed differences among these groups and each group's reasoning of civil rights, state services and state-citizen interface are interpreted as reflecting each group's particular location within and commitment to the Zionist State and its medical institutions. The comparison shows Israeli-born Jewish women as having the strongest sense of entitlement for state funded ART and other forms of public support for parenting. More generally, the state is increasingly viewed as an instrumental service provider rather than a collective mission that the women are part of.

In the volume's last research chapter, Seeman takes us back, in a critical and innovative way, to probe Jewish religion and tradition as one of the major influences on the proliferation of RTs in Israel. Through textual analysis, ethnography and scrutiny of public ethical deliberation, Seeman asks whether there is anything distinctively Jewish or Israeli that has facilitated the smooth adoption of RTs in Israel. His suggestion is that the Jewish focus on positive law, namely the emphasis on discrete kinship prohibitions, which in principle licenses all practices that are not forbidden, allows an unusual degree of flexibility in setting ART policies.

Notes

1. As this chapter is being written, a group of US and Japanese researchers are announcing the production of stem cells from skin types, thereby probably rendering embryos unnecessary to further research and developments in this field (Henderson 2007).
2. CIA (N.D).
3. An indication of the contemporary significance of these statuses, at least in observant circles, was provided in 2004, when the PGD committee (that considers applications for non-medical sex selection) accepted the request of an ultraorthodox couple, who planned to undergo donor insemination, to have only female embryos transferred to the woman in order to avoid public exposure of the treatment in case they had a son who would not inherit the father's Cohen status (owing to the donation). The request was one of the few that was approved by the

committee, and it was repeatedly invoked in subsequent discussions of the subject in the Knesset committees (e.g., on March 16, 2005; July 5, 2005; and October 30, 2006).

4. An incidental illustration printed in Israel's widest read daily and titled, "Who Wants to be a Jew—the New Jews" (Palter and Mosgovoya 2007), presumably traced various tribes of Israel throughout the world.

5. We note that the situation in the Israeli Palestinian sector is quite similar. See for instance Mor et al. (2006: 31).

6. Mercer Human Resources Consulting (2007).

7. Social Security Online (2004).

8. Alexander von Humboldt Foundation (2006).

9. Forsakringskassan (2007).

10. The National Insurance Institute of Israel <(http://www.btl.gov .il/BENEFITS/CHILDREN/Pages/ירועיש%20הבצקה.aspx> (accessed March 25, 2009). The allowance for children born after May 31, 2003, will be further reduced to $ 40 (U.S.) each.

11. Citizens Information (N.D).

12. Cleiss (N.D).

13. HM Revenue and Customs (N.D).

14. Norway: The Official Site in the United States (N.D).

15. Indeed, in several Knesset discussions some experts seemed to be willing to compromise accepted medical knowledge in order to make their point. For example, one eminent practitioner claimed that "a five cycle limit per child would leave childless half the patients who could have conceived," which is a statement at odds with data showing a steep decline in pregnancy rates after three unsuccessful cycles (Jones 2005). On the other hand, in a private communication, the head of one IVF unit estimated that roughly 80 percent of treatment cycles in Israel are performed on women who keep repeating unproductive cycles, many of whom are over 40. A claim that in many cases treatment was continued primarily owing to doctors' economic motivation has also been mentioned to us informally, as well as doctors' growing financial interest in privately funded reproductive tourism for purposes of egg donation and sex selection.

16. For a recent illustration, see the BBC front page report (Roberts 2007) of "a huge advance" made by Israeli scientists who had extracted, matured, and frozen eggs from young cancer patients for possible fertility treatment in the future.

17. This exceptional starting point of Israel's gynecological research was part of a wider process that took place in the country at that time. This process began with the opening of the Hebrew University in Jerusalem in 1925, intensified with the Nazi rise to power, and continued with the emigration to Palestine of prominent Jewish scientists, intellectuals, and artists from central Europe, who set supreme professional standards in fields as diverse as mathematicians (Edmund Landau, Adolf Abraham Halevi Fraenkel and Mih´aly-Michael Fekete, who founded the Einstein Institute of Mathematics at the Hebrew University of Jerusalem [Katz 2004]),

sociology (Martin Buber was among the founders of Israeli sociology), Jewish philosophy (Gershon Sholem), and music (Bronislaw Huberman founded the Israeli Philharmonic Orchestra [Birenbaum-Carmeli 1991]).

18. Interestingly, we found some similarity between this understanding and Iran's population policy. In the last four decades Iran has reduced its TFR from roughly 6.0 to replacement level (Abbasi-Shavazi 2002; Tremayne 2004: 181–85). Among the various factors of successful intervention was the opening of dozens of fertility clinics that garnered the support of people who had objected to the government's primarily anti-natal stance (Tremayne).

19. A more comprehensive comparison of abortion statistics is complicated as it involves a variety of reasons for pregnancy termination. In an international comparison of the percentage of known pregnancies ending in legal abortions, Israel, with 12.3%, ranked lower than countries such as Sweden (25.3%), Canada (23.6%), New Zealand (23.3%), U.S.A. (23.29%), U.K. (21.8%), Denmark (19%), Germany (15.3%), and the Netherlands (13%). These figures do not provide, however, information regarding abortions on ground of embryopathy (Johnston 2007).

20. The other side of the coin can be observed in Israelis' intolerance towards bodily imperfections as manifested in popular perceptions (Remennick 2006), state policies (Rimmerman and Birenbaum-Carmeli; Mor 2006) and the life conditions of people with disabilities that have been found to be worse in Israel than in any Western country (Sinai 2007b).

References

Abbasi-Shavazi, Mohammad Jalal. 2002. "Convergence of Fertility Behaviours in Iran: Provincial Fertility Levels, Trends and Patterns in Iran." *Social Science Journal* 18: 201–31.

Alexander von Humboldt Foundation. 2006. "Child Benefit According to German Law or Child Allowance of the AvH." <http://www.avh.de/EN/PROGRAMME/STIP_AUS/doc/stp/merkblatt_kinderzulage.pdf> (accessed January 31, 2008).

Amir, Delila and Orly Benjamin. 1992. "Abortion Approval as a Ritual of Symbolic Control." In *The Criminalization of a Woman's Body*, ed. Clarice. Feinman. New York: Haworth Press.

Angel, Dvorit. 2007. "Press Release: Patterns of Fertility in 2006" [Hebrew] <http://cbs.gov.il/www/hodaot2007n/01_07_215b.pdf> (accessed February 3, 2008).

Azoulay, Yuval. 2007. "Sixty-Nine Professional Associations: Increase the Medication Basket." <http://www.haaretz.co.il/hasite/spages/925348.html> (accessed November 18, 2007).

Barkai, Haim. 1998. *The Evolution of Israel's Social Security System: Structure, Time Pattern and Macroeconomic Impact*. Aldershot: Ashgate.

Bates, Stephen R. 2006. "Making Time for Change: On Temporal Conceptualizations within (Critical Realist) Approaches to the Relationship between Structure and Agency." *Sociology* 40, no. 1: 143–61.

Beck, Ulrich. 1992. *Risk Society: Towards a New Modernity*. New Delhi: Sage

Bell, Catherine. 1992. *Ritual Theory, Ritual Practice*. Oxford: Oxford University Press.

Berkowitch, Nitza. 1997. "Motherhood as a National Mission: The Construction of Womanhood in the Legal Discourse in Israel." *Women's Studies International Forum* 20, nos. 5–6: 605–19.

———. 2000. "Eshet Hayil Mi Yimtza: Women and citizenship in Israel" [Hebrew]. *Israeli Sociology* 2, no. 1: 277–317.

Berman, Eli. 2000. "Sect, Subsidy, and Sacrifice: An Economist's View of Ultra-Orthodox Jews." *The Quarterly Journal of Economics* 115, no. 3: 905–53.

Birenbaum-Carmeli, Daphna. 1991. "Overtones: The Social World of the Israeli Philharmonic Orchestra." *International Review of the Aesthetics and Sociology of Music* 22: 81–98.

———. 1997. "Pioneering Procreation: Israel's First Test-Tube Baby." *Science as Culture* 6: 525–40.

———. 2003. "Reproductive Policy in Context: Implications on the Rights of Jewish Women in Israel 1945–2000." *Policy Studies* 24, no. 2: 101–14.

———. 2004a. "'Cheaper than a Newcomer': On the Political Economy of IVF in Israel." *The Sociology of Health and Illness* 26, no. 7: 897–924.

———. 2004b. "The Prevalence of Jews as Subjects in Genetic Research: Explanation and Potential Implications." *American Journal of Medical Genetic* 130A, no. 1: 76–83.

———. 2007. "Contested surrogacy and the gender order: an Israeli case study." *Journal of Middle East Women's Studies* 3: 21–44

Birenbaum-Carmeli, Daphna and Yoram S. Carmeli. 2002a. "Physiognomy, Familism and Consumerism: Preferences among Jewish Israeli Recipients of Donor Insemination." *Social Science and Medicine* 54, no. 3: 363–76.

———. 2002b. Hegemony and Homogeneity: "Donor Preferences of Recipients of Donor Insemination." *The Journal of Material Culture* 7, no. 1: 73–94.

Birenbaum-Carmeli, Daphna. and Martha Dirnfeld. 2007. "Women's Experiences Following Repeated IVF Treatments in Israel." *Annual Meeting of the European Society of Human Reproduction and Embryology (ESHRE) (Poster presentation)*. Lyon, France.

Birenbaum-Carmeli, Daphna, Yoram S. Carmeli and HaimYavetz. 2000. "Secrecy among Israeli recipients of donor insemination." *Politics and the Life Sciences* 19: 69–76.

Birenbaum-Carmeli Daphna and Marcia C. Inhorn. 2009. Introduction: Assisting Reproduction, Testing Genes: Global Encounters with New Biotechnologies. In *Assisting Reproduction, Testing Genes: Global Encounters with New Biotechnologies*, eds. Daphna Birenbaum-Carmeli and Marcia C. Inhorn. Oxford and New York: Berghahn Books.

Bradshaw, Jonathan and Naomi Finch. 2002. "A Comparison of Child Benefit Packages in 22 countries." <http://www.dwp.gov.uk/asd/asd5/rport174/Inside.pdf> (accessed February 1, 2008).

British Employment Law. 2007. "Paternity Leave/International Comparisons." <http://www.emplaw.co.uk/researchfree-redirector.aspx?StartPage=data % 2f20033221.htm> (accessed November 8, 2007).

Carmeli, Yoram S. and Daphna Birenbaum-Carmeli. 2000a. "Ritualizing the 'Natural Family': Secrecy in Israeli Donor Insemination." *Science as Culture* 9, no. 3: 301–25.

———. 2000b. "State Regulation of Donor Insemination: An Israeli Case Study." *Medicine and Law* 19, no. 4: 839–54.

Center for Disease Control and Prevention. 2003. "QuickStats: Average Age of Mothers at First Birth, by State—United States, 2002." <http://www.cdc.gov/mmwR/preview/mmwrhtml/mm5419a5.htm> (accessed January 28, 2008).

Central Bureau of Statistics. 2005a. "Immigrant Population from the Former USSR—Demographic Trends 1990–2001" [Hebrew]. <http://www.cbs.gov.il/www/publications/migration_ussr01/pdf/mavo_03.pdf> (accessed January 11, 2008).

———. 2005b. "Table: Divorce Rates, by Religion." <http://www.cbs.gov.il/shnaton58/diag/03_02.pdf> (accessed January 28, 2008).

———. 2006a. "Live Births—Selected Figures" [Hebrew]. <http://www.cbs.gov.il/reader/cw_usr_view_SHTML?ID=630> (accessed January 28, 2008).

———. 2006b. "Press Release: International Women's Day, March 7, 2007" [Hebrew]. <http://www.cbs.gov.il/reader/newhodaot/hodaa_template.html?hodaa=200711038> (accessed January 8, 2008).

———. 2006c. "Patterns of Fertility in 2006" [Hebrew]. <http://www.cbs.gov.il/www/hodaot2007n/01_07_215b.doc> (accessed January 31, 2008).

———. 2007a. "OECD Statistical Data." <http://www.cbs.gov.il/oecd/oecdisrn.htm> (accessed (accessed January 28, 2008).

———. 2007b. "Marriages, Divorces, Live Births, Deaths, Natural Increase, Infant Deaths and Stillbirths, by Religion." <http://www.cbs.gov.il/shnaton58/st03_01.pdf> (accessed January 28, 2008).

———. 2007c. "Press Release for Tu Be'av, July 29, 2007" [Hebrew]. <http://www.cbs.gov.il/www/hodaot2007n/11_07_137b.doc> (accessed January 28, 2008).

———. 2007d. "Family Day—Families and Households in Israel" [Hebrew]. <http://www.cbs.gov.il/www/hodaot2007n/11_07_021b.doc> (accessed January 28, 2008).

———. 2007e. "Press Release: Selected Data for International Child Day" [Hebrew]. <http://www.cbs.gov.il/reader/newhodaot/hodaa_template.html?hodaa=200711223> (accessed January 8, 2008).

———. 2007f. "Population in Israel by Numbers 2007" [Hebrew]. <http://www.cbs.gov.il/www/publications/isr_in_n07h.pdf> (accessed December 30, 2007).

———. 2007g. "Press Release: Social Survey 2006" [Hebrew]. <http://www.cbs.gov.il/reader/newhodaot/hodaa_template.html?hodaa=200719104> (accessed January 8, 2008).

———. 2007h. "Israeli Statistical Monthly 9/2007, Table 20/1, Population by Population Group" [Hebrew]. <http://www.cbs.gov.il/www/yarhon/b1_h.htm> (accessed February 4, 2008).

————. 2007i. "Fertility Rates, by Age and Religion (Table 3.12)." <http:// www1.cbs.gov.il/shnaton58/shnaton58_all_e.pdf> (accessed February 4, 2008).

CIA. N.D. *The World Fact Book.* <https://www.cia.gov/library/publications/ the-world-factbook/geos/us.html#People> (accessed January 28, 2008).

Citizens Information. N.D. "Child Benefit Monthly Rate from April 2007 to March 2008." <http://www.citizensinformation.ie/categories/social-welfare/social-welfare-payments/social-welfare-payments-to-families-and-children/child_benefit#rates> (accessed January 31, 2008).

Chambers, G. M., M. G. Chapman, N. Grayson, M. Shanahan, and E. A. Sullivan. 2007. "Babies Born after ART Treatment Cost More than Non-ART Babies: A Cost Analysis of Inpatient Birth-Admission Costs of Singleton and Multiple Gestation Pregnancies." *Human Reproduction* 22, no. 12: 3108–15.

Clalit HMO. 2007. "Pregnancy Tests Table." <http://www.clalit.co.il/HE-IL/ Family/pregnancy/exemlist/> (accessed November 29, 2007).

Cleiss. N.D. "The French Social Security System." <http://www.cleiss.fr/ docs/regimes/regime_france/an_3.html> (accessed January 31, 2008).

Collins, J. A. 2002. "An International Survey of the Health Economics of IVF and ICSI." *Human Reproductive Update* 8: 265–77.

Doron, Abraham. and Ralph M. Kramer. 1991. *The Welfare State in Israel: The Evolution of Social Security Policy and Practice.* Boulder, CO: Westview Press.

Douglas, Mary. 1966. *Purity and Danger.* London: Routledge and Kegan Paul.

————. 1999 [1975]. *Implicit Meanings: 2nd Edition: Selected Essays in Anthropology.* London: Routledge.

Drake, R.F. 1999. *Understanding Disability Politics.* London: Macmillan.

Ducker, Claire Louise. 2006. "Jews, Arabs and Arab Jews: The Politics of Identity and Reproduction in Israel." <http://biblio.iss.nl/opac/uploads/ wp/wp421.pdf> (accessed February 3, 2008).

EconStats. N.D. "GDP per Capita, Current Prices." <http://www.econstats. com/weo/V016.htm> (accessed February 3, 2008).

Editorial. 2006. "Cheap IVF Needed." *Nature* 442: 958.

ESHRE. 2006. "Three Million Babies Born Using Assisted Reproductive Technologies." <http://www.eshre.com/emc.asp?pageId=806> (accessed January 10, 2008).

Eurofound. N.D. "EurLIFE: Age of Woman at First Birth." <http://www. eurofound.europa.eu/areas/qualityoflife/eurlife/index.php?template=3 &radioindic=58&idDomain=5> (accessed January 28, 2008).

Eurofound. N.Db. "EurLIFE: Non-Marital Births." <http://www.eurofound. europa.eu/areas/qualityoflife/eurlife/index.php?template=3&radioindic =59&idDomain=5> (accessed January 28, 2008).

Europa. N.D. "Data on the Healthy Life Years in the European Union." (accessed January 28, 2008. <http://ec.europa.eu/health/ph_information/ indicators/lifeyears_data_en.htm>

Eurostat. N.Da. "Infant Mortality (per 1000 Live Births)." (accessed January 28, 2008. <http://epp.eurostat.ec.europa.eu/portal/page?_pageid= 1996,39140985&_dad=portal&_schema=PORTAL&screen=detailref&

language=en&product=Yearlies_new_population&root=Yearlies_new_
population/C/C1/C14/cba13072>

Eurostat. N.Db. "Marriages (per 1000 Persons)." (accessed January 28, 2008.
<http://epp.eurostat.ec.europa.eu/portal/page?_pageid=1996,39140985&_
dad=portal&_schema=PORTAL&screen=detailref&language=en&product
=Yearlies_new_population&root=Yearlies_new_population/C/C1/C13/
cab10000>

Fogel, Nir and Israela Friedman. 2006. "Orthodox in the Labor Market: Social Survey Findings for the Years 2002–2005." <http://www1.cbs.gov.il/
www/publications/pub52_h.pdf> (accessed January 8, 2008).

Forsakringskassan. 2007. "Child Allowance and Large Family Supplement."
(accessed January 31, 2008. <http://www.fk.se/fakta/andra_sprak/barn-
bidrag_eng/index.php>

Franklin, S. 1997. *Embodied Progress: A Cultural Account of Assisted Conception.*
London: Routledge

———. 2006. "The Cyborg Embryo: Our Path to Transbiology." *Theory Culture Society* 23: 167–89.

———. 2007. *Dolly Mixtures: The Remaking of Genealogy.* Durham, NC: Duke
University Press.

Franklin, Sarah and Susan McKinnon, eds. 2001. *Relative Values: Reconfigur-
ing Kinship Studies.* Durham, NC: Duke University Press.

Franklin, Sarah and Roberts Celia. 2006. *Born and Made: An Ethnography of
Preimplantation Genetic Diagnosis.* Princeton: Princeton University Press.

Friedlander, Dov. N.D. "Fertility in Israel: Is the Transition to Replacement Level in Sight?" <http://www.un.org/esa/population/publications/completing-
fertility/RevisedFriedlanderpaper.PDF> (accessed October 28, 2007).

Gammeltoft, Tine M. 2007. "Prenatal Diagnosis in Postwar Vietnam: Power,
Subjectivity, and Citizenship." *American Anthropologist* 109, no. 1: 153–63.

Glickman A. 2003. Marriage in Israel on the threshold of the 21st century
[Hebrew]. *Public Opinion [De'ot Ba'am]*, no. 7.

Gluzman, Michael. 2007. *The Zionist Body: Nationalism, Gender and Sexuality
in the New Hebrew Literature* [Hebrew]. Tel Aviv: Hakibbutz Hameuchad.

Gold, M. 1988. *And Hannah Wept: Infertility, Adoption and the Jewish Couple.*
Philadelphia: The Jewish Publication Society.

Goldscheider, C. 1996. *Israel's Changing Society: Population, Ethnicity and Development.* Boulder, Co: Westview Press.

Gonen, Amiram. 2005. Between Bible Learning and Breadwinning: Learning Earners Society in London" [Hebrew]. <http://www.fips.org.il/fips/
site/p_publications/item_he.asp?iid=733> (accessed January 8, 2008).

Government Decision No. 3551. 2005. "Cost of the Health Basket, April
17." (accessed December 16 2007. <http://www.pmo.gov.il/PMO/
Archive/Decisions/ 2005/04/des3551.htm>

Greenhalgh, Susan. 1990. "Toward a Political Economy of Fertility: Anthropological Contributions." *Population and Development Review* 16, no.
1: 85–106.

Gurovich, Norma and Eilat Cohen-Kastro. 2004. "Ultra-Orthodox Jews: Geographic Distribution and Demographic, Social and Economic Characteristics

of the Ultra-Orthodox Jewish Population in Israel 1996–2001." <http://www. cbs.gov.il/www/publications/int_ulor.pdf> (accessed January 8, 2008).

Hashash, Yali. 2004. "Ethnicity, Class and Gender in Israel's Fertility Policy, 1962–1974" [Hebrew]. Masters thesis, Haifa University.

Hashiloni-Dolev, Y. 2007. *A Life (Un)Worthy of Living: Reproductive Genetics in Israel and Germany.* Secaucus, NJ: Springer.

Hasson, Nir. 2007. "For the First Time: Parents of a Deceased Soldier are Allowed to Use His Sperm to Fertilize a Woman He Has Not Known" [Hebrew]. *Ha'aretz*, January 15.

Henderson, Mark. 2007. "Breakthrough as Stem Cells are Produced from Skin, not Embryos." (accessed November 28, 2007. <http://www.time-sonline.co.uk/tol/life_and_style/health/article2908408.ece>

Heyd, David. 1992. *Genethics: Moral Issues in the Creation of People*, Berkeley, CA: University of California Press.

HM Revenue and Customs. N.D. "How Much Child Benefit Will I Get?" <http://www.hmrc.gov.uk/childbenefit/cb-key.htm#h> (accessed January 31, 2008).

Inhorn, Marcia and Daphna Birenbaum-Carmeli. 2008. "Male Infertility, Chronicity, and the Plight of the Palestinian Men in Israel and Lebanon." In *Chronic Conditions, Fluid States: Globalization and the Anthropology of Illness*, eds. Lenore Manderson and Carolyn Smith-Morris. New Brunswick, NJ: Rutgers University Press.

Institute for the Study of Civil Society. 2006. "Family Does Best When Governments Don't Try to Nationalise Child-Rearing." (accessed January 28, 2008. <http://www.civitas.org.uk/press/prcs43.php>

Israel Women's Network. N.D. "The Exceptionality of Fertility Treatment in Israel" [Hebrew]. <http://www.iwn.org.il/inner.asp?newsid=52> (accessed February 3, 2008).

Jewish Agency for Israel. 2007. "40 Years of Struggle for the Soviet Union Jewry" [Hebrew]. <http://www.jewishagency.org/JewishAgency/Hebrew/Education/Compelling+Content/Jewish+World/Diaspora/Russia/> (accessed January 8, 2008).

Johnston, William Robert. 2007. "Percentage of Pregnancies Aborted by Country." <http://www.johnstonsarchive.net/policy/abortion/wrjp333-pd.html> (accessed January 8, 2008).

Jones, C. A. 2005. "Cost-effectiveness of the Single Embryo Transfer." Presentation given at the Reproductive Disruption Conference, Ann Arbour, Michigan.

Kanaaneh, Rhoda Ann. 2002. *Birthing the Nation: Strategies of Palestinian Women in Israel.* Berkeley, CA: University of California Press.

Kahn, S.M. 2000 *Reproducing Jews: a Cultural Account of Assisted Conception in Israel.* Durham and London: Duke University Press.

———. 2002. Rabbis and reproduction: the uses of new reproductive technologies among ultraorthodox Jews in Israel. In *Infertility around the Globe: New Thinking on Childlessness, Gender, and Reproductive Technologies*, eds. Marcia C. Inhorn and Frank Van Balen, 283–97. Berkeley, CA: University of California Press.

Katz, Jacob. 1971. *Tradition and Crisis: Jewish Society at the End of the Middle Ages*. New York: Schoken Books.

Katz, Shaul. 2004. "Berlin Roots—Zionist Incarnation: The Ethos of Pure Mathematics and the Beginnings of the Einstein Institute of Mathematics at the Hebrew University of Jerusalem." *Science in Context* 17, no. 1/2: 199–234.

Khazoom, Aziz. 2003. "The Great Chain of Orientalism: Jewish Identity, Stigma Management, and Ethnic Exclusion in Israel." *American Sociological Review* 68: 481–510.

Koivurova, S., A.L. Hartikainen, M. Gissler, E. Hemminki, R. Klemetti and M.-R. Järvelin. 2004. "Health Care Costs Resulting from IVF: Prenatal and Neonatal Periods." *Human Reproduction* 19, no. 12: 2798–2805.

Landau, R. 2004. "Posthumous Sperm Retrieval for the Purpose of Later Insemination or IVF in Israel: An Ethical and Psychosocial Critique." *Human Reproduction* 19, no. 9: 1952–56.

Leach, Edmund. 1969. "The Legitimacy of Solomon." In *Genesis as Myth and Other Essays*. London: Jonathan Cape.

Lerner-Geva, L., E. Geva, J.B. Lessing, A. Chetrit, B. Modan and A. Amit. 2003. "The Possible Association between In Vitro Fertilization Treatments and Cancer Development." *International Journal of Gynecological Cancer* 13: 23–27.

Meiselman, Moshe. 1978. *Jewish Woman in Jewish Law*. New York: Yeshiva University Press.

Mercer Human Resources Consulting. 2007. "Cost of Living Survey—Worldwide Ranking 2007." <http://www.mercer.com/costofliving> (accessed January 31, 2008).

Ministry of Finance. 2007. "Ministry of Health Budget—2005." <http://www.mof.gov.il/budget2006/fbudget.htm?/budget2005/budget.htm> (accessed November 8, 2007).

Ministry of Health. 2005. "Program for the Prevention of Congenital Anomalies and Genetic Diseases in Israel in the Year 2003" [Hebrew]. <http://www.health.gov.il/download/forms/a2670_momim2003.pdf> (accessed February 3, 2008).

Ministry of Industry, Commerce and Employment. N.D. "The Mother's Rights in Israel." (accessed February 3, 2008. <http://www.moit.gov.il/NR/exeres/EAD58FC4-F826–43B5–890D-3E17452313C0.htm>

Mishori Dery, Anat, Rivka Carmi and Ilana Shoham Vardi. 2007. "Different Perceptions and Attitudes Regarding Prenatal Testing among Service Providers and Consumers in Israel." *Community Genetics* 10, no. 4: 242–51.

Mor, S. 2006. Between Charity, Welfare, and Warfare: A Disability Legal Studies Analysis of Privilege and Neglect in Israeli Disability Policy." *Yale Journal of Law and the Humanities* 18, no. 1: 63–137.

Mossawa Center Staff. 2006. "The Palestinian Arab Citizens of Israel: Status, Opportunities and Challenges for an Israeli-Palestinian Peace." <http://www.mossawacenter.org/files/files/File/The%20Palestinian%20Arab%20Citizens%20of%20Israel_Status...2006.pdf> (accessed January 11, 2008).

Mosse, George L. 1985. *Nationalism and Sexuality: Respectability and Abnormal Sexuality in Modern Europe*. New York: Howard Fertig.

Nahman, M. 2005. "Israeli extraction: an ethnographic study of egg donation and national imaginaries." PhD thesis, Lancaster University, UK.

Nahmias, Petra. 2004. Fertility Behaviour of Recent Immigrants to Israel: A Comparative Analysis of Immigrants from Ethiopia and the Former Soviet Union." *Demographic Research* 10: 83–120. <http://www.demographic-research.org/volumes/vol10/4/10–4.pdf> (accessed January 8, 2008).

National Center for Health Statistics. 2007 [2006]. "Table 27. Life Expectancy at Birth, at 65 Years of Age, and at 75 Years of Age, by Race and Sex: United States, Selected Years 1900–2004." In *Health, United States, 2006*. <http://www.cdc.gov/nchs/data/hus/hus06.pdf#027> (accessed on January 28, 2008).

National Center for Health Statistics. 2007. "Infant Health." (accessed January 28, 2008. <http://www.cdc.gov/nchs/fastats/infant_health.htm>

National Center for Health Statistics. 2007b. "Births, Marriages, Divorces, and Deaths: Provisional Data for March 2007." (accessed January 28, 2008. <http://www.cdc.gov/nchs/data/nvsr/nvsr56/nvsr56_04.pdf>

National Center for Health Statistics. 2007c. "Unmarried Childbearing." <http://www.cdc.gov/nchs/fastats/unmarry.htm> (accessed January 28, 2008).

Nelkin, Dorothy and Susan M. Lindee. 2004. *The DNA Mystique: The Gene as a Cultural Icon*. Ann Arbor: University of Michigan Press.

Nimwegen, Nico van, Gijs Beets, Jørgen Mortensen, Anna Ruzik, Ulrich Schuh, and Erika Schulz. 2006. "Europe at the Cross Roads: Demographic Developments in the European Union." <http://ec.europa.eu/employment_social/spsi/docs/social_situation/2006_exec_sum_demo.pdf> (accessed January 8, 2008).

Norway: The Official Site in the United States. N.D. "Family Allowance." <http://www.norway.org/policy/family/allowance/allowance.htm> (accessed January 31, 2008).

Nyboe Andersen, A, V. Goossens, L. Gianaroli, R. Felberbaum, J. de Mouzon and K.G. Nygren. 2007. "Assisted Reproductive Technology in Europe, 2003. Results Generated from European Registers by ESHRE." *Human Reproduction* 22, no. 6: 1513–25.

Nyboe Andersen, A., L. Gianaroli and K.G. Nygren. 2004. "Assisted Reproductive Technology in Europe 2000. Results Generated from European Registers by ESHRE." *Human Reproduction* 19, no. 3: 490–503.

Okun, B. 1997. "Innovation and Adaptation in Fertility Transition: Jewish Immigrants to Israel from Muslim North Africa & the Middle East." *Population Studies* 51: 317–35.

Ophir, M., and T. Eliav. 2005. "Child Allowance in Israel: Historical and International Perspectives" [Hebrew]. <http://www.btl.gov.il/NR/rdonlyres/D225ED4F-6EDA-4280–84E3-E30FF1DF6D0E/0/mechkar_91.pdf> (accessed January 8, 2008).

Palter, Nurit and Natasha Mosgovoya. 2007. "Who Wants to be a Jew—the New Jews" [Hebrew]. *Yediot Aharonot*, September 16.

Portuguese, J. 1998 Fertility Policy in Israel: The Politics of Religion, Gender and Nation. Westport, CT: Praeger.

Prainsack, Barbara. 2006. "'Negotiating Life': The Regulation of Human Cloning and Embryonic Stem Cell Research in Israel." *Social Studies of Science* 36, no. 2: 173–205.

———. 2007. "Research Populations: Biobanks in Israel." *New Genetics and Society* 26, no. 1: 85–103.

Prainsack, Barbara and Gil Siegal. 2006. "The Rise of Genetic Couplehood? A Comparative View of Premarital Genetic Testing." *BioSocieties* 1: 17–36.

Prainsack B. and O. Firestine. 2006. "'Science for survival': biotechnology regulation in Israel." *Science and Public Policy* 33, no. 1: 33–46.

Prime Minister's Office. 2007. "Social Economic Agenda for Israel 2008–2010" [Hebrew]. <http://www.pmo.gov.il/NR/rdonlyres/4835300C-FB14–457E-9376–59EC0DC64DF0/0/Agenda.ppt#2> (accessed January 11, 2008).

Rabinerson, D., A. Dekel, R. Orvieto, D. Feldberg, D. Simon. 2002. "Subsidised Oocyte Donation in Israel (1998–2000): Results, Costs and Lessons." *Human Reproduction* 17: 1404–06.

Raz, A. 2004. "'Important to Test, important to Support': Attitudes toward Disability Rights and Prenatal Diagnosis among Leaders of Support Groups for Genetic Disorders in Israel." *Social Science and Medicine* 59, no. 9: 1857–66.

Rebibo, Joel. 2002. "The Road Back from Utopia" [Hebrew]. *Tchelet [Azure]*. http://www.tchelet.org.il/magazine/magazine.asp?id=174 (accessed February 3, 2008.

Remennick, Larissa. 2000. "Childless in the Land of Imperative Motherhood: Stigma and Coping among Infertile Israeli Women." *Sex Roles* 43, no. 11/12: 821–41.

———. 2006. "The Quest after the Perfect Baby: Why Do Israeli Women Seek Prenatal Genetic Testing?" *Sociology of Health and Illness* 28, no. 1: 21–53.

Rimmerman, A. and Daphna Birenbaum-Carmeli. "Disability and Policy in Israel: An Overview" (unpublished paper).

Riskin-Mashiach, Shulamit. 2007. The Vision, the Preparations and the Pregnancy." <http://www.clalit.co.il/HE-IL/Family/pregnancy/preparing+pregnancy/articles/וירה+סינכתמ.htm> (accessed November 29, 2007.

Roberts, Michelle. 2007. "IVF Hope for Child Cancer Cases." http://news.bbc.co.uk/2/hi/health/6259864.stm (accessed July 2, 2007).

Romano- Zelicha, Orly, Keren Serr and Tammy Shohat. 2002. "Uptake of Prenatal Genetic Tests by Pregnant Women in Israel." http://www.health.gov.il/download/icdc/genetics2002.pdf (accessed November 30, 2007).

Roseberry, William. 1989. "Balinese Cockfights and the Seduction of Anthropology." In *Anthropologies and Histories: Essays in Culture, History, and Political Economy*. 17–29. New Brunswick: Rutgers University Press.

Rosenblum, Sarit. 2008. "The Heavy Price of Fertility Treatments" [Hebrew]. *Yediot Aharonot*, January 22.

Safir, P. Marilyn. 1991. "Religion, Tradition and Public Policy Give Family First Priority." In *Calling the Equality Bluff*, eds. Swirski Barbara and Marilyn P. Safir, 57–65. New York: Pergamon.

Schenker, J.G. and A. Shushan. 1996. "Ethical and Legal Aspects of Assisted Reproduction Practice in Asia." *Human Reproduction* 11, no. 4: 908–11.

Schtrassler, Nehemia. 2008. "It's the Allowance, Idiot" [Hebrew]. *Ha'aretz*, January 15.

Science and Technology Knesset Committee. 2005. "PGD for Sex Selection and Other Purposes." <http://www.knesset.gov.il/protocols/data/html/mada/2005-03-16.html> (accessed February 4, 2008).

Shadmi, Erella. 2000. "Between Resistance and Compliance, Feminism and Nationalism—Women in Black in Israel." *Women's Studies International Forum* 23, no. 1: 23–34.

Shalev, C. and B. Lev. 1999. "Public Funding for IVF in Israel—Ethical Aspects" (working paper).

Shenhav, Y. and S. Melamed. 2006. "Beyond Nationalism: Neo-Malthusianism and the Formation of Fertility Policy in Pronatalist Contexts" (paper presented at the annual meeting of the American Sociological Association, Montreal Convention Center, Montreal, Quebec, Canada).

Shepard, Jonathan. 1998. "The Khazars' Formal Adoption of Judaism and Byzantium's Northern Policy." *Oxford Slavonic Papers, New Series* 31: 11–34.

Shohat, Mordechy and Roni Levy. 2007. "Before You Jump into Bed: The Genetic Screening Guide" [Hebrew]. (accessed November 29, 2007. <http://www.clalit.co.il/HE-IL/Family/pregnancy/preparing+pregnancy/articles/genetic.htm>

Shuval, J.T. and Anson, O. 2000. *Social Structure and Health in Israel*. Jerusalem: Magnes Press [Hebrew].

Siegel-Itzkovich, Judy. 2003. "Israel Allows Removal of Sperm from Dead Men at Wive's Request." *British Medical Journal* 327:1187.

Sinai, Ruth. 2007a. "Survey: A Third of Jewish Israelis and Half the Arabs Think that Developmentally Impaired People are Dangerous" [Hebrew]. *Ha'aretz*, June 3. (accessed December 2, 2007. <http://www.haaretz.co.il/hasite/spages/866345.html>

———. 2007b. "Report: The Economic Situation of People with Disabilities in Israel—The Most Difficult in the Western World" [Hebrew]. *Ha'aretz*, December 3.

Social Security Online. 2004. "Social Security Programs Throughout the World: Europe, 2004—Belgium." (accessed January 31, 2008. <http://www.ssa.gov/policy/docs/progdesc/ssptw/2004-2005/europe/belgium.html>

Stern Z., N. Laufer, R. Levy, D. Ben-Shushan, S. Mor-Yosef. 1995. "Cost Analysis of In Vitro Fertilization." *Israel Journal of Medical Science* 31: 492–96.

Stoler-Liss, Sachlav. 2003. "'Mothers Birth the Nation': The Social Construction of Zionist Motherhood in Wartime in Israeli Parents' Manuals." *Nashim* 6: 104–18.

Strathern, M. 1992a. *Reproducing the Future: Essays on Anthropology, Kinship and the New Reproductive Technologies*. New York: Routledge.

———. 1992b. *After Nature: English Kinship in the Late Twentieth Century*. Cambridge, UK: Cambridge University Press.

———. 2005. *Partial Connections*. Landham, MD: AltaMira.

Swirski, Barbara. 2007. "The 2008 Budget: The Health Chapter" [Hebrew]. (accessed December 16, 2007. <http://www.adva.org/view.asp?lang=he&catID=8&articleID=485>

Swirski, S., E. Konor-Attias, B. Swirski and Y. Yecheskel. 2001. *Women in the Labor Force of the Israeli Welfare State* [Hebrew]. Tel-Aviv: Adva Center.

Swirski, S. 1976 Community and the Meaning of the Modern State: The Case of Israel, *The Jewish Journal of Sociology* 18: 123–40.

Tremayne, Soraya. 2004. "'And Never the Twain Shall Meet': The Reproductive Health Policies of the Islamic Republic of Iran." In *Reproductive Agency, Medicine and the State: Cultural Transformations in Childbearing*, ed. M. Unnithan-Kumar. New York, London: Berghahn Books.

———. Forthcoming. "Law, Ethics, and Donor Technologies in Shi'a Iran." In *Assisting Reproduction, Testing Genes: Global Encounters with New Biotechnologies*, eds. Daphna Birenbaum-Carmeli and Marcia C. Inhorn. Oxford and New York: Berghahn Books.

United Nations Statistics Division. 2005. "Divorces and Crude Divorce Rates by Urban/Rural Residence: 2001—2005." <http://unstats.un.org/UNSD/demographic/products/dyb/dyb2005/Table25.pdf> (accessed January 28, 2008).

University of Helsinki. N.D. "Women and the Family in Europe: Who or What Constitutes a Family." <http://www.helsinki.fi/science/xantippa/wee/weetext/wee233.html> (accessed January 28, 2008).

US Department of State. 2006. "European Union Economic Overview." <http://www.state.gov/p/eur/rls/fs/58969.htm> (accessed 28 January, 2008).

Vizner, Yafa. 2007. "'Dor Yeshorim'—Genetic Counseling in the Orthodox Community from a Sociological Perspective" [Hebrew]. Master's thesis, Ben Gurion University, Beer Sheba.

Wahrman Miriam Z. 2002. *Brave New Judaism: When Science and Scripture Collide*. Hanover, NH: Brandeis University Press.

Weiss, M. 2002. *The Chosen Body: The Politics of the Body in Israeli Society*. Stanford, CA: Stanford University Press.

Wertz, D. 1998. "Eugenics is alive and well: A survey of genetics professionals around the world." *Science in Context* 3–4: 493–510.

Wyatt, Sally. 2007. "Technological Determinism Is Dead; Long Live Technological Determinism." In *The Handbook of Science and Technology Studies*. 3rd ed. Eds. Edward J. Hackett, Olga Amsterdamska, Michael Lynch and Judy Wajcman. Cambridge, MA: MIT Press.

Yogev, Y., Y. Simon, A. Ben-Haroush, D. Simon, R. Orvieto, B. Kaplan. 2003. "Attitudes of Israeli Gynecologists Regarding Candidate Screening and Personal Responsibility in Assisted Reproductive Technologies versus Adoption in Israel." *European Journal of Obstetrics and Gynecology and Reproductive Biology* 110, no. 1: 55–57.

Yuval-Davis, Nira and Floya Anthias, eds. 1989. *Woman—Nation—State*. London: MacMillan.

Part I

KIN:
REPRODUCTIVE TECHNOLOGIES
AND THE QUEST FOR
BIOGENETIC PARENTHOOD

Chapter 1

THE CONTRIBUTION OF ISRAELI RESEARCHERS TO REPRODUCTIVE MEDICINE: FERTILITY EXPERTS' PERSPECTIVES

Shlomo Mashiach, Daphna Birenbaum-Carmeli, Roy Mashiach and Martha Dirnfeld

This chapter explores historical landmarks and more recent Israeli contributions to the science of human reproduction and outlines their socio-political contexts. It is based on written descriptions and interviews with six senior Israeli gynecologists and researchers and represents their perspectives on the subject at this point in the history of the field. Being aware of the personal component that imbues such perspectives we tried to approach experts form a range of geographical locations, professional generations, and subfields of specialty.

All the experts who were interviewed for this chapter have unanimously traced the high local standard in fertility research to Professor Bernhard Zondek, whom they considered the preeminent figure in the field. Zondek was a physician-in-chief in the Department of Obstetrics and Gynecology at the municipal hospital of Berlin-Spandau at an exceptionally young age. In his early Berlin years, Zondek played a leading role in major research projects that would soon distinguish him as an outstanding scientist. However, with the rise of the Nazi regime in the 1930s, Zondek, a Jewish man, had to leave Germany. He spent short periods of time in Sweden and France and eventually, like other Jewish scientists, intellectuals and artists, arrived in Jerusalem in 1940, where he headed the Obstetrics and Gynecology Department at the Hebrew University, and the Obstetrics and Gynecology Ward at the Hadassah Medical Center. One of the doctors we spoke to has described Zondek as the greatest gynecologist of his time, if not of all times. His contribution was described as consisting of several main parts.

Zondek's early work, which was conducted in Germany, furnished the basis of his depiction by contemporary gynecologists as the founding father of gynecological endocrinology. He was a leader in the group that explained the role of the pituitary hormones, the gonadotropins, in the regulation of the menstrual cycle. According to one of the senior Israeli gynecologists we talked to, Zondek's understanding of the hypothalamic–pituitary–ovarian axis virtually paved the way to modern treatment of infertility. Already in the mid 1920s (Zondek 1926), Zondek implanted anterior pituitary glands from adult animals and humans into immature animals, and observed the rapid development of sexual puberty. This pioneering experiment, essential in revealing the role of the pituitary gland in ovarian function regulation, led Zondek to the perception that the pituitary secretes two hormones that stimulate the gonads (Zondek 1929). He named these biological substances "Prolan A" and "Prolan B," after the Latin "proles," which designates "descendant," thus probably implying that these substances were the "spiritus movens" of sexual function, the master hormones that control all the gonadal sex hormones, which were eventually seen as responsible for maintaining the species.

Zondek further expanded his mapping of the female monthly cycle. He postulated that Prolan A stimulated follicular growth, that in conjunction with Prolan B it stimulated the secretion of "foliculin," and that Prolan B induced ovulation, the formation of the corpus luteum and the secretion of lutein and foliculin. These two hormones induced the glandular transformation of the endometrium, with endometrial proliferation, and also caused changes in the vaginal epithelium. Zondek realized that the dynamics of Prolan A secretion by the anterior pituitary and the correct timing of Prolan B discharge were responsible for the rhythm of ovarian function. This in turn controlled the proliferation and function of the endometrium to create optimal conditions for nidation of the fertilized oocyte. If we just change the names of Prolan A and Prolan B to FSH and LH, and the names of foliculin and lutein to estrogen and progesterone, we can see that by 1930 Zondek had described the pituitary-gonadal relationship as gynecologists understand it today.

In addition to these foundational insights, Zondek demonstrated that the blood and urine of postmenopausal women contained gonadotropins (Zondek 1930). Together with Ascheim (Ascheim and Zondek 1927) he also showed that the blood and urine of pregnant women contained a gonad-stimulating substance: When they injected this substance subcutaneously into intact immature female mice, the mice produced follicular maturation, luteinization, and haemorrhage into the ovarian stroma. This procedure, which became known as the Ascheim-Zondek pregnancy test, was the first of its kind, confirming pregnancy by testing the woman's urine. Ascheim and Zondek believed that this gonadotrophic substance was produced by the anterior pituitary.

Another foundational discovery of Zondek's was that of human chorionic gonadotropin and ways to measure its presence. This new understanding revolutionized the monitoring of early pregnancy and various related pathologies (e.g., primarily hydatidifom mole).

Zondek continued his scientific work in Palestine in the 1940s, and later in Israel. In his important monograph, published in 1942, *The Antigonadotrophic Factor with Consideration of the Anti-hormone Problem* (Zondek and Sulman 1942), Zondek claimed that gonadotropins from animal origin produced "anti-hormones," which decreased ovarian responsiveness in humans. The researchers wrote: "It was noted in 1930, during chronic treatment with gonadotrophic hormone, that the. . . ovary maintains its response only in a limited period of time, at the end of which the response becomes increasingly weaker and finally disappears" (Zondek and Sulman 1942). They further stated, "Chronic treatment of animals with gonadotrophic hormones evokes in them the formation of a new blood substance, called an anti-hormone. This is capable of inactivating gonadotrophin hormone both in vivo and in vitro." Thus, more than two decades before the immunological system and related phenomena were fully recognized, Zondek had actually described the formation of antibodies to animal gonadotropins in women.

One Israeli gynecologist, a former student of Zondek's, has claimed that it was Zondek who had first reported the performance of an amniocentesis test. According to this narrative, in the mid 1950s, being aware that an Australian team was developing the test, Zondek, who was himself immersed in the same pursuit, used his overarching connections to have his own report of the procedure become the first ever professional report of amniocentesis. This claim has been keenly rejected by other younger doctors, who claimed that Zondek never approached the subject. According to these doctors, Zondek was indeed open enough to innovative ideas to encourage his student Professor David Serr to explore the new test, thus helping Serr to become one of the world's first experts in the field. Our own web search on the history of amniocentesis has indeed not retrieved Zondek's name in the context of amniocentesis.

Probably not as foundational but still of substantial influence were several other gynecologists who were working on and researching fertility during the 1940s. These experts, too, launched their scientific careers in pre-war Europe and, after immigration, continued in Israel. Prominent among them was the Czech-born gynecologist Professor Joseph Asherman, who later immigrated to Israel, Asherman, an avid opponent of abortion, had researched and described the association between traumatic curettage postpartum or postabortal and subsequent amenorrhea, recurrent miscarriages, and infertility (Asherman 1948). The syndrome became known as "Asherman's syndrome," rendering his name probably the best known of all Israeli fertility experts worldwide.

A more locally anchored contribution to fertility research emerged from the mass immigration of Jews from Muslim countries to Israel in the early 1950s. The prevalence of severe tubal infertility caused by tuberculosis in this population had led Israeli gynecologists Rabau and Halbrecht to investigate the condition. In their works, conducted within the slightly more established local medical research, these researchers presented a comprehensive picture of this type of infertility and suggested new diagnostic and therapeutic modalities.

The following years, from 1953 to 1961, saw the "maturation" of Zondek's groundbreaking work on gonadotropins. Though the research was not fully conducted in Israel, an Israeli scientist played a key role in its development. Between 1949 and 1953, post-doctorate researcher Dr. Bruno Lunenfeld worked in Geneva with Dr. Hubert De Watteville. Being aware of Zondek's discoveries of "antibodies," their team concentrated its efforts on identifying a human source for gonadotropins. Somewhat surprisingly, they found it in the urine of post-menopausal women. At first, the group succeeded in isolating menopausal gonadotropins from the urine of menopausal women and stimulating ovaries of hypophysectomized female immature rats with this preparation (Borth et al. 1954). At a later stage, the group also stimulated spermatogenesis in immature hypophysectomized male rats, and subsequently had their discovery published in a professional journal (Borth et al. 1957). Important as it was scientifically, this publication ruled out the patenting options of human menopausal gonadotropins (hMG), thus reducing pharmaceutical company interest in the potential drug. It was Lunenfeld who was sent by De Watteville to the then small pharmaceutical company, Serono, to try and market the breakthrough. Though at first deterred by the idea, the company eventually agreed to embark on what would become the Pergonal project.

In the mid 1950s, already back in Israel, Lunenfeld's personal acquaintance with the company's directors paved the way for a unique agreement between Serono and the State of Israel: Israel would provide urine, collected by female residents of old age homes, and in exchange, would receive Pergonal nearly free of charge. Ben Gurion, then Prime Minister, who was an avid proponent of the "internal immigration" concept—namely the encouragement of Jewish natality, a theme that runs through this volume in many different ways—supported this arrangement, and for many years funded the Pergonal program straight out of the Prime Minister's office budget. This unusual arrangement lasted until the 1970s, when Pergonal funding was transferred to the Ministry of Health. Still, for many more years, Israel would buy Pergonal at an exceptionally low price. Serono's exceptional ties with Israel also led the company to fund Lunenfeld's research laboratory at the Sheba Medical Center.

In retrospect, Lunenfeld pointed towards a "Jewish aspect" in these special ties and gestures. Serono's director at the time had been imprisoned in a concentration camp during World War II as one of the officers who tried to rebel against Mussolini. An even earlier personal encounter with a Jewish person who had helped him during World War I was also mentioned as a likely influence. Lunenfeld himself moved from menopause research to fertility research, following a comment by the rabbi who wed him in the 1950s that he should help "make up for the one and a half million Jewish children murdered by the Nazis" (Lunenfeld 2004).

Lunenfeld continued with hMG research in Israel. Together with Rabau, he conducted the first experimental treatments of unovulatory women using Pergonal. In 1960, the team reported their first successful induction of ovulation, followed by pregnancies in hypogonadotrophic anovulatory women using a sequential step-up/step-down regime. This breakthrough was later followed by a series of collaborative studies in which Lunenfeld, together with numerous Israeli gynecologists (Oelsner et al. 1978) further developed the treatment of infertility diagnosed as hypopituitaric-hypogonadotropic amenorrhea (WHO type I patients), which had been untreatable until that time. Pergonal, the new drug, proved to be tremendously effective for the induction of ovulation and thus enabled pregnancies in this category of women. Later on, it also proved efficient in the treatment of Polycystic Ovaries Syndrome patients (PCOS; WHO type II patients).

The Pergonal protocols that were devised by the Israeli research-ers were rapidly adopted worldwide by leading fertility experts and became the mainstay of infertility treatment. About a decade later, this drug and subsequent recombinant gonadotropins had formed the basis for ovulation induction in IVF.

Pergonal and related substances continued to be the heart of sub-sequent contributions of Israeli researchers to reproductive medi-cine. Concepts like "FSH effective daily dose" and "latent phase and active phase," which have become basic terms in clinical infertility discourse, were developed by local practitioners (e.g., Insler et al. 1968). The classification of patients selected for gonadotropin ther-apy, which had been developed by Vaclav Insler in the 1960s (Insler et al. 1968), has been adopted by the World Health Organization (WHO Technical Report Series, No. 514, 1976) and is widely used until today, as is Insler's "Cervical Score" (Insler 1972). The latter, which estimates the physical properties of cervical mucus, enabled the monitoring of gonadotropin treatments at a time when neither ultrasound nor accurate laboratory tests were available. The severe complications that may occur after stimulation of the ovaries with gonadotropins (Ovarian Hyperstimulation Syndrome) were initially described by Rabau David, Serr, Mashiach, and Lunenfeld (in 1967) and later modified and adopted by the World Health Organization (WHO Technical Report Series, No. 514, 1973). This syndrome was later analyzed by Professor Joseph Schenker and the finer details of ovulation induction were studied, developed, and described by other senior Israeli researchers (e.g., Lunenfeld, Insler, David, and Mashiach). In the 1980s, these early studies become a cornerstone in IVF research.

Steptoe and Edwards' accomplishment of the first IVF pregnancy in 1978 in the U.K. stirred great commotion in Israel's gynecologi-cal community. In 1980, Mashiach, as the head of the division of obstetric and gynecologic at the Sheba Medical Center, realized the importance of IVF for the treatment of infertility and sent the young Dr. Joshua Dor to Edinburgh, Scotland to master this new technol-ogy. During his training, Dor met Dr. Edwina Rudak, one of the leading experts in the animal experimentation that paved the way to human IVF. Rudak agreed to come to Israel and establish the first IVF laboratory in the country. Her contribution to the early success of IVF in Israel has been mentioned by doctors as vital. In 1982, the Israeli team, headed by Mashiach and Dor, achieved Israel's first "test tube baby," making Israel the fifth country in the world to achieve pregnancy following an IVF procedure. IVF soon attracted the coun-try's best gynecologists who began to apply, study, and contribute to this new field. As an instructive illustration of the country's unique international standing at that time, Israeli doctors described the 1987 annual conference of the prestigious European Society for Human Reproduction and Embryology (ESHRE). In these early days of IVF, when treatment outcomes were a major finding, figures were reported at the ESHRE conference by the following categories: USA, Europe, Australia and South Africa, and Israel. While Israel's separateness could be partly explained, according to the doctors, by its exclusion from geographically-defined professional organizations, the single-country category of a country as small as Israel still illustrates the volume of local IVF activity in these early years as well as the interest of the international community in its doctors' work.

Throughout the same period, but with a lower profile, Professor Amnon Makler also made a unique contribution to the practice of infertility (Makler 1980). Makler's device for determining the amount of spermatozoa and their motility parameters has become a basic appliance in virtually all IVF laboratories worldwide. One doctor stressed that despite numerous attempts to "overtake" this relatively old appliance, it is still a standard piece of equipment in all IVF laboratories from the early 1980s to the present day. It is noteworthy that the same doctor emphasized that many professionals who use the Makler Counting Chamber on a daily basis are unaware of its Israeli origin.

Thinking of the lack of awareness of the Israeli origin of some reproductive medicine accomplishments, one of the doctors we talked to mentioned a renowned Israeli scientist who was recently awarded a highly prestigious international prize for his life-long contribution to the molecular study of infertility. In his inaugural talk, the scientist chose to highlight the American institute in which he had conducted one particular research, while listing his Israeli home university, where he had been working for decades, merely by its name, without specifying that it was located in Israel. The gynecologist's obvious pain while telling this anecdote may itself be taken as indicating a sense of generalized national pride that Israeli practitioners do hold regarding their collective contribution to global fertility research.

Israeli experts continued to probe the boundaries of IVF also in subsequent years. Among their major contributions, local doctors have counted the preparation of the uterus lining for oocyte donation in women without ovaries (Laufer and Shenker); the first pregnancy and birth by a woman in the absence of ovarian function (Laufer); the first pregnancy and birth by a woman with XY Dysgenesis (Swyer) Syndrome (Dirnfeld); the world's first reimplantation of ovarian tissue in a chemotherapy-treated cancer survivor that led to pregnancy and delivery; and, the first baby born from an implanted ovary (Meirow et al. 2005).

In the domain of male infertility, the researchers highlighted as their main accomplishments laser drilling of the oocyte to allow sperm penetration, which paved the way for micromanipulation (currently known as ICSI) that is now routinely applied to resolve most types of male infertility (Laufer and Gordon); testicular fine needle sperm aspiration that is also used for micromanipulation (Laufer); and coining the term "OTA syndrome" (oligo-terato-asthenospermia), which designates the frequent concurrence of low sperm concentration with abnormal morphology and impaired motility (Glezerman).

Israeli experts have also made substantial scientific contributions in other areas of infertility. Using preimplantation genetic diagnosis (PGD), Israeli physicians developed detection methods for several cystic fibrosis mutations as well as for typically Jewish genetic diseases like familial dysautonomia. The conservative treatment of ectopic pregnancy (Mashiach et al 1982), and of torsion of the ovaries while avoiding surgery and retaining the ovaries (Shalev et al 1989), were also developed in Israel and went on to become standard practice in many countries. Israeli scientists have also made major, world renowned contributions to the study and treatment of polycystic ovary syndrome (Homburg 2005). In the domain of perinatology, too, fetal lung maturity testing (Barkai et al. 1982), fetal heart rate monitoring, scalp PH sampling and fetal ultrasonography were substantially advanced by local experts whose works became landmark studies worldwide.

In two other scientific fields that go beyond reproductive medicine Israeli researchers have made principal contributions. The first is the field of human embryonic stem cell research, in which Israeli scientists stood out through their exceptional participation in the early days of the evolving field (see chapters 9 and 10, this volume). The second contribution is in basic science research, where the insights of Nobel Prize laureates Avram Hershko and Aaron Ciechanover on cell proliferation and death have inspired new lines of exploration on embryonic invasiveness and implantation.

To demonstrate the international standing of Israeli fertility experts, the doctors we spoke to listed the prestigious titles that some of them have earned. Homburg was ranked seventh in an international survey grading the "most influential leaders in the world, in the field of reproductive medicine" (Organon Internal Company Survey 2006). Lunenfeld served as a consultant and member of various expert committees at the World Health Organization (WHO) and was an honorary member of the main European and American Societies of Gynecology and Obstetrics. In 1972, Lunenfeld chaired the WHO meetings that developed guidelines for the diagnosis and treatment of infertile couples (WHO Technical Report Series, No. 514 1973) and for gonadotropin preparations (International Units IU, Technical Report Series, No. 565 1975). Schenker, the former head of the Division of Gynecology and Obstetrics at the Hadassah Medical Center, chaired the Ethics Committee of the World Federation of Gynecologists and Obstetricians and was president of the International Academy of Reproduction.

From this brief historical description then, fertility emerges as an important and innovative field of research in Israel. At several crucial points in time, primarily in the 1940s and in the early 1960s, a few Israeli researchers had substantial funding for research, which helped established them as eminent figures in the field and bestowed increased visibility on the local scientific and expert community. Whereas some of these contributions have not always been fully associated with Israel, a generally high level of participation has positioned Israel and its fertility researchers as prominent contributors to the field internationally.

References

Ascheim, S. and B. Zondek. 1927. "Hypophysenvorderlappen Hormone und Ovarialhormone im Harn von Schwangeren." *Klin Wochenschr* 6: 13–21.

Asherman, J. G. 1948. "Amenorrhea Traumatica (Atretica)." *Journal of Obstetrics and Gyanecology of the British Commonwealth* 53: 23–30.

Barkai, G., S. Mashiach, D. Lanzer, Z. Kayam, M. Brish and B. Goldman. 1982. "Determination of Fetal Lung Maturity from Amniotic Fluid Microviscosity in High-Risk Pregnancy." *Obstetrics and Gynecology* 59: 615–23.

Borth, R., B. Lunenfeld and H. de Watteville. 1954. "Activité Gonadotrope d'un Extrait D'urines de Femmes en Menopause." *Experientia* 10: 266–70.

———. 1957. "Le Dosage des Gonadotrophins—Méthode et Intérêt Clinique." *Bulletin de la Société Royale Belge de Gynécologie et d Obstétrique* 27: 639.

Homburg, R. 2005. *Ovulation Induction and Controlled Ovarian Stimulation—A Practical Guide*. London and New York: Taylor & Francis Group.

Insler, V., H. Melmed, S. Mashiach, M. Monselise, B. Lunenfeld and E. Rabau. 1968. "Functional Classification of Patients Selected for Gonadotropin Therapy." *Obstetrics and Gynecology* 32: 620–25.

Insler, V., H. Melmed, I. Eichenbrenner, D.M. Serr and B. Lunenfeld. 1972. "The Cervical Score." *International Journal Obstetrics and Gynecology* 10: 223–28.

Lunenfeld B. 2004. "Historical Perspectives in Gonadotrophin Therapy." *Human Reproduction Update* 10, no. 6: 453–67.

Makler, A. 1980. "The Improved Ten-Micrometer Chamber for Rapid Sperm Count and Motility Evaluation." *Fertility & Sterility* 33: 160.

Mashiach, S., G. Barkai, J. Sack, E. Stern, M. Brish, B. Goldman and D.M. Serr. 1979. "The Effect of Intra-Amniotic Thyroxine Administration on Fetal Lung Maturity in Man." *Journal of Perinatal Medicine* 7, no. 3: 161–70.

Mashiach, S, H.J.A. Carp, D.M. Serr. 1982. "Nonoperative Management of Ectopic Pregnancy." *Journal of Reproductive Medicine* 27, no. 3: 127–32.

Meirow D, Levron J, Eldar-Geva T, Hardan I, Fridman E, Zalel Y, Schiff E, Dor J. 2005. "Pregnancy after transplantation of cryopreserved ovarian tissue in a patient with ovarian failure after chemotherapy." *New England Journal of Medicine* 21;353(3):318–21.

Oelsner G, D.M. Serr, S. Mashiach, J. Blankstein, M. Snyder and B. Lunenfeld. 1978. "The Study of Induction of Ovulation with Menotropins Analysis of Results of 897 Treatment Cycles." *Fertility and Sterility* 30, no. 5: 538–44.

Rabau, E., David, A., Serr, D.M., Mashiach, S. and Lunenfeld, B., 1967. Human menopausal gonadotropins for anovulation and sterility. Results of 7 years of treatment. *American Journal of Obstetrics and Gynecology*, 98: 92–98.

Shalev, J., M. Goldenberg, G. Oeslner, Z. Ben-Rafael, D. Bider, J. Blankstein and S. Mashiach. 1989. "Treatment of Twisted Ischemic Adnexa: Preservation and Revival of Normal Ovary by Detorsion." *New England Journal of Medicine* 321: 546.

Zondek, B. 1926. "Ueber die Funktion des Ovariums." *Zeitschr Geburtsh Gynakol* 90: 327.

Zondek, B. 1929. "Weitere Untersuchungen zur Darstellung. Biologie und Klinik des Hypophysenvorderlappenhormons (Prolan)." *Zentralbl Gynakol* 14: 834–48.

Zondek, B. 1930. "Ueber die Hormone des Hypophysenvorderlappens." *Klin Wochenschrift* 9: 245–48.

Zondek. B. and F. Sulman. 1942. *The Antigonadotropic Factor*. Baltimore: Williams and Wilkins.

Chapter 2

The Regulation of Preimplantation Genetic Diagnosis for Sibling Donors in Israel, Germany, and England: A Comparative Look at Balancing Risks and Benefits

Yael Hashiloni-Dolev and Shiri Shkedi

Introduction

PGD is an early form of prenatal diagnosis. Couples opting for PGD undergo in vitro fertilization (IVF). The pre-embryos are biopsied and genetically screened in vitro. Only those which have the desired genetic profile are transferred to the uterus, using standard IVF procedures (Sermon 2002). During the years since its introduction in the 1990s, PGD has been used predominantly to avoid the birth of children affected by identified incurable genetic diseases, such as monogenic disorders[1] (i.e.: cystic fibrosis, hemophilia), or chromosomal aberrations[2] (Geraedts et al. 1999; Harper et al. 2006). Thus, the technique is mainly used (where allowed) by couples for one or more of the following purposes: high risk of having a child affected by a monogenic disease; recurrent miscarriages; religious or moral objections to selective abortions. In some cases (mainly in the U.S.) it is also used for social sex selection, a highly controversial purpose. Recently, PGD has been used not only to test embryos for genetic anomalies, but also to test them for tissue matching so that they can later serve as cord blood or bone marrow donors to an existing affected sibling (Van de Velde et al. 2004; Bielorai et al. 2004). This procedure is commonly refereed to as PGD for SDs. The SDs themselves can be at risk for the condition to be treated in the existing child (e.g., Fanconi anemia and thalassaemia both involve hematological complications which can be overcome by using bone marrow transplantation from a matched donor), or not at risk themselves, but selected for tissue matching with siblings who have sporadic conditions requiring bone marrow transplantation. In recessive transmitted genetic disorders[3] (such as Fanconi anemia or thalassaemia), theoretically only 3 out of 16 embryos would be free of the disease and tissue matched, making the procedure's success rate relatively low. Consequently, several treatment cycles may be necessary in order to establish a pregnancy of a healthy offspring.

Ethical debate concerning PGD for SDs

There are three main sets of ethical objections to PGD (as well as to other NRTs) whose themes overlap and intertwine: The first is held by people who believe that the embryo should be treated like a person holding rights, even at a very early developmental stage, and therefore oppose the selection of pre-embryos which necessarily involves destroying undesired ones (Robertson 2003). In that regard it is important to mention that while standard repro-genetics (testing for conditions such as CF, Trisomy 21 or Tay-Sachs) selects embryos for their own future health, PGD for SDs involves destroying pre-embryos who are believed to be perfectly "healthy" just because they do not match the needs of a sick sibling. The second line of argumentation has to do with the fact of selection itself. Believing that human reproduction should stay a "natural" process, and that any form of selection turns the child into a "manufactured good" (Kass 2000, 2002; President's Bioethics Commission 2002), these people fear that genetic screening of prospective children will move us towards a eugenic world in which "designing" children will become an uncontested routine (King 1999). This argument is often linked to fears of interfering with God's creational plans, or of "playing God" (Prainsack and Spector 2006; Evans 2005). The third line of argumentation has to do with the future rights of the unborn and its human dignity, as well as with the generational relationship (Prainsack and Spector 2006). Stemming from the logic of Kantian philosophy, a child should always be treated as an end in itself, and never merely as a means. Consequently, it is feared that the selection of future children will instrumentalize them, deprive them of their ability to choose whether they wish to live up to their parents' plans and expectations—or not—and irreversibly change the relationship between them (the "produced") and their parents (the "producers"). It is hence argued that no human being is allowed to determine the genetic traits of another, whether born or unborn (Habermas 2003).

On the other hand, bioethicists in favor of PGD argue that since prenatal diagnosis in general is widely accepted, there is no reason to single out PGD and ban it (Penning et al. 2002). Another counterargument is that failure to implant an embryo is morally preferable to the killing of a more developed fetus (Robertson 2003; Draper and Chadwick 1999).

On top of these arguments concerning PGD in general, PGD for SDs raises more specific concerns that have to do with how family relations are viewed, such as: What can families rightly expect of their future children? Are the present family's needs synonymous with those of the future child, or do they conflict? Should it be permissible to create a child not merely for her own sake but to save the life of another child (Devolder 2005)? What unique emotions may the relationship between the future siblings involve (Landau 2003; Terry 2002)? And finally, should the transplantation fail, would the donor child be loved anyway (Pennings et al. 2002)?

Comparing public policies concerning PGD for SDs

Legal, social, and ethical concerns regarding PGD for SDs differ among countries[4]. The Israeli case is quite exceptional. In contrast to many other societies where PGD for SDs raised various concerns, and where a thorough ethical discourse preceded its approval (if approved at all), this new technique was endorsed with hardly any hesitation in Israel. Aiming to understand the uniqueness of Israeli policy-making concerning PGD for SDs, we will follow the technology-in-practice approach. This dynamic approach, in contrast to social essentialist or technological determinist approaches, probes what become relevant "social" or "technological" categories in the development and usage of technology, instead of assuming that the technical or the social predetermine either the development or application of medical innovations (Timmermans and Berg 2003).

In order to shed light on Israel's approach to PGD for SDs, we chose to compare the ethical discourse in Israel with two other

Western societies—Germany and England—each of which employ two extreme points on the continuum of Western policies regarding NRTs. Germany is known for its restrictive policy compared to most other advanced liberal societies (Hashiloni-Dolev 2007; Krone and Richter 2004). England, with its famed "Warnock Report" and later its HEFA, has led the way for many other Western countries in terms of setting liberal standards for embryo research and the use of NRTs (Van Balen and Inhorn 2003). Our comparative method of analysis will allow us to demonstrate how the meaning of the studied biomedical technology was assigned locally according to unique interplays between the medical, ethical, and social categories that became relevant in the process of the procedure's evaluation and regulation. More specifically, we will analyze how the risks and hopes (both medical and ethical) raised by the technology were understood in the three different studied societies.

First, we will briefly describe the materials our research builds upon.

Methodology

While ethical debate in Germany and England regarding PGD is both widespread and dense, such a debate hardly exists in Israel. This difference is part of the phenomenon analyzed in this paper, and the reason why our empirical data from the three countries is dissimilar. In Israel our empirical materials include: (i) An ethics committee's report regarding PGD (Advisory Bioethics Committee Israel National Academy of Sciences and Humanities and the Helsinki Committee for Genetic Experiments on Human Beings 2003; hereafter ABC 2003), which is only 5 pages long; (ii) a Science and Technology Committee Parliament Report, *PGD for Sex Selection and Other Medical Purposes* (Science and Technology Committee 2005); (iii) the official guidelines issued recently by the Israeli Ministry of Health (Ministry of Health 2006), which are mainly technical; and (iv) a position paper regarding the use of PGD for detecting embryos at high risk for late onset diseases (such as cancer and Huntington's disease), *PGD Guidelines for Late Onset Diseases and Susceptibility Genes for Cancer* (Israeli National Bioethics Council 2007).

Since the official guidelines published by the Ministry of Health do not touch upon the ethical and social aspects of PGD, we will mainly use in our analysis the position paper prepared in 2003 (ABC 2003).

Concerning SDs, the ethical as well as public discourse in Israel is very much entwined with the personal story of the Harari family. Sharon Harari and her husband Yavin Atzmon were the second couple in the world who succeeded using PGD for SD in order to save their child, who was suffering from Fanconi anemia. Consequently, Harari, who meanwhile has published a book describing her personal experience (Harari 2005), became an advocate for PGD. Being invited to tell her story in regulatory committees and professional conferences, she played an important role in shaping the Israeli policy regarding SDs. For this reason, Harari's story as depicted in her book, and the way it was presented in the media and in reports from the Israeli parliament, and not only the writings of ethics committees, will serve our analysis of the Israeli case.

Our comparison with England and Germany builds on much lengthier official materials, of which there are plenty. In Germany, our analysis is mainly focused on two governmental reports, each hundreds of pages long: *Law and Ethics in Modern Medicine*, initiated by the German Parliament in March 2000 (German Bundestag 2002), and the final report of the National Ethics Council, initiated by the German Chancellor in June 2001, titled *Genetic Diagnosis Before and During Pregnancy* (National Ethics Council 2003). These two reports deal with different clinical, social, and ethical issues regarding prenatal diagnosis and PGD.

In England, we follow the discussion of the subject by the Human Fertilization and Embryology Authority (HFEA) as well as the House of Lords' position papers and legislation from 1999 to 2007. These include: *Preimplantation Genetic Diagnosis* (Human Fertilization and Embryology Authority 1999); *HFEA to Allow Tissue Typing in Conjunction with Preimplantation Genetic Diagnosis* (Human Fertilization and Embryology Authority 2001a); *Outcome of the Public Consultation on Preimplantation Genetic Diagnosis* (Human Fertilization and Embryology Authority 2001b); *Preimplantation Tissue Typing* (Human Fertilization and Embryology Authority 2004a; see also McLean 2006); and *New Guidance on Preimplantation Tissue Typing* (Human Fertilization and Embryology Authority 2004b).

The regulation of PGD in England, Germany and Israel

While Germany is renowned for its restrictive policy concerning NRTs, both England and Israel are famous for being at the forefront of bio-technological research and application, equally allowing PGD and PGD for SDs. Yet, the regulation processes in England and Israel are very different. We will now describe the regulation process in the three societies, starting with England.

England

The legal situation regarding PGD for SDs in England is especially interesting since it shifted throughout the years from disapproval to acceptance. Regulation of fertility treatments and human embryo research in England is determined by the HFEA statutory body, which was founded in 1991 under the 1990 Human Fertilization and Embryology Act (Office of Public Sector Information 1990).

PGD has been allowed in England since 1999, when the HFEA set up a working group to develop specific interim guidance for the use of PGD. According to that first report, PGD could be carried out after receiving the HFEA license committee's approval. In reaching its decision, the committee had to consider whether the proposed treatment was lawful under the Act (Human Fertilization and Embryology Authority 1999). At first, PGD for SDs was not specifically mentioned. Obliged to consult with the general public during the year of 2000, consultation questionnaires were sent by the HFEA to both individuals and organizations, under the categories of "clinical," "disability," and "other," asking their opinions concerning PGD. The majority of all respondents were in favor of PGD in principle, and in favor of restricting the use of PGD to serious conditions evaluated on a clinical judgment based on general guidance, such as termination of pregnancy criteria (Human Fertilization and Embryology Authority 2001). At that time, PGD for SDs was not yet discussed. It was only after the birth of the first SD, Adam Nash, in the U.S. in 2000, that the controversial issue of PGD for SDs was discussed in England. At first, Dr. Vivienne Nathanson, head of ethics and policy for the British Medical Association, supported prohibiting this use of PGD in England (McLean 2006). However, shortly after that, on November 2001, HFEA agreed that PGD with tissue matching may be permitted under the following criteria: the condition of the affected child should be severe or life threatening; the embryos conceived following use of this technology should be themselves at risk for the condition by which the existing child is affected; the technique should only be allowed for treating a sibling and not a parent; the intention should be to take only cord blood and no other tissues or organs from the child; all other possibilities of treatment and tissue sources should have been explored; and embryos should not be modified to create a tissue match. In addition, each and every case should receive the approval of HFEA before the procedure is performed (Human Fertilization and Embryology Authority 2001; see also Human Fertilization and Embryology Authority 2004a).

Following a court appeal in which HFEA was asked to approve the procedure for a family with a child affected with a sporadic condition in cases where the future child would not be at risk, HFEA once again asked its Ethics and Law Committee (ELC) to review its policy on the subject matter. The course of the review included research evaluating the procedure's psychological and physical risks to the future child, reviewing case laws relating to authorization of procedures involving minors, as well as U.K. and international ethics and advisory body decisions and public opinion. A revised policy was published in 2004, allowing PGD for SDs on a case-by-case basis where the future child is not herself at risk of the condition for which cord blood donation is needed (Human Fertilization and Embryology Authority 2004a, 2004b). The Science and Technology Committee of the House of Commons took this decision a step further when it stated in its fifth report (2004–2005) that PGD for tissue typing can also be used to benefit other family members, not only siblings (McLean 2006).

Thus, it can be concluded that in England, the issue of PGD and PGD for SDs has been evaluated almost on a yearly basis since its first authorization in 1999. HFEA's approach to PGD for SDs has gradually become less restrictive, subsequent to a constant evaluation of the procedure's risks and legitimacy.

Germany

The legal situation regarding PGD in Germany is very much influenced by the Embryo Protection Act (EPA), legislated in 1990, which defends the human rights of the embryo (German Bundestad 1990). According to the EPA, an embryo is defined as the fertilized ovum after the fusion of two nuclei, and every single totipotent cell derived from the embryo (Krones and Richter 2004). As a result of this stance, the embryo is entitled to legal protection from early developmental stages, and the vast majority of the currently available NRTs are prohibited in Germany. Although there is no explicit law in Germany that bans PGD, the very techniques involved in performing PGD (embryo cryopreservation; testing a single [controversially] totipotent cell) are interpreted as contradicting the EPA, and therefore prohibited. Two commissions that have attempted to generate regulations concerning PGD have been appointed in Germany: the German Parliament Commission (GP) and the National

Ethics Council (NEC). The majority (16 against 3) of the parliament commission's members recommended that the German Bundestag should not approve PGD in Germany (German Bundestag 2002). On the other hand, two thirds of the members of the NEC recommended permitting PGD for couples who are: (i) at high risk of having a child with a severe genetic condition or a disability that cannot be effectively treated; or (ii) at high risk of transmitting a chromosomal aberration; or (iii) infertile and undergoing IVF treatments (National Ethics Council 2003: 96). PGD for SDs is presented in this report as debatable, with no concrete recommendations. However, in the absence of a law explicitly permitting PGD, no center in Germany currently offers this procedure. The public discourse in Germany regarding PGD is composed of two alternative voices: that of the supporters (liberal scientists, physicians, and politicians), and that of the opponents, who think in a more categorical way (intellectuals, politicians, feminists, organizations of disabled people, and the pro-life lobby) (Krones and Richter 2004). For now, the German law reflects the opponents' point of view.

Israel

Despite the mass demand for NRTs in Israel, there is no inclusive parliamentary legislation on medically assisted conception, except for surrogacy, which has been allowed by law since 1996 (State of Israel 1996), and human reproductive cloning, which is banned by a moratorium at least until 2009 (State of Israel 1999). Thus, most guidelines regarding NRTs are set by secondary legislation determined by the Ministry of Health, the legal strength of which is somewhat dubious (Schenker 2003). The practice of NRTs in Israel often precedes the ethical and legal debate, as the policy is usually determined following medical and public demand, and even personal stories (like the one of the Harari family), and not in advance.

PGD was first performed in Israel in the early 2000s. Currently there are five medical centers performing PGD in Israel (out of thirteen large hospitals in the country). In the year of 2003, a position paper regarding guidelines for the use of PGD was prepared by a joint committee combining the Advisory Bioethics Committee of the Israel National Academy of Sciences and Humanities, and the Helsinki Committee for Genetic Experiments on Human Beings (ABC 2003). This paper examines ethical aspects of PGD and was submitted to the Israeli Ministry of Health.

However, only in December 2006, following the joint recommendation of the Israeli National Bioethics Council and the Israeli

Committee for Medical Experiments on Human Beings, the Israeli Ministry of Health issued new guidelines regarding PGD in Israel. These guidelines were explicitly issued "in order to organize the *already* operating PGD activity" (Ministry of Health 2006: 1; emphasis added). According to these guidelines, which mainly focus on technical aspects of the procedure, PGD is allowed for the same prerequisites as prenatal diagnosis. Hence, PGD may be used by couples for three main categories: a risk of having a child affected by a severe monogenic disease expressed in childhood (from 10 percent risk in diseases with partial penetrance and up to 50 percent in dominant or sex-linked inherited diseases), a chromosomal aberration carried by one of the parents, and double diagnosis of both a monogenic disease and tissue matching for SDs. Regarding disorders that do not follow these criteria, a separate consideration should take place, in which criteria of severity of the disease, recurrence risk, treatment options, and age of onset need to be evaluated. In March 2007, a position paper regarding the use of PGD for detecting embryos at high risk for late onset diseases was issued by the Israeli National Bioethics Council (Israeli National Bioethics Council 2007).

The Ministry of Health's official guidelines (2006) declare that conclusions regarding ethical, social, philosophical, and medical aspects of PGD will be published shortly. Thus, the official guidelines have in fact been issued separately from any thorough ethical or social evaluation. Hopefully such a discussion will take place; yet it will only be post factum.

According to the ABC's report, PGD for SDs is allowed for parents of a child affected by a disease which can only be treated by transplanting cord blood or bone marrow from a tissue matched first-relative donor. It is stressed that the diagnosed embryo would not have any chance of being harmed by the procedure or by the donation (in cases where the donation may harm the donor, it should be postponed until the child can actively consent, and if not possible, any action should be in line with Israeli laws protecting the child), that the donor and the recipient will be first degree relatives, and that the excess embryos will be kept frozen in order to allow their future implantation in case the couple ever wishes to have another child. PGD for SDs was also endorsed without hesitation by the Israeli parliament's commission appointed to discuss PGD for sex selection and other medical conditions (Science and Technology Committee 2005). It is important to mention that PGD for the purpose of non-medical sex selection was authorized in Israel, for the first time in the world, in 2005 (Ministry of Health

2005; Yasur-Beit-Or 2006; Traubman 2005). However, approvals have been rare.

To conclude, PGD in general and for SDs in particular is understood as a non-debatable life saving procedure in Israel, and is thus widely accepted.

Having reviewed the regulatory status of PGD in the three studied societies, we now wish to elaborate on the dominant categories used in the discussion of PGD for SDs in England, Germany, and Israel. We will demonstrate that while similar ethical, social, and medical categories exist in each society, their interpretation and the balance between the salience of different categories in the discussion concerning the regulation of the technology largely varies.

Dominant categories in the regulation and ethical debate concerning PGD in England, Germany, and Israel

England: examining scientific (medical and psychological) knowledge about the possible risks of the procedure to the future child

In 2001, following the birth of Adam Nash in the U.S., HFEA's Ethics and Law Committee was asked to review the medical and psychological literature, as well as to consult with various experts, while reaching its decision regarding the approval of PGD for SDs. The guidelines issued in 2001 were immediately challenged in court, which led to their reconsideration. HFEA's final report (2004a) reviews the way of thinking that led to the initial restriction of PGD for SDs:

> In 2001, there was no evidence available about the possible health risks to the resulting child from embryo biopsy. This led the Authority to take a precautionary approach. The benefit of PGD, when it is performed both to avoid a particular genetic condition and to select for tissue type, is that it brings about the birth of a child without a particular genetic condition. This benefit outweighs any concerns about the possible risks associated with embryo biopsy. However, when PGD is performed for tissue typing alone, the procedure does not bring about the birth of an unaffected child where an affected one might have been born. In this circumstance, the theoretical risk of embryo biopsy to the resulting child was enough to convince the Authority that PGD for tissue typing alone would not be a desirable

use of the procedure. (Human Fertilization and Embryology Authority 2004a: 3)

The same report goes on to explain why the restrictions were moved:

> Issues relating to the psychological welfare of the child arising from knowledge of the circumstances of their conception were examined carefully. It was concluded, firstly, that there was no evidence that being conceived in this manner is necessarily injurious to the psychological welfare of the child and, secondly, that, in the absence of relevant empirical information, consideration of these concerns, whilst important, was merely speculative. . . the Authority found no evidence that was transferable or relevant to the issue of preimplantation tissue typing that adverse psychological effects would result from the procedure. (Human Fertilization and Embryology Authority 2004a: 5)

As we can see, the main categories which became relevant for the evaluation of the new technology in England were largely techno-medical or psychological, showing concern about the future medical and psychological welfare of the SD. Thus, when HFEA was convinced that according to present scientific (medical or psychological) knowledge, no potential harm exists, the procedure was approved on a large basis.

Germany: Threats to the status of future children as autonomous individuals, and to socially desired family relations

While "objective" scientific knowledge (either medical or psychological) served as the main category for thinking about the pros and cons of the new procedure in England, in Germany it was ethical categories regarding human dignity and ideal family relations which became dominant in the discussion regarding the usage of the new technology.

The dominant moral reasoning in Germany, and a main argument in the Western ethical discourse regarding PGD for SDs, is the deontological Kantian, emphasizing human dignity and the state of every human being as an end in itself, and never merely as a means (Krones and Richter 2004; Kass 2000, 2002). Accordingly, in the German debate regarding NRTs it is often claimed that children should never be intentionally designed to fulfill society's or their parents' needs or expectations. Following this line of argumentation, opponents of PGD in Germany employ ethical categories having to do with the view of children as individual subjects, namely as ends in themselves, and not as parts of a social group, that is to say, their family. As a result, they argue that families or future parents should never be allowed to design their children in order to satisfy their own needs or desires. Such an act would violate the future child's rights as an individual subject. To give just a few examples, in 2003 members of the German National Ethics council wrote that "[b]y virtue of assisted reproduction for the purpose of PGD and as a result of the ensuing PGD itself, the future child inevitably becomes the object of decisions (determination of criteria, selection, or rejection) inconsistent with the acceptance of the child *for his own sake*" (National Ethics Council 2003: 71; emphasis added).

And, specifically concerning PGD for SDs and the "designed" child's status as an individual subject, they write, "[T]he same applies to the worry that a child's notion of his own identity and self-esteem might later be adversely affected when he learns that he owes his existence to a process of selection. . .the child subsequently comes to feel that he exists not for his own sake but only to serve as a donor of a particular tissue for a sick sibling" (National Ethics Council 2003: 85).

Related to the view of children as existing for "their own sake" is the view of family relations as highly prone to exploitation. The dominant German ethical discourse regarding reproductive medicine is based on the assumption that the interests of future children are potentially in conflict with those of their family members. This concern is very explicit in the PGD debate. For example, the opponents of PGD in the German National Ethics council do not primarily think of the family in terms of a unified body with a common good, but rather in terms of different individuals with competing interests. Thus, they cast doubt concerning the parents' true ability to make decisions in their children's best interests. Moreover, they argue that the child's status as a subject might be violated even by good intentions of the parents, and thus it must be protected by the state. This need to protect children from the possible exploitive tendencies of their parents is repeatedly stressed in the discussion concerning PGD for SDs. For example, opponents from the parliament committee view PGD for SDs as "... an *obvious exploitation* of children for a particular purpose" (German Bundestag 2002: 186; emphasis added).

Yet, it is not only the future child who is feared to be possibly exploited by its family members. Some opponents of PGD in Germany worry equally that allowing PGD for SDs might place pressure on the mother to become pregnant and have another child in order to save her sick child: "To produce a genetically compatible stem cell donor for a child affected by a hereditary blood condition, women must, given the availability of PGD, *wrestle* with the question of whether they wish to become pregnant for this purpose. In such a case, a woman is subject to intense pressure of expectation, which it is difficult for her to escape" (National Ethics Council 2003: 84; emphasis added).

Israel: PGD as a blessing for the entire family, as it brings and saves life simultaneously

The official guidelines of the Israeli Ministry of Health and the Israeli position paper regarding PGD were both issued long after the first English reports concerning PGD and PGD for SDs were published. In these years, hundreds of healthy babies were born following PGD. Therefore, it is difficult to compare the importance given to potential risks to the health of the future child in Israel and England. However, the fact that the performance of a new controversial technique was allowed in Israel without extended evidence of its safety and without official guidelines implies that evaluation of potential risks (medical or psychological) did not play a major role in the Israeli discourse regarding PGD. Indeed, the only reference to risks involved in PGD in the Israeli Ministry of Health's report (2006) states, "The fact that up until now more than a thousand healthy children were born following PGD (about 7000 PGD cycles), points to the fact that this technology is reliable. The long-term influence of this technology on children born after the biopsy of pre-embryos for PGD is not yet clear" (Ministry of Health 2006: 3; our translation).

Likewise, while discussing the stated undisputable uses of PGD (as described above), the Israeli position paper regarding PGD does not mention the potential risks of IVF and PGD. Evaluation of the potential risks involved in IVF as a criterion to the approval of PGD is mentioned only while discussing PGD for mild medical conditions. However, even then, priority is given to evaluating the family's previous experience and the parents' emotional condition, and only afterward is the risk discussed. Thus, although risk is taken into account while approving PGD, it is secondary to other considerations that have to do with the family's well-being. Only when the guidelines discuss the controversial (so far hypothetical) possibility of the use of PGD by couples who wish to perform the procedure in order to ensure the birth of a healthy child lacking a high risk factor in the family, or due to a fertility deficiency of the parents (ABC 2003: 2), are the risks of IVF and of PGD itself emphasized. Even in the guidelines concerning PGD for late onset diseases (Israeli National Bioethics Council 2007), the potential risk of IVF for the mother is downplayed. In a section discussing the differences between PGD for late onset diseases and other indications for PGD, it is argued that in case the parents chose PGD among all possible alternatives, it is justified since it "increases the mother's will to have another child" (Israeli National Bioethics Council 2007: 1; our translation). Once again, emphasis is placed on the desire to become a parent and to form a family, and not on the personal risks involved in the medical procedures. Regarding PGD for SDs, ABC's guidelines state that "all alternatives for treating the sick brother must be considered versus the risks (even small ones) involved in the process of IVF and PGD" (ABC 2003: 4; our translation). Yet, assuming that there is no other treatment and that the cord blood recipient is a first degree relative, this procedure is described as serving the benefit of all participants. Hence, while in England the future child's welfare is the main concern, in Israel it is the family as a whole which is at the focus of concern. According to the ABC's report, PGD for SDs is legitimate since it is advantageous to all family members: The mother "benefits since she avoids the mental distress of a dying child" (ABC 2003: 5; our translation). It is argued that the future child "has an interest in being born to a family without a sick brother/sister, or parent" (ABC 2003: 5; our translation). Obviously, the existing child also benefits, as her life is saved. Thus PGD for SDs is not only seen as morally acceptable; but rather it is considered "a double blessing, for it brings and saves life simultaneously" (ABC 2003: 5; our translation).

Furthermore, our findings concerning PGD suggest that achieving a pregnancy following ground-breaking fertility treatments is viewed as heroic and undisputable in the Israeli society. This can be illustrated by some of the responses to Sharon Harari's personal tale. The Israeli press coverage of her story laid emphasis on the procedure's advantages and the medical breakthrough, while representing Harari as a heroine mother who did everything possible to save her child. Little or no attention at all was given to potential physical or psychological damages to the future SD or to the mother (see Negev 2005; Limor 2002). Rather, the story of the Harari family was described as "[a]n Israeli precedent; parents saved their child's life. . . . it was the beginning of an exhausting, lengthy journey of parents determined to seek cure for their child's fatal disease, [a journey] which broke the conventional borders of science" (Negev 2005: 33; our translation).

In summary, while in England the dominant argument in favor of approving PGD for SDs was the *lack of evidence for potential risks to the future child* (medical or psychological), in Israel, the issue of safety was far less central in the discussion. In fact, the lack of knowledge regarding the safety of the procedure in the very early days of its application did not prevent the performance of PGD in Israel. Rather, emphasis was placed on the technology's potential benefits for the entire family.

Views of the family as a group with shared or conflicting interests are very prominent while comparing the ethical debate and regulations in Israel and Germany.

Compared with the German discourse, Israeli discourse of reprogenetics is based on the assumption that family members are mutually dependant, and thus none of them is seen as truly autonomous. In the Israeli-Jewish culture, an embryo/fetus obtains its status through relations with the members of the particular family it will be born into (if born at all), and its moral standing is not separated from its mother-to-be, but rather dependent on her condition, and the definition of the pregnancy situation (Hashiloni-Dolev and Weiner in press). Likewise, womanhood in Israel is understood as synonymous with motherhood (Berkowitch 1999), and women are not commonly referred to as autonomous and fully independent individuals, either by the state or by themselves. This bond between mother and child, which weakens the independent individuality (quite literally) of each of them, is illustrated in Sharon Harari's story about her personal experience with PGD for SDs:

> There is an unresolved question regarding the family's genealogical tree. Where do we end and where do they begin? Are there any clear boundaries in this continuum of parents and children? My margins were clear until I became a mother myself. . . . [at that point] the lines of the private body were blurred, and part of my inside was freed from my body. It had a figure, a name, and an identity of its own, but in fact, a complicated symbiotic connection had been created between us. (Harari 2005: 132–33; our translation)

Likewise, in an interview in Israel's most popular weekend newspaper, Harari was asked whether she and her husband would tell their girl, born as a result of the PGD procedure, that she was chosen in order to be a donor to her brother. Harari answered in a manner which once again pointed to her view of the family as a unified group, whose members are obligated to help each other without that endangering their personal/autonomous identity:

> "We don't see it like that," she said. "We would tell her what we told Amitai [the affected son], that his bone marrow was ill, and since in a family you do whatever you have to for one another, we made a cooperative effort to save him by finding the best bone marrow . . . and found that it exists in the cord blood, the combined blood of her

mother and father . . . and we are all connected in a blood tie."
(Negev 2005: 36; our translation)

Thus, Harari understood the PGD process to have been a collective family enterprise, representing family members' responsibilities toward each other, and not as an act which treated her daughter as mere means. While any mother around the world could very well have a similar understanding of such a situation, we wish to highlight that Harari's story is not just another personal point of view, and that similar opinions were also voiced by Israeli press and policy makers.

When appointed to discuss PGD for the purpose of sex selection and other medical purposes, the Science and Technology Committee of the Israeli Parliament invited Sharon Harari to tell her story. Following Harari's presentation, an attorney from the Israeli Ministry of Justice said: "[T]he second purpose [of PGD] is the case presented by Sharon; giving birth to a healthy child in order to help cure a sick brother. Also this issue is under debate and controversy [around the world. . .]. [However] the child is not an instrument; the child is a goal in itself, who in his birth brings cure to his family and to his sick brother, and by that helps. I think that the feelings towards him become even more precious, both as a human being, and as a person who helped his fellow-man, even before becoming intelligent (*"bar-daat"*). I don't think we should consider it improper" (Science and Technology Committee, 2005: 13; our translation).

Moving to the official Israeli position concerning PGD for SDs, it is interesting to note that the Israeli guidelines regarding PGD for SDs mention the Kantian imperative that is dominant in discussions of genetics and ethics in the West. However, this principle is interpreted differently than in Germany. While the opponents of PGD in Germany argue that PGD necessarily violates the future child's status as a subject, in Israel SDs are not considered as either a mean or an end. Rather they can supposedly be both, as "instrumentalization," and having and loving a child on its own merit, or as an end in itself, are not seen as contradictions. Thus, the Israeli guidelines regarding PGD for SDs state, "Parents who wish to save the life of one of their children are certainly parents who love all their children, and one should not fear that they will have another child who will serve as a mere 'mean'" (ABC 2003: 5; our translation).

Accordingly, parents who use PGD in order to select a SD are considered to act in a loving and responsible manner, for the sake of all their children. In fact, their use of PGD in order to help their sick child is understood as a sign of their love and devotion to all their children, sick or healthy, "designed" or not. While the Israeli guidelines do demand a psychological evaluation of parents who wish to use PGD for SDs in order to make sure that the future child is wanted for her own sake, the guidelines also state that there is "no moral fault in choosing a healthy child, who is simultaneously a potential donor" (ABC 2003: 4; our translation).

Thus, while in England as well as in Germany concern is given primarily to the good of the future child herself, regardless of the family's wants and needs, in Israel emphasis is placed on the needs of the family as a whole. In the same vein, the child's benefit is believed to stem from and intertwine with the benefit of other family members.

Conclusion

In spite of the common technological background and cooperation of scientific centers world wide, there is no broad international consent as regards the regulation of different NRTs. Reviewing the ethical discussion and regulation of PGD for SDs in Israel, Germany and England, we have shown that PGD for SDs was approved with no genuine opposition in Israel, limited but later on widely permitted in England, and banned for the time being in Germany. Furthermore, we have demonstrated that while both German and English discussions placed the future SD at the focus of their concern, emphasizing either its potential medical and/or psychological risks (in England), or risks to its freedom and autonomy (in Germany), the Israeli discussion centers on the welfare of the entire family.

Looking for the complex historical, political, and cultural background of the official positions of the three studied societies, or answering the question of why is it that different categories became dominant in the discourse regarding PGD for SDs, is beyond the scope of this paper. However, we would like to suggest that by comparing the regulation and ethical discussion regarding PGD for SDs in Israel, Germany and England, a salient feature of the common reasoning embedded in the regulation of NRTs in Israel came to the fore. In contrast to Germany and England, in which despite all their differences, the social category placed at the center of attention was the individual child, in Israel the welfare of the entire family was the category demanding concern. One possible explanation for this disparity is the fact that Israel is a more familistic society in comparison to most other advanced liberal societies, in which interfamilial involvement and assistance (from baby sitting to major financial help) are the norm (Birenbaum-Carmeli 1999). Israeli familism has been attributed to a complex matrix of reasons. For example, questioning why in Israel, a modern society by economic, political, and cultural criteria, the family retains a degree of centrality typical to non-western societies, Peres and Katz (1981) claim that the fact that Israel faces a permanent security threat increases its inhabitant's need for intimate affiliation. Another optional explanation is that since Israel is a small country, family members often live in close geographic proximity and can therefore have frequent personal contact. The central role that family has in Jewish life has been offered as another explanation, as even among the secular population, major life events and holidays are celebrated according to Jewish tradition (e.g., marriage, adolescence, and birth). Moreover, according to Jewish thought, although it is important to ensure the maintenance and development of selfhood, the self is not defined in isolation, but rather in relation to a community (Wolpe 1997).

Accordingly, the findings of this study suggest that, in Israel, it is considered far more legitimate for parents to "design" or select their children as an expression of their parental love, care, and responsibility toward the future child and its entire family. This view is aligned with thinking of children not solely as individual subjects, but rather as members of a unified body, consisting of different members whose interests are imagined to be mainly in concert, and whose welfare cannot be measured separately. This highlighting of the well-being of the entire family goes hand in hand with a disregard for the potential risks to either the future child, or its mother, who is expected to take upon herself a complex medical treatment. (Similarly, highlighting the rights of the SD goes hand in hand with less attention given to the welfare of the parents or the existing sick child.)

While it has been formerly argued that the medical field of NRTs and the regulations accompanying it in Israel shed light on the Israeli attitude toward fertility and vice versa (Hashiloni-Dolev 2007; Birenbaum-Carmeli 2000; Shalev and Gooldin 2006), official positions concerning assisted reproduction have not often been linked to how family relations and obligations are ideally viewed in different societies, or to the effect of family concepts on the regulation of NRTs. We suggest that looking at the regulation and ethical debate regarding PGD for SDs in Israel and comparing it with other societies unveils the importance of particular understandings regarding family relations and obligations. It is thus an important component of any further discussion concerning the regulation of NRTs in Israel and beyond.

Appendix

Table 7   The main differences between Israel, England, and Germany

	Germany	England	Israel
General Status of PGD	Prohibited	Allowed	Allowed
PGD for SDs	Prohibited	Allowed	Allowed
Ethical discourse	Intense	Intense	Relatively scarce
Ethical bodies	German Parliament Commission on Law and Ethics in Modern Medicine, National Bioethics Council	HFEA Ethics and Law Committee (ELC)	Up to 2004: Israeli National Academy of Sciences & Humanities, Helsinki Committee for Genetic Experiments on Human beings. From 2004: Israel National Bioethics Council.
Main concerns regarding SDs	Violating the autonomy of the future child; Possible conflicts between family members	Medical and psychological risk to the future child	Family as a unified group with mutual interests. All members benefit from the procedure.

Notes

1. Genetic disorders caused by a mutation in a single gene.
2. Changes in the structure or number of the chromosomes carrying the genetic information (DNA).
3. Disorders that are expressed only when both copies of the gene are mutated.
4. In the United States, the Congress refuses to fund the use of PGD. Consequently, providers offering those services and patients who seek them are the ones who determine how and for whom PGD is used (Robertson 2003). In Europe, there is no applicable EU directive concerning PGD. Hence, different countries have different policies. In France and Finland the issue is under constant debate. In Portugal there is no specific applicable law, while in Italy, Ireland, Austria and Germany, PGD is illegal (Krones and Richter 2004).

References

Advisory Bioethics Committee Israel National Academy of Sciences and Humanities and the Helsinki Committee for Genetic Experiments on Human Beings (ABC). 2003. "Guidelines for Using PGD" [Hebrew]. Obtained from Professor Michele Revel, Head of the Israeli National Bioethics Council.

Berkowitch, N. 1999. "Women of Labor: Women and Citizenship in Israel." *Israeli Sociology* 2, no. 1: 277–317.

Bielorai, B., Hughes, M.R. Auerbach, A.D. Nagler, A. Loewenthal, R. Rechavi, and G. Toren. 2004. "Successful Umbilical Cord Transplantation for Fanconi Anemia Using Preimplantation Genetic Diagnosis for HLA-Matched Donor." *American Journal of Hematology* 77, no. 4: 397–99.

Birenbaum-Carmeli, D. 2000. "Our First 'IVF Baby': Israel and Canada's Press Coverage of Procreative Technology." *International Journal of Sociology and Social Policy* 20, no. 7: 1–38.

———. 1999. "Intergenerational Relations among Israeli Upper Middle Class Jewish Families in Israel." *The Jewish Journal of Sociology* 41, no. 1–2: 24–49.

Devolder, K. 2005. "Preimplantation HLA Typing: Having Children to Save Our Loved Ones." *Journal of Medical Ethics* 31, no. 10: 582–86.

Draper, H. and R. Chadwick. 1999. "Beware! Preimplantation Genetic Diagnosis May Solve Some Old Problems But it Also Raises New Ones." *Journal of Medical Ethics* 25, no. 2: 176–82.

Levinson, D., ed. 1995. *Encyclopedia of Marriage and the Family*. New York: Simon and Schuster.

Evans, J.H. 2005. *Playing God? Human Genetic Engineering and the Rationalization of Public Bioethical Debate*. Chicago: University of Chicago Press.

Fogiel-Bijaoui, S. 2003. "Familism, Postmodernity and the State: The Case of Israel." In *Israeli Family and Community*, ed. Hannah Naveh. London and Portland: V. Mitchell.

Gaziev, J and G. Lucarelli. 2003. "Stem Cell Transplantation for Hemoglobinopathies." *Current Opinion in Pediatr*ics 15, no. 1: 24–31.

Geraedts, J., A. Handyside, J. Harper, I. Liebaers, K. Sermon, C. Staessen, A. Thornhill, A. Vanderfaeillie, and S. Viville. 1999. "ESHRE Preimplantation Genetic Diagnosis (PGD) Consortium: Preliminary Assessment of Data from January 1997 to September 1998. ESHRE PGD Consortium Steering Committee." *Human Reproduction* 14, no. 12: 3138–48.

German Bundestag. 1990. *Embryo Protection Act*. <http://www.bmj.bund.de/enid/Publications/Embryo_Protection_Act_19u.html> (accessed October 6, 2007).

German Bundestag. 2002. *Final Report, Submitted by the Study Commission on "Law and Ethics in Modern Medicine."* Document 14/9020.

Habermas, J. 2003. *The Future of Human Nature*. Cambridge, U.K.: Polity Press.

Handyside, A., E. Kontogianni, K. Hardy, K. Winston, and R. Winston. 1990. "Pregnancies from Biopsied Human Preimplantation Embryos Sexed by Y-specific DNA Amplification." *Nature* 344: 768–70.

Harari S. 2005. *A Present for the Future* [Hebrew]. Or Yehuda: Kinneret Zmora-Bitan, Dvir Publishing House.

Harper, J.C., K. Boelaert, J. Geraedts, G. Harton, W.G. Kearns, C. Moutou, N. Muntjewerff, S. Repping, S. SenGupta, P. N. Scriven, J. Traeger-Synodinos, K. Vesela, L. Wilton, and K.D. Sermon. 2006. "ESHRE PGD Consortium Data Collection V: Cycles from January to December 2002 with Pregnancy Follow-up to October 2003." *Human Reproduction* 21, no. 1: 3–21.

Hashiloni-Dolev, Y.2007. *A Life (Un)Worthy of Living: Reproductive Genetics in Israel and Germany.* Dordrecht: Springer.

Hashiloni-Dolev, Y., and N. Weiner. 2008. "Reproductive Technologies and the Moral Status of the Embryo: A View from Israel and Germany." *Sociology of Health and Illness* 30(7): 1055–69.

Human Fertilization and Embryology Authority (HFEA). 1999. "Preimplantation Genetic Diagnosis (CE 13/08/1999)." October 12, 2007. <http://www.hfea.gov.uk/en/603.html>

———2001a. "HFEA to Allow Tissue Typing in Conjunction with Preimplantation Genetic Diagnosis". http://www.hfea.gov.uk/en/960.html (accessed October 18, 2007).

———. 2001b. "Outcome of the Public Consultation on Preimplantation Genetic Diagnosis." http://www.hfea.gov.uk/cps/rde/xbcr/SID-3F57D79B-42394002/hfea/PGD_outcome.pdf (accessed February 24, 2007).

———. 2004a. "Preimplantation Tissue Typing." 2007.http://www.hfea.gov.uk/docs/PreimplantationReport.pdf (accessed February 24, 2007).

———. 2004b. "New Guidance on Preimplantation Tissue Typing." http://www.hfea.gov.uk/en/599.html (accessed October 18, 2007).

Office of Public Sector Information. 1990. "Human Fertilisation and Embryology Act." http://www.opsi.gov.uk/ACTS/acts1990/ukpga_19900037_en_1 (accessed October 12, 2007).

Israeli National Bioethics Council. 2007. "PGD Guidelines for Late Onset Diseases and Susceptibility Genes for Cancer." Obtained from Professor Michele Revel, Head of the Israeli National Bioethics Council.

Kass, L.R. 2000. "Triumph or Tragedy: The Moral Meaning of Genetic Technology." *American Journal of Jurisprudence* 45: 1–16.

———. 2002. *Life, Liberty and the Defense of Dignity: The Challenge for Bioethics.* San Francisco: Encounter Books.

King, D.S. 1999. "Preimplantation and the New Eugenics." *Journal of Medical Ethics* 25, no. 2: 176–82.

Krones, T and G. Richter. 2004. "Preimplantation Genetic Diagnosis: European Perspectives and the German Situation." *Journal of Medicine and Philosophy* 29: 623–40.

Landau, R. 2003. "Ethical Aspects of PGD" [Hebrew] *Refua and Mishpat* 28: 77–83.

Limor, T. 2002. "Fluorescent Chromosomes: A New Technique Enables Genetic Testing of the Embryo, Prior its Implantation to the Uterus Through In Vitro Fertilization" [Hebrew]. *Ha'aretz* December 30.

McLean, S. 2006. *Modern Dilemmas: Choosing Children.* Edinburgh: Capercaillie Books.

Ministry of Health. 2005. "The National Committee to Sex Selection using PGD" [Hebrew]. http://www.health.gov.il/download/forms/a2692_mk21_05.pdf (accessed March 31, 2007).

Ministry of Health. 2006. "Guidelines for Preimplantation Genetic Diagnosis" [Hebrew]. http://www.health.gov.il/download/forms/a2930_mr50_06.pdf (accessed March 31, 2007).

National Ethics Council. 2003. "Genetic Diagnosis Before and During Pregnancy." http://www.nat-ethikrat.de/_english/press/Opinion_Genetic_Diagnosis.pdf (accessed April 5, 2007).

Negev E. 2005. "The Last Chance" [Hebrew]. *Yediot Aharonot,* 2 November 2005.

Penning, G., R. Schots, and I. Liebaers. 2002. "Ethical Considerations on Preimplantation Genetic Diagnosis for HLA Typing to Match a Future Child as a Donor of Haematopoietic Stem Cells to a Sibling." *Human Reproduction* 17, no. 3: 534–38.

Peres, Y and R. Katz. 1981. "Stability and Centrality: The Nuclear Family in Modern Israel." *Social Forces* 59, no. 3: 687–704.

Prainsack, B and T. D. Spector. 2006. "Twins: A Cloning Experience." *Social Science & Medicine* 63, no. 10: 2739–52.

President's Council on Bioethics. 2002. *Human Cloning and Human Reproduction: An Ethical Inquiry.* http://www.bioethics.gov/reports/cloningreport/overview.html (accessed October 12, 2007).

Remennick, L. 2006. "The Quest for the Perfect Baby: Why Do Israeli Women Seek Prenatal Genetic Testing?" *Sociology of Health and Illness* 28, no. 1: 21–53.

Robertson, J.A. 2003. "Extending Preimplantation Genetic Diagnosis: The Ethical Debate." *Human Reproduction* 18, no. 3: 465–71.

Schenker, J.G. 2003. "Legal Aspects of ART Practice in Israel." *Journal of Assisted Reproduction and Genetics* 20, no. 7: 250- 59.

Science and Technology Committee. 2005. "PGD for Sex Selection and Other Medical Purposes (Protocol No. 124)" [Hebrew]. <http://www.knesset.gov.il/protocols/data/html/mada/2005–03–16.html> at: http://www.knesset.gov.il/protocols/data/html/mada/2005–03–16.html (accessed March 8, 2007).

Sermon, K. 2002. "Current Concepts in Preimplantation Genetic Diagnosis (PGD): A Molecular Biologist's View." *Human Reproduction Update* 8: 1–10.

Shalev, C., and S. Gooldin. 2006. "The Uses and Misuses of In Vitro Fertilization in Israel: Some Sociological and Ethical Considerations." *Nashim* 12: 151–76.

State of Israel. 1996. "Knesset Law, Surrogacy" [Hebrew]. http://www.medlaw.co.il/imgs/uploads/hakika/nesiat%20obarim.doc (accessed October 12, 2007).

State of Israel. 1999. "Knesset Law, Prohibition of Human Cloning" [Hebrew]. http://www.academy.ac.il/bioethics/hebrew/documents/bioethics_law-h.pdf (accessed October 12, 2007).

Terry, L.M. 2002. "The Child That Might Be Born." *Hasting Center Report* 32, no. 3: 11–12.

Timmermans, S. and M. Berg. 2003. "The Practice of Medical Technology." *Sociology of Health and Illness* 25: 97–114.

Traubman, T. 2005. "Health Ministry: Parents Could Choose the Sex of Their Baby in Anomalous Cases" [Hebrew]. *Ha'aretz,* May 19, 2005.

Van Balen, F. and M.C. Inhorn. 2003. "Son Preference, Sex Selection, and the 'New' New Reproductive Technologies." *International Journal of Health Services* 33, no. 2: 235–52.

Van de Velde, H., I. Georgiou, M. De Rycke, R. Schots, K. Sermon, W. Lissens, P. Devroey, A. Van Steirteqhem, and I. Liebares. 2004. "Novel Universal Approach for Preimplantation Genetic Diagnosis of Beta-Thalassaemia in Combination with HLA Matching of Embryos." *Human Reproduction* 19, no. 3: 700–08.

Wolpe, P.R. 1997. "If I Am Only My Genes, What Am I? Genetic Essentialism and a Jewish Response." *Kennedy Institute of Ethics Journal* 7, no. 3: 213–30.

Yasur-Beit-Or, M. 2007. "For the First Time, a Committee Allowed a Couple to Choose the Sex of Their Child." http://www.ynet.co.il/articles/1,7340, L-3220136,00.html (accessed February 24, 2007).

Chapter 3

The Man in the Sperm: Kinship and Fatherhood in Light of Male Infertility in Israel

Helene Goldberg

Introduction

This article explores kinship and fatherhood in light of male infertility and artificial reproductive technologies (ARTs) in the Jewish-Israeli context. I became interested in the male reproductive experience in Israel through a backdoor interest in Jewish identity, and then came across Susan Kahn's groundbreaking study (2000) of single, secular Jewish women's reproduction in Israel with the use of sperm donation. It seemed that because of Israeli technological advances in reproductive technologies, the state's support of fertility treatment, national efforts to increase the Jewish population, and the concept that Jewish identity is passed through the mother, men could be removed from Jewish-Israeli reproduction and kinship. Kahn's study captured my attention and compelled me to consider Jewish-Israeli reproduction and kinship with a focus on men.

In the process of exploring possible research topics I realized that a severe silence surrounded male infertility, in Israel and in general, and that men had been crudely overlooked in studies of reproduction, if compared with the number of studies that have dealt with women and reproduction (Goldberg 2004; Inhorn et al. 2009).[1] Recently an increasing number of social scientists have begun to explore various aspects of the male experience of reproduction and infertility (Birenbaum-Carmeli et al. 1995; Inhorn 2003, 2004; Goldberg 2004; Inhorn et al. 2009). In terms of male reproduction and infertility, sperm donation is probably the best explored aspect (Tjørnhøj-Thomsen 1999a, 1999b; Becker 2002; Nachtigall et al. 1997; Inhorn 2006b), a subject which has been researched in the Israeli context by sociologists Yoram S. Carmeli and Daphna Birenbaum-Carmeli (1994, 2000a, 2000b).

As a response to infertility, ARTs challenge traditional thoughts about reproduction, moving it from the privacy of the house into the public clinical setting. ARTs let us visualize the body, its substances and conception in new ways, adding new choices and experiences of the body and of the self (Tjørnhøj-Thomsen 1999a, 1999b). The body is a subject of culture (Csordas 1990); body parts, even at the cellular level, serve as icons charged with the shifting cultural meaning of kinship, gender, religion, nationhood, and so on. The many new options of ARTs, such as surrogacy and gamete donation, both challenge and make explicit such cultural meanings (Strathern 1992) and also trigger new questions, such as how to define who the parents are as well as the legal/religious status of the child.

Thus, reproduction and the uses of ARTs transcend immediate family concerns. In the Israeli context national, religious, and personal demands are central to the legislation and practice of ARTs (Teman 2001; Shalev and Gooldin 2006) and answers to questions about who the parents are and what the basis of the relations between parent/child is depend upon the specific situation (Goldberg 2006).

Anthropologist Janet Carsten introduced the term "notions of relatedness" to emphasize possible variations in views of being related, to introduce questions about what being related does, and indicate what implications relatedness has in changing situations (Carsten 2000: 1). I find this term useful because of its openness and flexibility. In the course of my research on Jewish-Israeli reproduction I have encountered various notions of relatedness, which tie the individual to the collective and individual family in different ways: through the mother (matrilineally), through the father (patrilineally) or through both the mother and father (bilaterally). A brief look into these notions of relatedness, which are implicit in ideas of nationhood, Jewishness, citizenship, kinship, and the family in the Jewish-Israeli context (Goldberg 2006), will yield a later discussion about the stakes for individual men and for couples when they consider alternative ways to have children.

It is usually held that Jewishness is passed matrilineally through the mother, which stems from *halachah*, Jewish law.[2] In the light of ARTs, most rabbis argue that Jewishness is passed through pregnancy and birth—not through genetics, meaning that Jewishness is established through the womb (See Kahn 2000, 2002).[3] On a national level, Israel is defined as a state for Jews, and anyone born of a Jewish mother—anywhere in the world—is granted the right to citizenship in Israel.[4]

Meanwhile, in prayers and in biblical stories, children are referred to as the children of their father, and the father's last name is passed on to the whole family unit (Carmeli and Birenbaum-Carmeli 2000a: 304). Lineage is passed patrilineally and Jews are often called the children of Abraham—evoking the story of origin from Genesis. The lineage is traced back to Abraham's grandson, Jacob's son, though such status only has practical implications to religious Jews.[5] In light of ARTs, most, but not all, rabbis argue that lineage and fatherhood are passed on or established through the sperm (Gold 1988; Kahn 2000).[6]

Finally, relatedness is thought to be passed on by both the mother and father's genes, which is comparable to western understandings of kinship (Schneider1980; Tjørnhøj-Thomsen 1999a). Central to such bilateral notions of relatedness are the ideas that kinship comes from *law* (marriage) and from *nature*—through a conjugal sexual relationship where the man's and woman's "biogenetic half" ("blood" or genes) is passed to the child (Schneider1980; see also Carmeli and Birenbaum-Carmeli 2000a: 304).[7]

Using a lens of male infertility, I explore some aspects of male reproduction, kinship, and gender in this chapter. Male infertility is stigmatized cross-culturally (Mason 1993; Tjørnhøj-Thomsen 1999a; Inhorn 2003, 2004) because it challenges various aspects of masculinity and sexuality by conjuring ideas of failed sperm, failed intercourse, and failed virility (Goldberg 2009). Here however, I will focus on the man's role in the course of clinical treatment and the notions of relatedness passed through the man and the sperm in reproduction. By focusing on men, I do not intend to undermine women's experience of reproduction or the meanings of motherhood and matrilineality (see Teman 2001, 2003, 2006; Ivry 2004, Kahn 2000, Sered 2000, Haelyon 2006; Remennick 2006), but to forefront other, often overlooked aspects of Jewish-Israeli kinship and reproduction. After an introduction to my methods, I explore some dilemmas and paradoxes of male infertility and its treatment in the clinic. Then I explore how the substance—the sperm—is collected, following which I discuss interviewees' different reactions and thoughts about reproductive alternatives, and I examine the practice of hiding sperm donation.

Method

My research[8] in Israel was based on participant observation at two main locations. The first site was an in vitro fertilization (IVF) clinic based in a hospital in Jerusalem, which also does intracytoplasmic sperm injection (ICSI).[9] The second fieldwork site was a spermatology clinic outside Jerusalem, which does advanced semen analysis, selecting sperm to be used for ICSI. Additionally, I visited two sperm banks and spent a week in a fertility clinic that performs artificial insemination. All of these clinics were located in Jerusalem. I formally interviewed 35 people, including patients (men, women, and couples together), doctors, rabbis, social workers, biologists, lab workers, an infertility group counsellor, and a religious supervisor (a *mashgicha* who was working in the IVF clinic). The shortest interview took fifteen minutes; the longest five hours. Several patients were interviewed a number of times. Interviews were tape recorded and transcribed verbatim. During my everyday interactions in the clinics where I observed operations, consultations, meetings, etc., I had informal conversations with secretaries, nurses, doctors, biologists, and patients.

The study did not focus on a specific sub-group, but on the social construction of male infertility among Jewish-Israelis in the fertility treatment settings. Given the complexities of Jewish religious association, I use the terms that religious patients used to define themselves when giving examples that involve such patients. It is difficult to ascertain how my gender played into my ability to conduct the study; that is, if the male patients were more or less likely to talk to me. Indeed some medical staff appeared more concerned about my research topic than did the patients, and several compelled me to focus on women rather than men.[10] The male patients I finally interviewed, religious as well as secular, spoke openly about intimate details of the fertility treatment. I asked two religious men whom I came to know quite well, and they both insisted they would be more likely to talk to a woman about their fertility problem. In general, the men had never spoken to anyone else besides their partner and the medical staff about the problem, and many expressed that they enjoyed the opportunity to talk and reflect about *their* experiences and thoughts. I guess that I was ultimately able to conduct the study because I was a stranger committed to confidentiality (see Inhorn 2004: 165), and because I was located in clinics where I was able to make the initial contact with the patients.[11]

"All a man has is his sperm": Some paradoxes of male infertility

A dilemma of male infertility is that it manifests itself on the woman's body—by the woman not becoming pregnant, as anthropologist Marcia C. Inhorn writes (2003, 2004). Thus, married women who are not pregnant are more likely to be "socially diagnosed" for infertility while men may pass unmarked. It can be debated whether it is at all possible to talk about male infertility inseparable from the women's body or from the couple as a unit.

Sal, a religious man[12] employed in the air force who had been married a little over a year, explained, "I didn't know that I have a problem. It is not something that you feel. Only the lab test could show you what the problem is." Sal and his wife, as many others, only realized after the sperm test that he, and not she, had a fertility problem. While women experience male infertility physically, by not becoming pregnant, men do not. Male infertility is hidden in the testicles of men (Inhorn 2003, 2004). In fact, male infertility is a hidden "truth" in the sperm itself (Goldberg in press)—a condition that only becomes a social problem after being discovered and diagnosed in the clinic though sperm analysis (Inhorn 2004).[13]

The dilemma of infertility manifesting itself on the woman's body continues even after a diagnosis, suggesting that the infertility stems from a "male factor problem." It is women who are treated since there is still a lack of treatment options available for men (see Birenbaum-Carmeli et al. 1995; Tjørnhøj-Thomsen 1999b).[14] This imbalance of available options often seemed very frustrating to men. As the director of the spermatology clinic argued, "When the men come here, they ask, 'Why am I not being treated? I have a problem, I know. I didn't get any treatment, she is treated'." Men's exclusion was further emphasized by a single female patient's remark that husbands only escort their wives to treatment.

A central understanding of bilateral kinship, however, is that reproduction is a joint, conjugal project (Schneider 1980; Tjørnhøj-Thomsen 1999b). Clinical staff conceptualize infertility in this way by insisting that the treatment was equally the couple's, though in practice it was the woman's. During a consultation, a doctor told a woman that her husband had to be present also. "But he works," said the woman, defending her husband. The staff told me that at times it was difficult to convince men to join women in treatment. A doctor explained, "Many times the husband is busy. I ask the husband to come. I emphasize that it is a problem of both sides. For the follicle follow-ups. it is okay that she comes alone. I don't want him to miss work too much."[15] This quote again shows that although ideally the husband should be participating because reproduction is understood as a joint, conjugal project, is not necessary in the course of the treatment, since his physical presence is not integral to the treatment. As long as the husband's sperm has been recovered, he can skip many of the medical appointments.

With treatment focusing *on* and succeeding *in* the woman's body, men and women experience the treatment in radically different ways. Gabi, an engineer who had been married for two years, said, "For me it is not a physical effect but a mental one. The time of the treatment is very difficult. For men it is mentally hard, you have to support and understand." Other men echoed the idea that they have an unequal role in the treatment, on the sidelines as supporters. Jonathan, an Orthodox man, who worked in an ultra-Orthodox school and had been married to his wife Michal[16] for 17 years, said, "The abuse that she went through physically and mentally was torturing for me. I want to help out, but I can't! I can't because it is still her body. You might not be able to feel her pain, but you can comfort and you can try to understand."

Jonathan and Gabi agreed that women and men suffered from the treatment in different ways, because the women underwent physical treatment, while the men did not. Some men expressed frustration over not being in the treatment, which was necessitated owing to their fertility problem. Jonathan, who seemed especially troubled by his wife's treatment, took the argument as far as to claim that it is easier for women. When I asked him why he insisted, "All a man has is his sperm." Jonathan's claim highlights that, in practice, all that is physically left of the man in the treatment is his sperm, while the man himself is pushed to the margin. It could be argued that men are marginalized because it is the women who become pregnant and carry the child. However, there are some interesting similarities and contrasts between men whose wives are in fertility treatment and infertile women who use surrogates in Israel.

In surrogacy a woman is commissioned to carry a couple's genetic embryo to term.[17] Thus, infertile women using a surrogate are like infertile men, linked to the clinical reproduction only through the genes (their egg), while the surrogate undergoes the fertility treatment and pregnancy, as the partner of the infertile man. However, in surrogacy, the woman is included at *all* stages of the medical treatment, often serving as an intermediate between the doctor and the surrogate, taking responsibility for both the treatment and the pregnancy. She may even be hospitalized in the new mothers' ward after birth while the surrogate is hospitalized in the gynecology ward (See Teman 2010). Men are not required or invited to take responsibility for the treatment or for the pregnancy. Like the infertile women using surrogates, infertile men could easily be included in the treatment, yet their absence indicates that clinical actions and conduct are informed by different gendered ideologies and expectations. In short, it seems that men are marginalized in the clinical reproduction because *they are men*.

The treatment of male infertility is still a treatment of the women's body and the women take charge of it while the men are marginalized. However, men are central before they become absent or unnecessary because they *must* leave their sperm behind for clinical examination and manipulation.

Obtaining the sperm from the man

Before the fertility treatment can proceed, the man must provide a sperm sample to be used in the clinic. Usually sperm is obtained through masturbation in the clinic, which some of the men in this study and in others associated with discomfort and pressure (Mason 1993; Tjørnhøj-Thomsen 1999a, 1999b). In some cases a lab sperm test will reveal that there is no sperm (azoospermia) or no functional sperm in the ejaculation of a man—the worst diagnosis the staff could imagine conveying to a man (Goldberg 2009). In this case, in the Jerusalem IVF clinic the male body was in fact put on the operating table. The clinic specialized in fine needle extraction of sperm from the testicles. If no sperm were located during this operation, a new operation would be scheduled. In the IVF clinic they would conduct up to three operations, though the staff admitted that it is highly unlikely that sperm is found if the first operation is unsuccessful. "We do it more for psychological reasons, for the men to be absolutely sure [there is no sperm]," a nurse explained. This practice, which briefly moves the male body from the margin to the center of the medical gaze, illustrates the extensive efforts both men and physicians will go through to obtain sperm from the infertile men. It further illustrates that these men are also ready to "put their genitals on the operating table" and physically share the burden of infertility with their wives (see Inhorn et al. 2009).

Turning now to the religious context to explore the reality of some of the Israeli fertility patients, a layer of complexity is added in obtaining sperm for clinical evaluation or treatment. Jerusalem, where I was mainly located, is the center of Israel's ultra-Orthodox population, who are also frequent visitors to the fertility clinics (Kahn 2002). The staff in the fertility clinics, in general, proudly claimed their excellent collaboration with rabbis and with PUAH, an Orthodox fertility organization led by rabbis. Yet, the means of obtaining sperm is problematic because masturbation is seen as a serious sin in the Torah (see Kahn 2000). In the spermatology clinic, a mandatory form accompanying a sperm sample reflects such religious concerns. All patients had to indicate how the sperm they were handing over to the lab worker had been produced. Four options were given: masturbation, interrupted intercourse, condom, or post-coital test.[18] The patient would simply circle the way their sperm was collected, which for the orthodox men would be contingent upon the rabbi they had consulted.[19] A few ultra-Orthodox rabbis would not allow use of condoms because they categorically see birth control as wasting sperm—even when it is used with reproductive intent. However, I was told at the IVF clinic that using a condom to collect sperm during sexual intercourse is the most common way of obtaining a sperm sample from religious men. Still, it was sometimes impossible for men to produce sperm at the time it was needed, especially because, as the *mashgicha* explained, most of them were wearing a condom for the first time in their lives, and it was against everything they had ever learned.

Inability to produce sperm sometimes created great irritation among doctors in the IVF-clinic because the clinic's work was put on hold. This happened one day during an ultra-Orthodox couple's treatment. The women had her ovum surgically removed in the morning. Now the lab was waiting for her husband's sperm sample, in order to search for sperm and inject it into the wife's ovum (using ICSI). The sample, which was to be produced during intercourse with the man wearing a condom, did not arrive as planned because the husband was too nervous to have intercourse with his wife.[20] As the acting doctor walked down the hallway, in rage, he exclaimed, "I am so upset [listing a number of things that went wrong the last days]...and this one couldn't perform!" The doctor told me that he had advised the man to use an electric apparatus that stimulates ejaculation, which some Orthodox men agree to use, but this man had refused, citing religious concerns. The doctor continued, "It is not masturbation, but he didn't want to. He said, 'It is forbidden.' Instead, they have to have intercourse, and it is a huge pressure."

Though rabbis usually did not condone masturbation initially, it was permitted in rare cases. Jonathan's wife Michal told me that her husband had finally been advised by a rabbi to masturbate, after many failed attempts to have intercourse with a condom. Jonathan told me the first time we met, the hardest thing about treatment was that he had to produce sperm. In a later interview he elaborated:

> It is a little bit demeaning, because it is not a comfortable thing to go to a bathroom in the morning at six o'clock in the hospital, and they tell you, "Here, take the cup." I know that what I am doing may be not the rightful thing, religious-wise and all. But also we have the guidance from a, you know, rabbi. Guidance to tell you that "if there is no choice, if there is no other answer, if this is the only way, then you have to do this in a respectable way." It is not a dirty way, or a sexual way. So sometimes I feel a little bit sad, but I know that after it is over, it is over. I know that they take my sperm, and they have to do all these experiments and growth [IVF] so that way it can be injected into my wife's uterus. Our only goal is to have a beautiful child. . .

The religious objection to masturbation and "wasting" sperm may add guilt[21] and additional stress and discomfort to religious men's experience when producing sperm. Providing the sperm is the man's integral contribution to the clinical reproduction—and until the sperm is obtained, further clinical procedures are put on hold. But what if there is no sperm to be found, or if the husband's sperm is of such a quality that it may preclude conception?

Thoughts about alternative ways to have children

I asked couples—and men specifically—as well as medical staff, their thoughts about alternative ways of having children. Most couples and men did not consider having children in other ways: "It is too soon," and "There are no alternatives" were some of their responses.

Considering adoption, Jonathan replied, "Adoption is a wonderful thing. They say that if you adopt a child who doesn't have a parent, then you are his parent. But before we really came to that level, we wanted to try for our own. We would if we knew there was no more hope." Jonathan, who urged his wife to end the treatment, did not want to consider alternative ways to have children but hoped he would have his own child, with the help of God, he said. The couple already had two children, an older child they had "the natural way" and a two year old they had by IVF; however, being a religious couple they wished for more children. Michal had several miscarriages behind her as a result of the treatment. When we were alone, she told me that she would have adopted a long time ago, but that Jonathan would not hear of it. This couple appeared troubled by their internal disagreement on how to continue their quest for a larger family, and since Jonathan was not ready to adopt, the wife simply stayed in treatment.

In general, doctors insisted that it was always better to have a genetic child. One doctor who was also a rabbi insisted that in the case of adoption you only transfer some legal rights, "but you are not changing the idea of family." The idea of family in Jewish tradition is that of a natural family, he asserted. Another doctor said that he would not recommend that couples go straight for sperm donation: "I wait until the end of the road. It is not preferable and they will want to maximize their chances. Sometimes there is no choice. At least it will be a *semi-natural* baby." But donation would still be better than adoption, he argued, because, "In adoption you get the whole package." The idea of natural and semi-natural children—which is informed by the bilateral notions of relatedness—is also mentioned in other studies of ARTs and kinship (Tjørnhøj-Thomsen 1999a). Both Israeli doctors used an argument of placing "natural" [i.e. genetic] children at the top of the hierarchy. The first insisted that if the child were adopted, the family union would not be real, because it was not based on "nature." The second doctor argued that sperm donation was a better solution than adoption, because a donor child would be "semi-natural," that is, genetically related to one of the parents while an adopted child would be unrelated to both.

Sperm donation was outright rejected by most of the men and women I interviewed. Michal, who, as mentioned before had considered adoption, had never considered sperm donation, for religious reasons: "By the Jewish law you can't have it, especially if you are married. It means that the child is a bastard, because you are a married woman, and you have some other man's child." The understanding that paternity is passed through the sperm in sexual intercourse makes sperm donation to religious Jewish couples extremely problematic, because it not only jeopardizes fatherhood and patrilineality, but also invokes the notion of adultery[22] and illegitimate children (Gold 1988; Kahn 2000, 2002; Goldberg in press). This is also the case in the Muslim context described by Inhorn, where sperm donation is seen as even more problematic than in the ultra-Orthodox Jewish context—it is very rare and even prohibited some places, such as in Egypt (Inhorn 2006a; 2006b). However, in Israel sperm donation, even to ultra-Orthodox couples, is conducted as a very last solution to male infertility, being accepted by rabbis in some situations, as when the man is azoospermic. In such cases, only gentile sperm donors are used, for religious reasons (Carmeli and Birenbaum-Carmeli 2000a: 321; Kahn 2000, 2002).[23]

The couple Jacob and Ester illustrate how several ideas about kinship and reproduction may coexist and be expressed at different times depending on the circumstances. Jacob and Ester considered themselves to be traditional[24] and had been married for a little more than a year, after meeting and working on the same kibbutz for several years. When I first met the couple, Ester had thought about sperm donation, but Jacob, who was azoospermic, rejected the idea, insisting that the biggest *mitzvah* is to keep the family name and to have children. He said, "Some people will say it [sperm donation] doesn't matter. I don't accept it for a few reasons. The biggest reason for me is roots. We know where we come from for thousands of years. My family name goes back that far: It was from the first son of Judah who was the son of King David."

Jacob was here expressing the view that the sperm donation would break patrilineal relatedness, which he believed had not been broken for thousands of years. He continued by explaining that he also opposed sperm donation because he considered it *"unnatural,"* and because he did not want to share his wife with another man (the notion of adultery). Jacob further suggested that physical traits from his wife's family or his family would manifest themselves in the child, "like red hair." Now he was drawing on bilateral notions of relatedness, where the mother and father each contribute with their biogenetic half of the child, a half which can also be split into quarters to include the four grandparents, or even further (Schneider 1980).

In this, our first of many conversations, where Jacob strongly had emphasized bilateral and patrilineal notions of relatedness to explain why he could not accept sperm donation, he surprised me by concluding: "I can adopt, but I can't accept [sperm donation] from a stranger [. . .]. This is how I think now, but maybe we—I—will change my mind."

This potential openness to consider alternatives, however, did not develop further. Jacob had a successful testicular operation where some sperm was found, which was then injected into Ester's eggs by ICSI. Two embryos were transferred to Ester's uterus, and she became pregnant and eventually they had a child. Ester, who had initially considered sperm donation, changed her mind after she got pregnant, insisting that she could not stand to even think about it. Jacobs's reasons for wanting his own child and rejecting alternatives developed even further.

Genetic children certainly are the desired goal of fertility treatment. Yet we also see different opinions about alternative ways to have children within and between the couple, and a potential openness to a change of heart after couples feel that they have exhausted other options (Tjørnhøj-Thomsen 1999a, 1999b; Goldberg 2004).

Sperm donation is an alternative, and since it is practiced in the Israeli fertility clinics, I shall explore this option in more detail. Sperm donation to couples was, according to the doctors, a common last resort to male infertility, though neither patients nor doctors seemed to have favored it to begin with. Sperm donation to couples presents problematic issues around the globe. In the Lebanese setting described by Inhorn, sperm donation is rarely considered an option (2006b). Some Western countries are now displaying more openness on the legislative level, as in Sweden where donor children can obtain information about the donor's identity (Carmeli and Birenbaum-Carmeli 2000b). However, only a minority of Swedish parents have told their child about the sperm donation, which essentially makes the legislative change from 1985 ineffectual.[25] Thus, also in the West, donor insemination remains stigmatized, and studies of couples who use it in other countries, such as Denmark and U.S.A., show that they were ambivalent about it, and about whether or not to tell the child (Tjørnhøj-Thomsen 1999a, 1999b; Becker 2002).

In Israel, the concealment of sperm donation is encouraged by the state (See Carmeli and Birenbaum-Carmeli 2000b). Sperm donation is anonymous, and there are no official records kept of sperm donors and donor children in Israel (Kahn 2000: 79). Couples receiving sperm donation have to sign an informed consent document, which blurs whether the husband's or a donor's sperm will cause conception.[26] The document states that the sperm to be used will be either from the husband, from the husband and a donor, or from a donor alone.[27]

I asked the director of the IVF-clinic how many couples use sperm donation and his reply was that they do not talk about it, suggesting that I should not push this question any further. Birenbaum-Carmeli et al.'s (2000) survey of couples using sperm donation in Israel shows that a majority of couples plan not tell anyone about it, which is also what medical staff and biologists in sperm banks in my study insisted.[28] Overall, sperm donation in Israel is hidden from others, which explains some major difficulties I had in locating couples using sperm donation to interview, and in obtaining permission to do part of my research in sperm banks (Goldberg 2009).

I only interviewed one couple who admitted that they had finally chosen to use sperm donation as an alternative way to have a child, after having spent the last ten years trying to have a second child, and being in treatment for several years. The couple, Hagit and Simon, worked in high-tech, and had started the fertility treatment years ago while working abroad. It had been a long process and a very difficult decision to make, but finally they had made the decision when they felt the doctor could give them no more hope in Hagit conceiving with Simon's sperm. The largest difficulty, said Simon, was that "it will not be my child." On the other hand, they agreed that they wanted to have a larger family, and that their 12-year-old son should have a sibling. Hagit insisted, "Family is what you raise." In Lebanon, men also rejected sperm donation by arguing that "it won't be my son"—though a minority would still consider alternative ways to have a family (Inhorn 2006b). In Denmark, however, people who had children by adoption or sperm donation all restructured their ideas about children and family, emphasizing the relationship between parent and child rather than the genetic connection as defining relatedness in a family (Tjørnhøj-Thomsen 1999a, 1999b). Also, all the couples who had accepted sperm donation in Gay Becker's American study agreed that the man who raises the child is the "real" father (Becker 2002: 130). Whether Simon and other Israeli men in the same situation, having accepted sperm donation, will later change their ideas about family and emphasize *social relatedness*—seeing themselves as the father after the child is born and they develop a relationship—remains an unexplored question.

In the Israeli sperm banks, biologists insisted on social relatedness by holding that the man who raised the child was the father. Yet, in the course of our long conversations, they often mistakenly called the sperm donors the fathers. One biologist said, "They [the donors] never ask about their children." These "slips" suggest that it was very hard to divorce the concept of father from the knowledge of who provided the genetic material—the sperm. This occurred even when the staff had every intention of distinguishing the concepts. In the context of the emphasis on the natural family and notions of fatherhood and lineage as passed through the sperm, I would assume that the redefinition of fatherhood outside genetics might be somewhat harder in the Israeli context than in the Western. In the case of Hagit and Simon, they planned that no one, including the child, would ever know about the donation. This way the donation would not publicly challenge the idea of the natural family and Simon as the genetic father. As Carmeli and Birenbaum-Carmeli (2000b) have shown, in Israel, if a couple does choose sperm donation, they have every opportunity to hide it—thus rather than redefining fatherhood as social, as people may do in the West, the way to come to terms with sperm donation seems to be through concealment and upholding the ideal of genetic fatherhood.

The final example will demonstrate an unusual case: the extent to which a couple, supported by the state and the medical team, went to hide sperm donation and uphold patrilineal notions of relatedness. While I was in Israel, the Ministry of Health granted an ultra-Orthodox couple the right to select a donor-conceived child's sex in order to conceal the sperm donation with sperm from a non-Jewish donor. The husband was a *Cohen*, meaning that he belonged to the priestly lineage, which was passed to him patrilineally (see note 4). *Cohenim* (pl.) men have specific religious obligations. Therefore, in order to keep the donation secret, the couple did not want to have a boy, and supported by the doctors, the couple received special permission from the Ministry of Health to select the sex of the child because of their "specific religious circumstances." The lab used Preimplantation Genetic Diagnosis (PGD) to select only female embryos before inserting them into the wife's uterus, and she became pregnant with a girl. It was the first time PGD was used not for medical, but for religious reasons, and it caused much attention.[29] With the sex selection the couple avoided the risk of having a son and deciding whether to publicly announce to their community that the man was infertile and the son was not the father's genetic child, and thereby not a *Cohen*.[30] The issue of the couple's grandchildren's status as *Cohenim* was also circumvented, since women do not pass on lineage to their children. It is passed patrilineally, and the couple's potential grandchild would therefore acquire the lineage of the couple's unborn girl's future husband. This incident took place in the very IVF clinic in which I conducted my research, but it was so concealed that I did not learn about it until the media revealed the story. Only then could I interview the staff, who were horrified that this secret had become public news.

In short, consideration of reproductive alternatives is a very last resort, since people hope and persist in having a genetic child (i.e., the husband providing the sperm as the genetic father). Alternative ways of having children that exclude use of the husband's sperm challenge notions of fatherhood, lineage, and the natural family. Having said this, however, individuals may choose different strategies to come to terms with their infertility and childlessness; sperm donation may be used secretly as an alternative. As Carmeli and Birenbaum-Carmeli have argued (2000a, 2000b), sperm donation is concealed at all levels in Israel: by the state, clinical staff, and the couples. These practices make it possible for couples to conceal male infertility by the use of sperm donation and uphold the image of the natural family and genetic fatherhood.

Conclusion

In this chapter I have explored some gendered expressions of male infertility in Israel. Traditional gender understandings, which associate the woman's body with reproduction, seem reproduced in the clinic. The clinic could give room to a redefinition of such traditional understandings by including men in new ways. Presently, the men are central yet absent in the treatment—the man is in the sperm. The husband's sperm must be recovered from his body for the fertility treatment to proceed, but he is peripheral to the actual treatment.

The infertile man's potential as a father who passes on the patrilineal and bilateral notions of relatedness depends on fertility treatment. The availability and use of ARTs in Israel supports men's and couple's wishes to pursue fertility treatment using the infertile man's sperm. When it was impossible to use the husband's sperm to achieve conception and sperm donation was used, it was carried out in such secrecy that I hardly knew it went on in the clinics. The concepts of fatherhood, natural family, patrilineality, and bilateral relatedness are embodied in sperm. Therefore, even in a clinic that offers extensive fertility treatment, sperm donation is concealed. Male infertility certainly challenges notions of relatedness, but in the end, rather than renegotiating and changing the ideas and the importance of the natural family, genetic fatherhood, and genetic descent, these notions of relatedness are emphasized, accentuated, and reinforced by the use of ARTs to overcome male infertility.

Some final reflections

ARTs, as medical technologies, are products of specific cultural understandings. ARTs are developed and used in societies in which having children who are genetically connected to the parents is considered the "right way" to have children. The ways the technologies are used in medical settings are also intertwined with specific cultural ideas of kinship, gender, sexuality, and religion, as we have seen. The somewhat homogeneous kinship understandings, highlighted in this discussion, must be seen in the context of the fertility clinic where religious and secular couples come sharing one wish—they want to have *their own* children. Had the focus been on couples who already had children alternative ways, and who were open about it, it is possible that traditional kinship understandings would have been undermined, and that other understandings would have been emphasized.

Acknowledgements

The title of this chapter is inspired by that of Emily Martin's (1987) book *The Woman in the Body: A Cultural Analysis of Reproduction*. I am grateful to all the people in Israel who talked to me and made this project possible. I am grateful to Tine Tjørnhøj-Thomsen, Elly Teman, and Lisbeth S. Jensen for their unlimited support throughout my fieldwork and for important contributions in analyzing my data, and to Lisa Brando for editorial assistance and important suggestions to this chapter. I am grateful to Dansk-Israelsk Studiefond, who provided financial support.

Notes

1. Though social scientists have been critical of the biological and reproductive essentialization of women's lives (Inhorn 2006a), an overwhelming amount of studies have focused on women, reproduction, and kinship. As mentioned by Inhorn (2006a), more than 150 ethnographic volumes have been devoted to women, reproduction, and women's health in the past 25 years (a few are Inhorn 1994; Ragoné and Franklin 1996; Franklin 1997; Inhorn and van Bailen 2002). Also in Israel, a large number of studies have focused on women and reproduction (some are Sered 2000; Kahn 2000; Teman 2001, 2003; Ivry 2004; Haelyon 2006; Remennick 2006). By this one-sided focus on women, social scientific studies may even reproduce gendered stereotypes of women's predestined roles as mothers and reproducers, while leaving the male experience in silence and open to unquestioned stereotypes (Goldberg 2004; Inhorn et al. 2009).

2. This idea is now being challenged by different kinds of Reform Judaism, especially from the United States, where men can father Jewish children with non-Jewish women. In early Judaism, the status of the child followed the father (Hyman 1998).

3. Some rabbis, however, argue in favor of a biogenetic understanding of motherhood, i.e., that maternity stems from the egg, says Kahn (2000: 129).

4. Israeli citizenship is, in accordance to the "Law of Return" (5710) of 1950, given to Jews. In amendment 4B (5730–1970) from 1970, a Jew is defined as "a person who was born of a Jewish mother or has become converted to Judaism and who is not a member of another religion" (Israel Ministry of Foreign Affairs 1998).

5. The tribes are traced back to Jacob's twelve sons: Reuben, Simeon, Levi, Judah, Isahar, Zeulun, Dan, Naphtali, Gad, Asher, Joseph, and Benjamin. The tribes had different roles in the temple; however, later ten of them were said to be lost (Bridger 1962: 284, 486, 495). Today, two of them, the priestly tribe (*Koheym*, Cohen, or *Kohen*) and the priests' helpers *Layvee* (*Levi*), are recognized, and *Cohen* men are given explicit roles (e.g., in the religious service). Those who are neither *Cohen* nor *Levi* are recognized as *Yisrael* (Kolatch 1985: 29). Today, DNA Y-chromosome testing is used to provide evidence for patrilineal relatedness, and it is argued that *Cohen* descent can be traced back 3,180 years (Skorecki et al. 1997; Thomas et al. 1998). The new DNA testing is increasingly used as proof in different ethnic group claims to be Jewish, and may place increasing emphasis on patrilineal descent and "genetics" as aspects of Jewish kinship in the future (Goldberg N.D.)

6. According to Kahn, other rabbis argue that paternity is established through sexual intercourse, not genes. Again others argue that paternity can be established "through the intentions and actions" when a man seeks to be fruitful and multiply (Kahn 2000: 110).

7. Bilateral notions of relatedness also seem to be behind the redefinition of who has the right to citizenship in Israel. See amendment A to the 1970 "Law of Return" (Israel Ministry of Foreign Affairs 1998). Here it is declared that children and grandchildren of a Jew, their spouses, and spouses of a Jew are entitled to citizenship. The notion of nature or genes as a central aspect of kinship seems reinforced with the increased use of genetic testing in Israel (Weiss 2002; Ivry 2004; Remennick 2006).

8. The data was collected from September 2002 to February 2003 and analyzed in my MA thesis, which was accepted at the Institute of Anthropology, University of Copenhagen 2004. All names used in this article are pseudonyms.

9. In ICSI and IVF the woman's body is in treatment with hormones and her follicles are removed surgically. In IVF, the ovum and sperm are placed together in a lab test tube. After two to three days, fertilized eggs, or embryos, are transferred to the woman's uterus. In ICSI, a single sperm cell is injected directly into the surgically removed ova, and upon fertilization, the embryos are transferred to the women's uterus. ICSI has been a new revolutionary method since the 1990s, allowing men with low sperm quality to become genetic fathers (Berger et al. 2001).

10. For a discussion about such methodological challenges see Goldberg (2009).

11. The fieldwork was conducted mostly in English. Medical terms in the clinics are all in English, and together with my basic Hebrew, I was able to understand the general content of consultations. Many patients spoke very good English, and some were native English speakers. It often happened that conversations in Hebrew, even in patient consultations, would shift from Hebrew into English because of my presence. All interviews were conducted in English, thus non-English speakers

were excluded. The people who were interviewed volunteered in the clinics.

12. Sal's religious standing was also indicated by the knitted *kipa* he wore along with his air force uniform.

13. The male fertility potential is defined according to a sperm test. Irvine (1998) notes that male infertility primarily involves low sperm count *(oligospermia)*, poor semen motility *(asthenospermia)*, defective sperm morphology *(teratospermia)* or no sperm in the ejaculation *(azoospermia)*.

14. The lack of treatments available for men has its roots historically in the focus on women's bodies. Research and financial resources are directed towards examining female reproduction rather than male. Consequently, it is then harder to solve the problem of male infertility (Mason 1993; Birenbaum-Carmeli et al. 1995; Tjørnhøj-Thomsen 1999a, 1999b). A reason for this imbalance is surely based on cultural biases connecting women with children, reproduction, and infertility. Much research has been carried out to understand female ovulation in order to provide birth control for women, and such research has also provided information toward female fertility treatment. Relatively few resources have been spent on inventing a "male pill." Andrology—the male equality to gynecology, is not a well-established or respected medical profession in most places in the world (Manson 1993; Tjørnhøj-Thomsen 1999b); only now we are beginning to witness increased medicalization of the male sexual and reproductive body and the marketing of a "male pill" (Oaks in press).

15. Carmeli and Birenbaum-Carmeli (1994: 669) point out that an extra financial burden is placed on men who often end up working extra hours, because women work less or give up working entirely in the course of the treatment.

16. This couple sometimes referred to themselves as religious and sometimes as Orthodox. They lived in the Jerusalem religious neighbourhood, *Meah Shearim*. Jonathan grew up in the United States. They dressed in an Orthodox manner and kept many of the religious rules. Michal's hair was covered, and she always wore long dresses. Jonathan had a long beard and wore a *kipa* and *tzitzit*. They had a rabbi involved in their fertility treatment.

17. According to the Israeli Law of Carrying Fetuses, surrogacy is only an option for heterosexual couples in Israel, and it is only used in the case of female infertility. It is stated that the surrogate mother must not contribute her own egg as in traditional surrogacy. The egg may come from the mother to be, i.e., the commissioner, or from a third donor. However, the sperm *must* come from the father to be, not from a donor (Teman 2001: 14).

18. A post-coital test requires regular intercourse, after which, a doctor removes the sperm sample from the woman's vagina.

19. What kind of treatment is given to the couple, and how it is conducted, is influenced by differing rabbi opinions in the evaluation of different factors pertaining to the couple's situation (Kahn 2002: 287–88). When

I asked a rabbi how he dealt with male infertility, he made clear, "There is no one press-button solution. I need to see their age, what they have been through, the pressure they are under, medical history, and their reactions. We see what the problem is, and then it can be treated." Rabbinical debate and disagreement is not unusual. Rabbinic decision-making is decentralized, yet binding, and there exist various opinions on topics ranging from how many hours one must wait between eating meat and drinking milk, to how sperm must be obtained for medical analysis (Kahn 2002: 289).

20. It is highly relevant, but beyond the scope of this article, to consider the pressure on the woman to have intercourse with her husband in order to collect his sperm for treatment or analysis, especially right after the ovum pick-up surgery.

21. In fact, the guilt over wasting sperm may also come later. One religious man claimed that God was playing with him and causing his infertility to make him realize the wrongness of his former "wasting of sperm." "It is forbidden," and now when he needed the sperm for reproduction, "you have to look for it [the sperm] in the dark with a candle," he explained.

22. This concern is often related to the quote, "thou shall not implant thy seed into thy neighbor's wife" (Leviticus 18:20) (see also Gold 1988; Kahn 2000).

23. Rabbis draw on a number of reasons to explain the use of non-Jewish sperm (See Kahn 2000). Some argue that since Jewish fatherhood and lineage are passed through the sperm, paternity can be totally erased if non-Jewish sperm is used (Kahn 2000: 110). To test a rabbi on this matter, I asked him if he would consent to the marriage of two people who were children of the same gentile donor. He said he didn't know how he would react, because it would be a medical problem, since they would have the same genes, but less of a *halachic* problem.

24. The couple dressed in modern clothes but kept what they defined as the three most important rules in Jewish law: kosher, *Shabbat* and sexual abstinence when Ester was *niddah*: menstruating. Ester was a convert from Eastern Europe.

25. A recent survey among parents who used donor sperm in Sweden showed that only 10% told the child about the sperm donation—though 40% said they intended to tell the child. Furthermore, an increased number of Swedes traveled to other countries such as Spain, Holland, and Denmark to use anonymous sperm donation (BIOSAM Informerer 2004).

26. This informed consent seems inspired by a clause from the Ministry of Health's Memorandum from 1992, which formalized donor insemination in Israel. It requires that "whenever possible the husband's or partner's sperm may be mixed with that of the donor's" (For more details see Carmeli and Birenbaum-Carmeli 2000b).

27. Though couples receiving sperm donation still have to sign this informed consent, sperm mixing is not done in "high tech" IVF and ICSI, according to the doctors interviewed. However, in the fertility clinic,

in which only artificial insemination was done, a doctor told me that he would always mix donor sperm with the husband's, "to give him the feeling that he could become the father." Carmeli and Birenbaum-Carmeli (2000a) encountered sperm mixing as a common practice in Israeli fertility clinics that did artificial insemination. They even met a doctor who would try to convince couples that the child had been conceived from the husband's sperm in the mixture instead of the donor's (Carmeli and Birenbaum-Carmeli 2000a: 316).

28. In this survey 22.1% of married Israeli women and 10.6% of the men told someone about the sperm donation (Birenbaum-Carmeli et al. 2000).

29. Kahn (2002: 291, 2000: 207–08) reports of a very similar situation told to her by a fertility doctor where an ultra-Orthodox woman underwent embryo reduction and had the male embryos aborted after they were placed in the woman's uterus for the same reason, her husband being a *Cohen*. The differences between the two cases are that the couple in the IVF clinic had permission to use PGD from the Ministry of Health, and sex selection was done prior the embryo transfer.

30. A director of a sperm bank told me, with much amusement, about a situation where a lesbian couple had concern about *Cohen* descent. The couple wanted to use Jewish donor sperm, but wanted to ensure that their donor was not a *Cohen*, because they were concerned about raising a *Cohen* son without a *Cohen* father.

References

Becker, Gay. 2002. "Deciding Whether to Tell Children about Donor Insemination: An Unresolved Question in the United States." In *Reproduction around the Globe: New Thinking on Childlessness, Gender and Reproductive Technologies*, eds. Marcia C. Inhorn and Frank Van Balen. Berkeley: University of California Press.

Berger, Gary with Marc Goldstein and Mark Fuerst. 2001. *The Couple's Guide to Fertility*. 3rd ed. New York: Broadway Books.

BIOSAM Informerer. 2004. "Æg og Sæd—med eller uden afsender.". <http://www.biosam.dk/biosam/biosaminformerer/biosam-informerer> (accessed 13 September 2007).

Birenbaum-Carmeli, Daphna with Yoram S. Carmeli and Robert F. Casper. 1995. "Discrimination Against Men in Infertility Treatment." *The Journal of Reproductive Medicine* 40(8): 590–594.

Birenbaum-Carmeli, Daphna, with Yoram S. Carmeli, and Haim Yavetz. 2000. "Secrecy Among Israeli Recipients of Donor Insemination." *Politics and the Life Sciences* 19, vol. 1: 69–76.

Bridger, David. 1962. *The New Jewish Encyclopedia*. New York: Behrman House.

Carmeli, Yoram S. and Daphna Birenbaum-Carmeli. 2000a. "Ritualizing the 'Natural Family': Secrecy in Israeli Donor Insemination." *Science as Culture* 9, vol. 3: 301–24.

———. 2000b. "State Regulation of Donor Insemination: An Israel Case Study." *Medicine and Law* 19, vol. 4: 839–54.

———. 1994. "The Predicament of Masculinity: Towards Understanding the Male's Experience of Infertility Treatments." *Sex Roles* 30, vol. 9/10: 663–77.

Carsten, Janet, ed. 2000. *Cultures of Relatedness: New Approaches to the Study of Kinship*. Cambridge: Cambridge University Press.

Csordas, Thomas J. 1990. "Embodiment as a Paradigm for Anthropology." *Ethos* 18, vol. 1: 5–47.

Franklin, Sarah. 1997. *Embodied Progress: A Cultural Account of Assisted Conception*. London and New York: Routledge.

Gold, Michael. 1988. *And Hanna Wept*. Philadelphia, New York, Jerusalem: The Jewish Publication Society.

Goldberg, Helene. 2004. *The Man in the Sperm: A Study of Male Infertility in Israel*. M.A. Thesis. Institute of Anthropology, University of Copenhagen.

———. 2006. "Kampen for overlevelse: demografisk bevidsthed og forestillinger om forbundethed i den israelsk-jødiske familie." *Tidsskriftet Antropologi*, 50: 13–30.

———. n.d. "'Jewish Genes': Kinship, Identity and Geneticization." Unpublished manuscript.

———. 2009. "The Sex in the Sperm: Male Infertility and its Challenges to Masculinity in an Israeli- Jewish Context." In *Reconceiving the Second Sex: Men, Masculinity, and Reproduction*, eds. Marcia C. Inhorn, Tine Tjørnhøj-Thomsen, Helene Goldberg and Maruska la Cour Mosegaard. Oxford: Berghan Books.

Haelyon, Hilla. 2006. "'Longing for a Child': Perceptions of Motherhood Among Israeli-Jewish Women Undergoing In Vitro Fertilization Treatments." *Nashim: A Journal of Jewish Women's Studies and Gender Issues* 12: 177–202.

Hyman, Meryl. 1998. *"Who is a Jew?" Conversations Not Conclusions*. Woodstock, Vermont: Jewish Lights Publishing.

Inhorn, Marcia C. 2006a. "Defining Women's Health: A Dozen Messages from More Than 150 Ethnographies." *Medical Anthropology Quarterly* 20, vol. 3: 345–78.

———. 2006b "'He won't be my son': Middle Eastern Muslim Men's Discourses of Adoption and Gamete Donation." *Medical Anthropology Quarterly* 20, vol. 1: 94–120.

———. 2004. "Middle Eastern Masculinities in the Age of New Reproductive Technologies: Male Infertility and Stigma in Egypt and Lebanon." *Medical Anthropology Quarterly* 18, vol. 2: 162–82.

———. 2003 "'The Worms Are Weak': Male Infertility and Patriarchal Paradoxes in Egypt." *Men and Masculinities* 5: 236–56.

———. 1994. *Quest for Conception: Gender, Infertility, and Egyptian Medical Traditions*. Philadelphia: University of Pennsylvania Press.

———. 2009. "Male Genital Cutting: Masculinity, Reproduction, and Male Infertility Surgeries in Egypt and Lebanon." In *Reconceiving the Second Sex: Men, Masculinity, and Reproduction*, eds. Marcia C. Inhorn, Tine Tjørnhøj-Thomsen, Helene Goldberg and Maruska la Cour Mosegaard. Oxford: Berghahn Books.

Inhorn, Marcia C. and Frank Van Balen, eds. 2002. *Reproduction Around the Globe: New Thinking on Childlessness, Gender and Reproductive Technologies.* Berkeley: University of California Press.

Inhorn, Marcia C., Tine Tjørnhøj-Thomsen, Helene Goldberg and Maruska la Cour Mosegaard, eds. In press. *Reconceiving the Second Sex: Men, Masculinity, and Reproduction.* Oxford: Berghahn Books.

Irvine, D.Stewart. 1998. "Epidemiology and Aetiology of Male Infertility." *Human Reproduction* 13, vol. 1: 33–44.

Israel Ministry of Foreign Affairs. 1998. *Acquisition of Israeli Nationality.* http://www.mfa.gov.il/mfa/go.asp?MFAH00mz0 (accessed 13 September 2007).

Ivry, Tsipy. 2004. "Pregnant with Meaning: Conceptions of Pregnancy in Japan and Israel' (PhD dissertation, Department of Sociology and Social Anthropology, Hebrew University).

Kahn, Susan Martha. 2002. "Rabbis and Reproduction: The Users of New Reproductive Technologies among Ultraorthodox Jews in Israel." In *Reproduction Around the Globe: New Thinking on Childlessness, Gender and Reproductive Technologies,* eds. Marcia C. Inhorn and Frank Van Balen. Berkeley: University of California Press.

———. 2000. *Reproducing Jews: A Cultural Account of Assisted Conception in Israel.* Durham and London: Duke University Press.

Kolatch, J. Alfred.1985. *The Second Jewish Book of Why.* New York: Jonathan David Publishers, Inc.

Martin, Emily. 2001 [1987]. *The Woman in the Body: A Cultural Analysis of Reproduction.* Boston, Massachusetts: Beacon Press.

Mason, Mary-Claire. 1993. *Male Infertility—Men Talking.* London and New York: Routledge.

Nachtigall, R.D., J.M. Tschann, S.S. Quiroga, L. Pitcher, and G. Becker.1997. "Stigma, Disclosure, and Family Functioning among Parents of Children Conceived through Donor Insemination." *Fertile Sterile* 68: 83–9.

Oaks, Laury. 2009. "Manhood and Meaning in the Marketing of the 'Male Pill'." In *Reconceiving the Second Sex: Men, Masculinity, and Reproduction,* eds. Marcia C. Inhorn, Tine Tjørnhøj-Thomsen, Helene Goldberg and Maruska la Cour Mosegaard. Oxford: Berghan Books.

Ragoné, Helena, and Sarah Franklin, eds. 1996. *Reproducing Reproduction: Kinship, Power and Technological Innovation.* Philadelphia: University of Pennsylvania Press.

Remennick, Larissa. 2006. "The Quest for a Perfect Baby: Why Do Israeli Women Seek Prenatal Genetic Testing?" *Sociology of Health and Illness* 28, vol. 1: 21–53.

Schneider, David M. 1980. *American Kinship: A Cultural Account.* 2nd ed. Chicago and London: The University of Chicago Press.

Sered, Susan. 2000. *What Makes Women Sick: Maternity, Modesty and Militarism in Israeli Society.* Hanover and London: Brandeis University Press.

Shalev, Carmel and Sigal Gooldin. 2006. "The Uses and Misuses of In Vitro Fertilization in Israel: Some Sociological and Ethical Considerations." *Nashim: A Journal of Jewish Women's Studies and Gender Issues* 12: 151–76.

Skorecki, Karl, Sara Selig, Shraga Blazer, Bruce Rappaport, Robert Bradman, Niel Bradman, P.J. Waburton, Monic Ismajlowitcz and Michael F. Hammer. 1997. "Y Chromosomes of Jewish Priests." *Nature* 385: 32–35.

Strathern, Marilyn. 1992. *After Nature: English Kinship in the Late Twentieth Century*. Cambridge: Cambridge University Press.

Teman, Elly. 2001. "Technological Fragmentation and Women's Empowerment: Surrogate Motherhood in Israel." *Women's Studies Quarterly* 3/4: 11–34.

————. 2003. "The Medicalization of 'Nature' in the 'Artificial Body': Surrogate Motherhood in Israel." *Medical Anthropology Quarterly* 17, vol. 1: 78–98.

————. 2006. "Birthing a Mother: the Mythology of Surrogate Motherhood in Israel" (PhD dissertation, Department of Sociology and Social Anthropology, Hebrew University).

————. Birthing a Mother: The Surrogate Body and the Pregnant Self. Berkeley: University at California Press.

Thomas, Mark G., Karl Skorecki, Haim Ben-Ami, Tudor Parfitt, Neil Bradman and David B. Goldstein. 1998. "Origin of Old Testament Priests." *Nature* 394: 138–40.

Tjørnhøj-Thomsen, Tine. 1999a. "'Det føles ikke-rigtigt mandigt på en måde.' Mænd og infertilitet." *Kvinder, køn og Forskning* 8, 3: 71–89.

Tjørnhøj-Thomsen, Tine. 1999b. "Tilblivelseshistorier. Barnløshed, slægtskab og forplantningsteknologi i Danmark" (PhD dissertation, Institute of Anthropology, University of Copenhagen).

Weiss, Meira. 2002. *The Chosen Body: The Politics of the Body in Israeli Society*. Stanford: Stanford University Press.

Chapter 4

The Last Outpost of
the Nuclear Family:
A Cultural Critique of
Israeli Surrogacy Policy

Elly Teman

Introduction

Surrogate motherhood,[1] a practice in which a woman agrees to carry
a child to term for a couple who will then keep the child as their own,
has emerged from the academic literature as an extreme case study
for feminist, ethical, legal, and social concerns. With respect to matters
of ethics, scholars have asked if there is not something intrinsically
immoral about surrogacy (Brennan and Noggle 1997), and some have
denounced the practice as depersonalizing or even dehumanizing of
women's reproductive labor and mutating it into a form of alienation
(van Niekerk and van Zyl 1995). In the radical feminist literature,
surrogacy has been interpreted as the ultimate form of medicalization, commodification and technological colonization of the female
body (Rothman 2000). It has also been compared to prostitution
and slavery (Corea 1985; 1987) and associated with the economic
exploitation of women and their subjugation to patriarchal authority (Farquhar 1996). On a social level, surrogacy has been perceived
as changing the cultural meanings of motherhood (Snowden et al.
1984) and kinship (Macklin 1991), and as jeopardizing women's and

children's basic human rights (Brennan and Noggle 1997). In general, the literature concerning the practice seldom veers far from the view that surrogacy invariably equals subjugation.

Because of its controversial nature, the common theme that emerges from the decisions of policy makers and legislators on surrogacy in different jurisdictions is the "sense of profound anxiety and ambivalence" that has pervaded their thinking on the subject (Cook 2003). As a result, the majority of governments around the world have felt justified in banning the practice entirely, and those countries that do allow surrogacy do not explicitly endorse such contracts, but sanction them to varying degrees (ibid.). Those few countries and few American states that allow surrogacy agreements do so grudgingly, and the lack of comprehensive regulation makes it difficult to determine whether these agreements will be upheld in courts of law if disputed (Weisberg 2005; Markens 2007).

The Israeli government's unique approach to surrogacy was to formally legalize surrogate motherhood agreements. The law, formally titled the "Embryo Carrying Agreements Law" (hereafter "the surrogacy law"), was passed by the Israeli Knesset on March 7, 1996. This law made Israel the first country in the world to legalize surrogacy arrangements under a law devoted entirely to this practice, as well as the only country in the world to implement a form of state-controlled surrogacy in which each and every contract must be approved directly by the state (Benshushan and Schenker 1997: 1832). The state-appointed surrogacy approvals committee has the solitary right to permit, refuse, or demand revisions of any contract according to the law's directives. Feminist legal scholar D. Kelly Weisberg (2005: 4) calls the Israeli surrogacy law a "revolutionary legislation," noting that "no other nation or American state goes so far in permitting surrogacy."[2]

In its present form, the Israeli surrogacy law makes it very clear which categories of persons it will grant permission to reproduce through surrogacy arrangements. Surrogacy is permitted only to infertile Israeli couples who are married or heterosexually, legally paired. Single women, single men, and homosexual couples are not permitted to contract a surrogate; and it is only single, divorced, or widowed women that are able to become surrogates. This dichotomic attitude towards the creation of alternative vs. classic nuclear families emerges within a cultural milieu which has otherwise been regarded universally pronatalist and overwhelmingly "liberal" and supportive towards the creation of alternative families.

This article addresses this incongruity through a cultural critique of the Israeli surrogacy law, focusing specifically on developments that have occurred in relation to contestations of this particular directive. I ask what is particular to surrogacy that made the state take such a restrictive stance towards the practice and in turn, convey such a conservative message about the type of family that surrogacy can legally aid to create. In the following, I compare surrogacy to other reproductive technologies, suggesting that surrogacy symbolically assaults the traditional definitions of motherhood and family in ways that the other NRTs do not. I suggest that in response the categories of mother and family are singularly designated within the law and preserved through the surrogacy committee's regulatory practices. In conclusion, these findings are related to the gatekeeping practices of the nation and the ways in which the nation is constructed and maintained through the bodies and families of its citizens.

My thoughts on this subject have developed in the framework of my larger ongoing study of Israeli surrogacy, for which I interviewed surrogates, intended mothers and fathers, doctors, and other professionals involved in these arrangements. This chapter, however, emerges from ideas that I have developed during my research regarding the surrogacy law and the government's regulation of surrogacy in practice over the past ten years. It also presents a cultural critique of Israeli social policy on surrogacy, drawing upon my textual analysis of the surrogacy law, Knesset debates surrounding its legislation, protocols of court cases relating to the law, and over 200 articles on surrogacy that have appeared in Israeli newspapers between 1995 and 2006. My findings from my interviews and fieldwork from the "natives'" point of view are explored elsewhere (Teman 2001; 2003a; 2003b; 2006a; 2006b; 2010).

The Israeli surrogacy law

The surrogacy law is unique to Israeli legislation on medical technological procedures because it is the only reproductive technology to be regulated through its own law. All other NRTs are legalized in Israel through regulations included in the Health Law [*chok bruit mamlachtit*] and Ministry of Health regulations. While Knesset bills on other controversial techniques, such as ova donation and organ donation, have been stuck in the legislative process for five and three years respectively, the issue of surrogacy was addressed with an urgency not replicated in these other cases.[3] In fact, the Israeli surrogacy bill passed from draft to law in what one might consider to be incomparable haste.

On November 16, 1994, a group of 25 infertile couples petitioned the High Court to cancel government regulations that prevented surrogacy arrangements in Israel (Bagatz 1994). The state responded positively but asked the court to keep the regulations in place until the government could pass new legislation on the issue (Gordon 1995). Health Minister Ephraim Sneh garnered public support for the law through the media (Gordon 1995) and met with the chief rabbis of the country to make sure that the law would not be delayed by religious opposition (Siegel 1995). He successfully pushed the surrogacy bill through all three Knesset readings within nine months by convincing Knesset members in his address on the topic that "[t]here is urgency in passing this law because if it is not approved as soon as possible. . . [without a law] the existing regulations will be cancelled, there will be no law, and a situation of chaos and trouble [*tohu va'vohu v'hefkerut*] will ensue" (Protocol A 1995: 33). The surrogacy bill was met by uncharacteristically unanimous approval by both religious and secular party officials, who are normally contentious on nearly any issue, approved with a majority of 44 to 12, with three abstentions (Siegel 1996). It was passed at the last minute before the High Court cancelled the previous regulations, and it was the last bill to be passed under Shimon Peres' Labor government.

The law's history is indicative of the general attitude of the State towards surrogacy. On the one hand, the government's choice to legalize surrogacy rather than outlaw it as many other countries have done testifies to the value of motherhood and childbearing in Israel. Even though surrogacy promised to help far less than 1 percent of the population become families, Knesset members who voted for the legalization of surrogacy expressed the sentiment that as long as surrogacy held the promise of "giving the childless family a chance to have her own children" (Nava Arad in Protocol A 1995: 54), then "it is our duty, as long as the technique and medical technology enable it, to solve their problem" (Ephraim Sneh, Protocol A 1995: 34–35).

On the other hand, the government's choice to restrict surrogacy under very strict state surveillance can be interpreted as a defensive act against what was understood to be the potential social anarchy that could result from permitting surrogacy without regulation (Teman 2006a). The official attitude was not to encourage surrogacy agreements, but to provide the opportunity to pursue this reproductive route for normative, heterosexual, legally paired couples among whom the woman could not carry a pregnancy herself. As the words of the late former chairwoman of the approvals committee reveal, "the assumption was that this extraordinary measure would be reserved for the extreme cases of childless couples for whom the experience of parenthood has been prevented due to their condition and that it would not turn into a routine solution for all cases of infertility" (Negev 2002).

The resulting law was of a very restrictive nature, which can partially be explained by the lawmakers' attempt to make it compatible with the widest possible range of the various *halachic* views on surrogacy. Among these efforts was the attempt to prevent cases of bastardry, which according to Jewish law results from a married woman carrying another man's child (see Kahn 2000). The law thus strictly limits the population of women who can become surrogates to unmarried, divorced, or widowed women. Moreover, there are some rabbis who view the marriage of two children born from the same woman's womb as incestuous, even if they are not genetically related as in the case of the surrogate's own children and the couple's child she gestates. Thus, the law directs that the surrogate cannot be related to either of the intended parents.

However, beyond these and other halachically influenced directives, the Israeli surrogacy law exhibits many additional restrictions that can better be explained as expressions of a very careful scheme of the social control of reproduction. The most obvious display of this social control is that the law calls for the establishment of a government committee to directly supervise all surrogacy agreements in Israel. This regulatory body (hereafter "the surrogacy approvals committee") meets regularly to determine if the applications that it receives accord with the highly specific criteria for approval set out in the law. The committee includes a specialist in internal medicine, two gynecologists, a state social worker, a clinical psychologist, a lawyer, and a rabbi, as well as a priest and a Muslim *kadi* who are called upon in cases where the applicants are not Jewish. In the past ten years since the committee began its work, it has added numerous additional criteria which serve to make Israeli surrogacy an even more limited and controlled practice than the law originally directed.

These criteria include the order that all parties to the agreement must be Israeli citizens or permanent residents and share the same religion. The parties must not be blood relatives to one another. The intended father must provide the sperm and the intended mother (IM), or an anonymous egg donor, must supply the egg. In no event may the surrogate supply the egg, thereby eliminating traditional surrogacy, and forcing all agreements to conform to the gestational type, which is dependent upon IVF technology. The intended parents must be married or legally, heterosexually partnered and present medical proof that the IM cannot carry a child to term because of prolonged infertility, the absence of a uterus, or severe risk to her health.

The IM must be aged 22 to 45 if providing the ova, and 22 to 51 if using donor eggs. The surrogate, on the other hand, must be between the ages of 22 and 38, single, divorced, or widowed, yet must be raising at least one child of her own. The surrogacy law also cloaks all surrogacy agreements in extreme secrecy: All meetings of the surrogacy approvals committee are closed to the public; all transcripts of the meetings are inaccessible; and there is a penalty of imprisonment of one year if a person publicly divulges details of contracts or names of surrogates, couples, or children born of surrogacy.

The restrictive nature of these guidelines can only be fully appreciated when they are compared to those of other countries that permit surrogacy. In California, where the majority of the world's surrogacy births occur, the approximately 1,000 annual surrogacy births are primarily managed by private, commercial agencies that screen, match, and regulate agreements according to their own criteria and without state intervention. Motivated by financial considerations, California agencies extend this option to persons of any age, nationality, marital status, sexual identity, and degree of infertility, and they assist with altruistic surrogacy within families. This non-interventionist climate has made California a popular destination for the pursuit of surrogacy contracts by homosexual couples, single men, foreign nationals who live in countries where surrogacy is prohibited, older heterosexual couples in which the wife is no longer fertile, and celebrity couples who choose surrogacy for fear that pregnancy will render the female star less marketable.

Alternatively, in the U.K., where an estimated 500 births by surrogacy had occurred as of 2005 (COTS 2005), state regulations are mainly intent on keeping surrogacy from becoming a commercial venture by ensuring that no private agencies profit from the agreements. In fact, intra-familial arrangements are actually preferred there because they tend not to involve financial incentives (Morgan 2003: 81). While surrogacy guidelines in some other countries and American states do include more stringent restrictions, such as age limitations and marital requirements that favor genetic ties with at least one parent (Cook et al. 2003), the Israeli law and guidelines remain arguably more restrictive.

Contested conceptions

At the surface level, Israel's legalization of surrogacy appears as just one more route made available to Israeli women to contribute to the nation through their wombs. As a nation-state (Berkowitz

1997), Israel's legislation is influenced by a nationalist discourse that frames women's central role as "biological reproducers" of the collectivity (Yuval-Davis and Antheas 1989). Berkowitz (1997) has suggested that women's gendered citizenship is set out in Israeli legislation from the earliest laws onwards as dependent upon their dutiful embrace of the "national mission" of motherhood, while Amir and Benjamin (1997) have argued that women's belonging to the Jewish-Israeli collective is dependent upon their disciplined sexual and reproductive conduct. Accordingly, one might imagine that enabling women to rent out their wombs in service of making other women into mothers would be consistent with the nation's values. Moreover, the willingness of women to lend their bodies to the cause of transforming other women into mothers would be viewed as docile citizenship. Indeed, one might go so far as to imagine that every Israeli woman might be encouraged to become a surrogate, and that any infertile Israeli woman might be permitted to hire a surrogate, all in the name of the nation's supposedly over-arching demographic goals.

Yet the Israeli surrogacy law also makes the state accountable for each and every family formed through local surrogacy arrangements, which makes monitoring the practice a difficult terrain to manage. Unlike other NRTs, which the state permits under the relatively lenient regulation of private and public physicians and hospitals, the surrogacy law requires the direct "stamp of approval" of a state-appointed committee on each and every contract. Thus, while the state is not directly involved in the creation of families through other reproductive routes, each endorsement of a surrogacy contract by the state committee can be viewed as an explicit public statement about who can and cannot reproduce with the state's help and approval. This accountability might be behind the persistent rigidity of the state in regard to the surrogacy law's prohibition of single women from hiring surrogates and of married women from becoming surrogates. Over the past ten years since the legalization of surrogacy in Israel, proposals to amend these restrictions have surfaced repeatedly, yet the law has remained unchanged.

The most well-known contestation of the surrogacy law in this respect occurred in 2002 when a single woman petitioned the High Court of Justice in Jerusalem to enable her to hire a surrogate (Bagatz 2001). The woman, who had lost her reproductive organs to cancer several years earlier, had first undergone IVF to produce ova, which were then fertilized with anonymous donor sperm and cryopreserved for a later date. Ironically, although state regulations enabled her to create the embryos for the sole purpose of enabling her future motherhood through state-subsidized procedures, the surrogacy law stood in the way of her having those same embryos implanted in a surrogate mother's womb. In response to her petition to the High Court, state legal council argued in defense of the law that a single parent family was not preferable and therefore its establishment prohibited in surrogacy: "The accepted social perception is that in general it is best for a child to be raised in a household with two parents, father and mother, loving and devoted, than in a single parent family, as loving and devoted as it may be" (Negev 2002).

A panel of seven High Court justices eventually unanimously rejected the single woman's petition on the grounds that it was not the court's place to intervene in the current legislation. A recommendation was made to the Health Ministry to consider changing the law, and a public-professional committee was formed to examine widening the eligibility for surrogacy applicants to include those currently excluded from the law. This committee published a report in late 2004 recommending "to delay at this time any deliberations on changing the surrogacy law until we acquire further experience in the law's operation" (Insler 2004: 11).

Then, in November 2005, the Knesset Committee on the Advancement of Women held a meeting devoted to discussing the surrogacy law's tenth year. At the meeting, the legal council of the Health Ministry, Mira Hibner, explained why the Health Ministry opposes changing the law: "From the moment that there is the option of opening [the law] to single women, I do not see any way to prevent it from same-sex family units. . ." She warned against "endangering the law," then adding that there may be room for change in the future, but added:

> that time has not yet come [*adayin lo bashla ha'et*]. Let's leave things as they are. I hinted that it is not just single women that will be able to enter this process. Other family units that we know of today will be able to enter the process and that is already a social revolution that we should not rush in to. . . The right to parenthood exists and people will come and say that it is their right. There is no end to this slope. So for now let's decide that this is the boundary and that it isn't final.

The meeting concluded with the recommendation to leave the law in its current form.

In a more recent case, in 2006, a couple who could not afford to hire a surrogate petitioned the surrogacy approvals committee to allow them to contract the services of a married friend who had offered to become their surrogate free of charge. Although the law prohibits married women from becoming surrogates, it specifies that in "special cases" a married woman may be permitted if the couple has exhausted all other avenues for finding an unmarried surrogate. Believing this to be a rabbinical obstacle, the couple turned to Israel's Chief Rabbi Shlomo Amar. After contemplating the case at length with several other prominent Rabbinical figures, including Rabbi Ovadia Yosef, who is known to have a severe view of surrogacy, Rabbi Amar sent a letter to the approvals committee giving *halachic* approval and justification for permitting the couple to hire a married surrogate. On June 11, 2006 Rabbi Amar's "breakthrough ruling" was announced on all local Israeli news stations (Levinson 2006). Yet, despite the rabbinical barrier having been removed, the surrogacy approvals committee has continued to refuse this and other applications involving a married surrogate.

In August 2006 the Knesset committee on work, welfare, and health held a meeting to discuss Rabbi Amar's ruling. Knesset member Yakov Margi of the Shas (Sephardic Ultra-Urthodox) party opened the session asking why the surrogacy approvals committee still refused to implement the ruling. Discussion of the issue produced the understanding that if the committee were to allow a married surrogate in this specific case, then it would have to allow all couples to hire married surrogates. It was unanimously agreed upon that this would not be preferable and therefore further inquiry into the potential consequences of Rabbi Amar's ruling was called for before its implementation.

This hesitancy of the Israeli government to enable single women to hire surrogates or to allow married women to become surrogates stands out in a country where intervention into natal issues is usually recognized as pronatalist and public policy on reproductive technologies is otherwise regulated with a "liberal hand" (Birenbaum-Carmeli 2004). The reason behind this hesitancy cannot be related to any obstacles in Jewish law[4]; although different rabbinical groups may offer different opinions, there is no apparent major *halachic* problem with single motherhood by choice (see Kahn 2000), and the ruling of Rabbi Amar, the Chief Rabbi and highest authority of the Israeli Rabbinate, should have resolved the government's doubts over the potential *halachic* complications of married women becoming surrogates.

Moreover, the hesitancy to amend the law cannot be explained in terms of bureaucratic difficulties in changing legislation; since I began my fieldwork on surrogacy in Israel in 1998, I have witnessed the regulations appended to the surrogacy law amended and successfully contested in many cases. It cannot even be successfully argued that the hesitancy to amend the surrogacy law stems from the controversial nature of the practice itself, since Israeli legislation permits other reproductive techniques that one might consider equally or more controversial than surrogacy. This includes stem cell research, pre-implantation genetic diagnosis and sex selection of embryos, and even practices that border on cloning. Israel even has formal regulations allowing bereaved widows to ask for the removal of sperm from their husband's body immediately after death (Siegel-Itzkovich 2003), and the Knesset has debated giving parents of combat soldiers the same option to produce grandchildren posthumously from their dead son's sperm.

Finally, the explicit references to the potential uptake of the surrogacy option by homosexual and single persons also does not explain the government's hesitancy to amend the law, since Israeli legislation on reproductive technologies has proven to be otherwise open to the creation of same sex and single parent families. Indeed, reproductive procedures including IVF, ICSI, AI, DI, and IVF with donor gametes are open to persons of any marital status and sexual preference and subsidized by the state, regulated only at the discretion of the medical professionals who administer them. Other kinship routes are also locally permitted to single men and women, such as inter-country adoption, and the Israeli High court approved a lesbian co-mother's legal adoption abroad of her partner's biological child in 2000.

Surrogacy, in fact, is the only reproductive technique that is restricted to married or legally-paired heterosexual couples. Single women can therefore potentially become pregnant through state-subsidized IVF with an embryo created from both egg and sperm of anonymous donors—until recently most of them non-Jewish, foreign donors (see Kahn 2000; Reznik 2000)—but they cannot hire a surrogate. A single man, or a man in a homosexual relationship, can adopt a child through inter-country adoption, but cannot hire a surrogate. And a married woman can partake in any of the reproductive options mentioned above, but she cannot become a surrogate.

Why then, fourteen years after passing the surrogacy law, and after over 350 children have been born from surrogacy arrangements, is the Israeli government still unwilling to allow single women to hire surrogates, or to allow married women to become surrogates?

Preserving traditional categories

I suggest that the restrictive social control of surrogacy in Israel and the unbending stance of the Israeli body politic in the two cases presented above stems from the direct challenge that surrogacy poses to two central concepts: *family* and *motherhood*. Surrogacy challenges these categories in ways that other NRTs and reproductive practices do not, and the Israeli government's consistently restrictive approach to surrogacy, including the hesitation to change the law, can to a large extent be read as the state's attempt to preserve traditional definitions of *mother* and *family*. While arguments can be made regarding the influence of the different rabbinical prohibitions and their effect on regulating different practices (see Shalev 1998; Kahn 2000; Weisberg 2005), I see Jewish law serving in this case as an "excuse" for the state to implement restrictions that actually end up serving other social and nationalistic goals.

In terms of *motherhood*, surrogacy assaults the concept of motherhood in ways that other NRTs do not. Surrogacy differs from IVF, egg donation, or even egg and sperm donation, for those practices result in only one woman being publicly identifiable as the child's *mother*: the woman who gestates and later raises the child. A triad of sources also protects the anonymity of third-party donors so that any threat to the one-mother fiction is eliminated: Jewish law, Israeli public policy, and the local medical regulation of egg and sperm donation. Kahn (2000) argues that rabbinic decisions regarding NRTs "erase" the kin-making power of genetics by privileging the womb and gestation as the main determinants of motherhood, and consequently of Judaism. Israeli public policy also symbolically erases the genitors in cases of egg and sperm donation through the secrecy enacted in state regulations and through local medical practices that ensure anonymity of the genitors (Birenbaum-Carmeli 2004). In the case of adoption as well, whether local or international, Israeli regulations also ensure anonymity of the birthparents so that only the adoptive parents are recognized as the child's parents. The "erasure" of the genitors in these cases makes certain that parental identity—and in particular, maternal identity—is singular and unambiguous.

By comparison, the social construction of kinship categories is exposed in surrogacy. First, the provider of the sperm cannot be "erased" because he will necessarily be raising the child. Likewise, it is the intended who usually provides the ova, so the ova cannot be "erased," nor can the mother's contracted role as future social mother of the child. Moreover, the surrogate cannot be "erased" because it is her gestational contribution that makes the child Jewish and an Israeli citizen. Even if donor ova are used, there are still two women who potentially fit the title of *mother* and whose links to the child are connected to criteria used to determine maternity in Jewish religious law and in Israeli law.

Consequently, the surrogate who gestates the child is just as entitled to the social label as women who conceive their children through IVF with donated ova, and the IM who contracted the surrogate with the commitment to raise the child is just as entitled to the title as an adoptive mother. The personhood of each of these women must therefore be recognized; neither of them can be "ignored" or made anonymous, making the anomaly of two potential mothers unavoidable. This makes the ambiguity of the concept of *mother* an inevitable part of surrogacy as a whole and an issue that Israeli surrogacy regulations take pains to resolve.

The effort at maintaining a clear designation of motherhood is evident in many aspects of the government's regulation of surrogacy. This categorization is evident first and foremost in the formal and lay Hebrew terminology for surrogacy. The law deems the woman who will raise the child the *intended mother* and the surrogate the *carrying mother*, thus specifying that only one of them is officially recognized as a parent and the other woman is merely fulfilling a temporary role. The informal, more popular terminology used in the Hebrew media, courts, and among professionals, surrogates, and couples involved with the agreements, refers to the intended mother as the *biological mother*, or simply as *the mother*. Unlike the English term surrogate, which literally means substitute, Israeli surrogates are popularly referred to as *pundekait*, meaning innkeeper. Israeli surrogates are thus linguistically constructed from the start in public consciousness as temporary hostesses who develop, feed, and care for the couple's fetus before it returns to its "real" parents.

The law consistently preserves the idea that only one woman is the official mother of the child by limiting the surrogate's rights to the child. While she is pregnant she has the right to abort, but following the birth, she has no claim on the child. A surrogate can contest the contract within the first seven days after the birth, but only on grounds that she thinks the intended parents are manifestly unsuitable for raising the child, not because she wants to retain custody herself. In such an event, which has yet to occur in Israel, custody would likely not go to the surrogate but to the emergency guardians appointed by the couple in the original surrogacy contract.

Further categorical recognition of the intended mother is embedded in the directive that the surrogate should be hospitalized in the gynecological ward after delivery rather than in the maternity ward, and in the now routine practice instituted by most Israeli hospitals, on recommendation of the Health Ministry, to hospitalize the intended mother in the maternity ward (Teman 2003b). It is furthermore only to the intended mother that the state grants maternity leave; surrogates are granted sick leave for recovery from the birth. However, in recognition of both women's contribution to the nation, they are both awarded a maternity grant. This continuous effort to sort out the two-mother anomaly and to categorically designate only one woman as the mother of the child results in the surrogate being alternately classified as carrier/hostess/innkeeper/woman/sick.

In terms of the *family*, surrogacy challenges the traditional family form in ways that other NRTs do not, for with other NRTs, only one *official family* is created: the nuclear family or the single-parent family that will raise the child. Surrogacy, on the other hand, involves two families—the surrogate's own, and the family being created through surrogacy—and thus renders the concept of *family* ambiguous. Surrogacy potentiates questions about which family the resulting child belongs to, and whether the surrogate's children are to be considered siblings of the surrogate child. Moreover, surrogacy has the potential of complicating the traditional concept of *family* by allowing for the upheaval of traditional family hierarchies and structures.

In the state of California, where most surrogacy agreements currently occur, the ambiguity of familial relationships produced through surrogacy is often celebrated rather than seen as threatening, with private agencies advertising their services by boasting of the unique familial situations they have helped to create.[5] In Britain, legislators preferred that surrogacy arrangements should remain within families or that they should be of a purely altruistic nature (Morgan 2003) so that it is more preferable for aunts to carry their nieces and nephews and grandmothers to gestate their grandchildren than for surrogacy to occur within strangers. Making surrogacy familial, even if it changes traditional meanings of family, has been positively featured in the British press in stories about British surrogates who describe their relationships with the families they have helped in familial terms, referring to the children they have birthed for different couples as siblings of one another and of their own children.

However, the Israeli government's response to surrogacy reveals a different attitude towards change in the family. Like many other Western countries, Israel too has experienced a growing divorce rate and increase in the numbers of alternative family forms, changing the concept of "family" significantly. In response to the uncertainty that surrogacy presents about the ties that bind individual parents to individual children (Stanworth 1987: 19), the surrogacy law's conservative approach ensures that families created through this practice replicate the heterosexual, married, nuclear family, and that the alternative family forms that surrogacy potentiates do not manifest.

The hetero-normative, nuclear family form is preserved in the law's prevention of homosexual couples and single women from hiring a surrogate. It is also ensured through the prevention of the upheaval of family hierarchies and relations since surrogates and couples cannot be related. In addition, the committee's hesitancy to allow purely altruistic agreements and its insistence on an official, commercial contract can be interpreted as a symbolic measure of the body politic to keep familial boundaries between the two parties clear and distinct. Money has a symbolic divisive quality (Friedland 2001), and in common with the US, families are culturally understood in Israeli society as giving to one another out of love, not for money (Layne 1999; Taylor et al. 2004). This frames Israeli surrogacy arrangements as business transactions and commodity exchange to the exclusion of gift, or familial exchange.

This approach can also explain, beyond the rabbinical reasoning, why the committee has been so hesitant to veer from the requirement that the intended parents are heterosexually paired and that surrogates are unmarried. These clauses distinguish two classifications of families: The family that is created through surrogacy is a normative, nuclear family, while the family that helps create that family is an alternative, single-parent family. This symbolic distinction privileges the two-parent, nuclear family as the official family; conversely, a married surrogate contracted by a married couple, or a single woman contracting a single surrogate would erase this distinction.

The resulting conclusion can only be that the state may be willing to aid single and lesbian women in becoming alternative families with the help of other NRTs, but in surrogacy, where the definitions of *mother* and of *family* are so extremely threatened, the state reverts to a conservative approach. Moreover, the state is not willing to directly endorse the creation of alternative families when its hand is involved in the approval of each and every contract, as in surrogacy. As the former secretary of the approvals committee told me: "Here the couple cannot naturally have children without the help of the state. Therefore we have the right to use our judgment on the matter."

Gate-keeping mechanisms of the nation

A number of conclusions can be elicited from the above. First, the restrictive governing of surrogacy in Israel puts the idea of Israeli pronatalism in perspective. On the one hand, the pronatalist impulse of lawmakers can explain why surrogacy was not entirely banned in Israel as it was in other countries. On the other hand, the restrictions in the original law and their continuous maintenance over the past eleven years shows that Israeli pronatalism has a limit: The state will not promote natal interests when the practice symbolically threatens the core concepts of motherhood and family. This finding adds to other critiques of the idea of Israeli *pronatalism* as blind towards the *selective* component of Israeli reproductive policies and practices. Morgenstern-Leissner's (2005) work on Israeli reproductive legislation has revealed the past encouragement of the Eastern-European [*Ashkenazi*] birthrate over the Oriental [*Mizrachi*] one. Moreover, Ivry (this volume) challenges the idea of pronatalism by citing the high rates of prenatal diagnoses and the high number of abortions—including very late abortions—when fetal abnormalities are discovered. She argues that Israel may have pronatalist policies, but that only "acceptable" births are encouraged. Weiss (2002) has also called attention to the selective component of Israeli reproductive policies, arguing that only *chosen bodies* are coveted.

A second conclusion we can make returns us to the scholarship on gender and nationalism, and to the argument that nations constitute themselves on the bodies of their female citizens (Yuval-Davis and Antheas 1989; Berkowitz 1997; Amir and Benjamin 1997). Aside from obviously serving as a case of the nation constructing itself on women's bodies, the surrogacy law reminds us that not just any body is considered appropriate for the "mission" of reproducing the classic nuclear family through surrogacy. Instead, it is only the bodies of unmarried women who have already fulfilled their national duty and are raising their own children who can lend their wombs to "incubate" other families.

Moreover, we are reminded that nations are not just "biologically reproduced" through women's bodies, but also through the institution of the family. This is doubly true in the case of the Jewish nation-state, for both Judaism and modern nationalism venerate the family as a cornerstone of their survival. The Jewish home has been considered the single most vital factor for the survival of Judaism and the preservation of the Jewish way of life, much more than the synagogue or school (Meiselman 1978: 16). Moreover, as Mosse (1985) maintains, the modern, nuclear family is at the cornerstone of the very cultural construct that we call the modern nation-state, and it is through this longstanding institution that the values of modern nations are preserved and reproduced. Accordingly, the Jewish collective in the Jewish State configures the territorial collectivity as a sacred space and the patriarchal family—with its capacity to discipline and contain sexuality and reproduction (Mosse 1985)—as the primary unit upon which the collectivity should be conceived and composed (Friedland 2001).

By limiting the surrogacy option to Israeli citizens who share the same religion, the surrogacy law ensures that only Jewish families are created through this practice, since Islam prohibits surrogacy. And as Carmeli and Birenbaum-Carmeli (2000) argue, the *natural family* can be seen as a microcosm of the *national family*, so that preserving its image becomes a measure of protecting the boundaries of the nation-state. The discussion above thus contributes to discussions of nationalism and gender by reminding us that the nation simultaneously constitutes itself on the bodies of its female citizens and through the social construction of the family.

Whereas Amir and Benjamin (1997) argue that the local hospital abortion committees they studied "educate" applicants and symbolically the entire social body that normative Israeli womanhood involves responsible and disciplined sexual and reproductive conduct, the surrogacy approvals committee and the social management of surrogacy in Israel in its entirety "educate" the social body that the nuclear family form and the traditional definition of motherhood are still to be regarded as sacred institutions, even when the state enables practices that lead to their so-called dissolution. Through its gatekeeping function the State symbolically expresses the hierarchy of Israeli reproduction, exposing that despite its "liberal" attitude, a hierarchy is still clear and that normative, nuclear families are still privileged above alternative family forms. As Kahn (2000) notes, it is better in the eyes of the state to be a single mother than just a single woman, therefore artificial insemination and gamete donation are available to single women. And as the recent lesbian "baby boom" in Israel instructs us, this rule seems to be applicable to same-sex families as well who have equal access to reproductive technologies, other than surrogacy, in service of their parenthood. However, the two-parent, hetero-normative nuclear family is still privileged above all other family forms.

In light of the tight state control of the surrogacy process, surrogacy emerges as what might be seen as the last outpost of the nuclear family; because surrogacy challenges this institution in an extreme form, the body politic has made it into an example. Afforded the ability to control which families are produced through this practice, the body politic ensures that only Jewish-Israeli citizens are born from these contracts to hetero-normative, two-parent, "natural" families.

Acknowledgments

I would like to thank Eyal Ben-Ari, Tsipy Ivry, Daphna Birenbaum-Carmeli and Yoram Carmeli for their comments on drafts of this article. I also appreciate the English editing expertise of my husband Avi Solomon and my mother Rhisa Teman.

Notes

1. Two types of surrogacy exist. The first, termed partial or traditional surrogacy, involves the surrogate being artificially inseminated with the intended father's sperm. The second, termed full, host, gestational or IVF surrogacy, is done through in vitro fertilization. The egg of the intended mother or of an anonymous donor is fertilized in a Petri dish with the sperm of the intended father or of a donor, and the embryo is transferred to the surrogate's uterus.
2. For a legal, historical and feminist analysis of the law, see Weisberg (2005), Shutz (2003) and Shalev (1998).
3. These bills were "stuck" in the legislative process for up to ten years despite the fact that the national shortage of eggs and organs has led to such dangerous practices as ova stealing by Israeli doctors (Reznick *Feb. 9*, 2000), international ova trafficking (Landau *Feb. 19*, 1999; Reznick *Sept. 25*, 2000), and active involvement of Israelis in international organ trafficking networks (Haaretz Service *June 10*, 2003; Reznick *Feb. 6*, 2005; Siegel-Itzkovich 2001).
4. For a discussion of the *halachic* issues surrounding surrogacy, see Schenker (2003) and Shifman (1993).
5. Surrogacy agencies often "sell" their services based on the same possibilities for new family formations that academics have written about with trepidation. The Center for Surrogate Parenting markets itself on its web site as the producer of "unique family combinations" that "have given a whole new meaning to the word 'family'" (Center for Surrogate Parenting 1993). What some might view with horror, they boast as their most "unique successes": "creating a family that included one homemade child, one adopted child, one surrogate-born child"; "fraternal quadruplets, born through gestational surrogacy from embryos implanted into two different surrogate mothers at the same time (One had triplets, the other a single baby)"; "twins, a boy and a girl, from the same egg retrieval, one embryo transferred to a gestational surrogate, the other embryo returned to the biological mother"; "one surrogate-born child and one child the result of an egg donated by the same surrogate mother but carried by the infertile wife"; "three surrogate-born children, two girls from the same surrogate mother, and a boy from a second surrogate"; and "Two children, a boy and a girl, born with the help of two different gestational surrogate mothers."

References

Amir, Delila and Orly Benjamin. 1992. "Abortion Approval as a Ritual of Symbolic Control." In *The Criminalization of a Woman's Body*, ed. C. Feinman. New York: Haworth Press.

———. 1997. "Defining Encounters: Who Are the Women Entitled to Join the Israeli Collective?" *Women's Studies International Forum* 20, vol. 5/6: 639–50.

Bagatz. 1994. "Michal Zabaro against the Health Minister." *Israeli High Court Petition Number 5087/94* [Hebrew].

Bagatz. 2001. "Anonymous against the Committee for the Approval of Embryo Carrying Agreements." *Israeli High Court Petition Number 2458/01* [Hebrew].

Benshushan, Abraham and Joseph G. Schenker. 1997. "Legitimizing Surrogacy in Israel." *Human Reproduction* 12, vol. 8: 1832–34.

Birenbaum-Carmeli, Daphna. 2004. "'Cheaper Than a Newcomer': On the Social Production of IVF Policy in Israel." *Sociology of Health & Illness* 26, vol. 7: 897–924.

Brennan, Samantha and Robert Noggle. 1997. "The Moral Status of Children: Children's Rights, Parents' Rights, and Family Justice." *Social Theory and Practice* 23, vol. 1: 1–26.

Carmeli, Yoram S. and Daphna Birenbaum-Carmeli. 2000. "Ritualizing the 'Natural Family': Secrecy in Israeli Donor Insemination." *Science as Culture* 9, vol. 3: 301–23.

Center for Surrogate Parenting, Inc. 1993. "Family Building Solutions." On file with the author (accessed June 19, 2001).

Chambers, Deborah. 2000. "Representations of Familialism in the British Popular Media." *European Journal of Cultural Studies* 3, vol. 2: 195–214.

Cook, Rachel, Shelley Day Sclater, and Felicity Kaganas. 2003. "Introduction." In *Surrogate Motherhood: International Perspectives*, eds. R. Cook, S.D. Sclater, and F. Kaganas. Oxford: Hart Publishing.

Corea, Gena. 1985. *The Mother Machine: Reproductive Technologies from Artificial Insemination to Artificial Wombs*. New York: Harper & Row.

———. 1987. *Man-Made Women: How New Reproductive Technologies Affect Women*. Bloomington: Indiana University Press.

COTS. 2005. *Childlessness Overcome Through Surrogacy*. <www.surrogacy.org.uk> (accessed September 13, 2007).

Farquhar, Dion. 1996. *The Other Machine: Discourse and Reproductive Technologies*. New York and London: Routledge.

Friedland, Roger. 2001. "Money, Sex and G-D: The Erotic Logic of Religious Nationalism." Paper presented at the Center for Comparative Studies and Sociology, University of California, Santa Barbara.

Gordon, Evelyn. 1995. "Surrogate Motherhood Soon to Be Legal." *The Jerusalem Post*, June 29.

Haaretz Service. 2003. "Bill to Set Compensation for Organ Donors." *Haaretz*, June 10.

Insler, Vatzlev. 2004. "Committee Report and Recommendations." *The Public Committee for the Examination of Eligibility for Surrogate Motherhood Arrangements, Health Ministry, Israeli Government* [Hebrew]. <www.health.gov.il/Download/pages/insler_internet.pdf> (access January 1, 2006).

Ivry, Tsipy. 2004. "Pregnant with Meaning: Conceptions of Pregnancy in Japan and Israel" (PhD dissertation, Department of Sociology and Social Anthropology, Hebrew University).

Kahn, Susan Martha. 2000. *Reproducing Jews: A Cultural Account of Assisted Conception in Israel*. Durham: Duke University Press.

Landau, Orna. 1999. "Rich Harvest." *Haaretz*, February 19.

Layne, Linda L., ed. 1999. *Transformative Motherhood: On Giving and Getting in a Consumer Culture*. New York: University Press.

Levinson, Haim. 2006. "Chief Rabbi: Married Woman Can Be Surrogate." *Ynet News*, June 11. http://www.ynetnews.com/articles/0,7340,L-3261249,00.html (accessed June 11, 2006).

Macklin, Ruth. 1991. "Artificial Means of Reproduction and Our Understanding of the Family." *Hastings Center Report* 21, vol. 1: 5–11.

Markens, Susan. 2007. Surrogate Motherhood and the Politics of Reproduction. Berkeley: University of California Press.

Meiselman, Moshe. 1978. *Jewish Woman in Jewish Law*. New York: Yeshiva University Press.

Morgan, Derek. 2003. "Enigma Variations: Surrogacy, Rights and Procreative Tourism." In *Surrogate Motherhood: International Perspectives*, eds. R. Cook, S.D. Sclater and F. Kaganas. Oxford and Portland: Hart Press.

Morgenstern-Leissner, Omi. 2005. "The Israeli Birth Law" (PhD dissertation, Department of Law, Bar Ilan University).

Mosse, George L. 1985. *Nationalism and Sexuality: Respectability and Abnormal Sexuality in Modern Europe*. New York: Howard Fertig.

Negev, Elat. 2002. "(Kept) out of the Womb [Michutz La'rechem]." *Sheva Yamim*, October 25 [Hebrew].

Protocol A. 1995. *Protocol of First Knesset Vote on Israeli Surrogacy Bill* [Hebrew]. December 11.

Reznick, Ran. 2000. "Facing Local Shortage, Israeli Women Go to Romania to Get Eggs Implanted." *Haaretz*, September 25.

———. 2000. "Health Ministry Suspects Doctors Sold Human Eggs." *Haaretz*, February 9.

———. 2005. "Still No Guidelines Covering Egg Donation." *Haaretz*, February 6.

Rothman, Barbara Katz. 2000. *Recreating Motherhood*. New Brunswick: Rutgers University Press.

Schenker, Joseph. 2003. "Legitimizing Surrogacy in Israel: Religious Perspectives." In *Surrogate Motherhood: International Perspectives*, eds. R. Cook, S.D. Sclater and F. Kaganas. Oxford and Portland: Hart Press.

Schuz, Rhona. 2003. "Surrogacy in Israel: An Analysis of the Law in Practice." In *Surrogate Motherhood: International Perspectives*, eds. R. Cook, S.D. Sclater and F. Kaganas. Oxford and Portland: Hart Press.

Shalev, Carmel. 1998. "Halakha and Patriarchal Motherhood: An Anatomy of the Israeli Surrogacy Law." *Israel Law Review* 32, vol. 1: 51–80.

Shifman, Pinhas. 1993. "A Perspective on Surrogate Motherhood in Jewish and Israeli Law." In *Frontiers of Family Law*, eds. A. Bainham, D. Pearl and R. Pickford. Chinchester: John Wiley and Sons.

Siegel- Itzkovich, Judy. 2001. "Israel to Allow Women to Donate Their Ova." *British Medical Journal* 322: 816.

———. 2003. "Israel Allows Removal of Sperm from Dead Men at Wife's Request." *British Medical Journal* 327: 1187.

Siegel, Judy. 1995. "News." *The Jerusalem Post*, July 18.

————.1996. "Surrogacy Bill Passes 3rd Reading." *The Jerusalem Post*, March 8: 22.

Snowden, Robert, E.M. Mitchell, and E. Snowden. 1984. *Artificial Reproduction: A Social Investigation*. London: George Allen and Unwin.

Stanworth, Michelle.1987. "Reproductive Technologies and the Deconstruction of Motherhood." In *Reproductive Technologies: Gender, Motherhood and Medicine*, ed. M. Stanworth. Cambridge, U.K.: Polity Press.

Taylor, Janelle S., Linda L. Layne, and Danielle F. Wozniak. 2004. *Consuming Motherhood*. New Brunswick: Rutgers University Press.

Teman, Elly. 2001. "Technological Fragmentation and Women's Empowerment: Surrogate Motherhood in Israel." *Women's Studies Quarterly* 31, vols. 3 and 4: 11–34.

————. 2003a. "The Medicalization of 'Nature' in the Artificial Body: Surrogate Motherhood in Israel." *Medical Anthropology Quarterly* 17, vol. 1: 78–98.

————. 2003b. "Knowing the Surrogate Body in Israel." In *Surrogate Motherhood: International Perspectives*, eds. Rachel Cook and Shelley Day Schlater. London: Hart Press, 261–280.

————. 2006a. "The Birth of a Mother: Mythologies of Surrogate Motherhood in Israel" (PhD dissertation, Department of Sociology and Social Anthropology, The Hebrew University of Jerusalem).

————. 2006b. "Bonding with the Field: On Researching Surrogate Motherhood Arrangements in Israel." In *Dispatches From the Field: Neophite Ethnographers in a Changing World*, eds. Andrew M. Gardner and David M. Hoffman. Long Grove, Illinois: Waveland Press.

Teman, Elly. 2010. Birthing a Mother: The Surrogate Body and the Pregnant Self. Berkeley: University of California Press.

van Niekerk, Anton, and Liezl van Zyl. 1995. "The Ethics of Surrogacy: Women's Reproductive Labour." *Journal of Medical Ethics* 21: 345–49.

Weisberg, D. Kelly. 2005. *The Birth of Surrogacy in Israel*. Florida: University of Florida Press.

Weiss, Meira. 2002. *The Chosen Body: The Politics of the Body in Israeli Society*. Stanford: Stanford University Press.

Yuval-Davis, Nira and Floya Anthias, eds. 1989. *Woman—Nation—State*. London: MacMillan.

Chapter 5

ADOPTION AND ASSISTED REPRODUCTION TECHNOLOGIES: A COMPARATIVE READING OF ISRAELI POLICIES

Daphna Birenbaum-Carmeli and Yoram S. Carmeli

Infertility affects some 8 to 14 percent of the fertility aged population worldwide (Bentley and Mascie-Taylor 2000). Many of the affected individuals seek medical assistance in their attempts to found families. Others, often after having exhausted and "failed" this option, opt for child adoption. Though popularly perceived of as the heart of one's private life, both these routes to family founding—fertility treatments and adoption—are tightly regulated by state policies.

State policies construct and mold the behavior of individuals and formal bodies, licensing some practices as acceptable, labeling others as not. But they go deeper than that. Initially imposed from the outside, policies also influence people's subjectivities and perceptions, so that they themselves eventually contribute, at times unconsciously, to a government's model of social order (Shore & White 1997). In so doing, state policies establish and reproduce local attitudes towards key social notions. Fertility treatments and child adoption, which are part of "[r]eproductive politics, are at the heart of questions about citizenship, liberty, family, and the nation" (Haraway

1997: 189). More concrete interests of professional groups and state agencies are also at stake.

At a more foundational level, policies contain implicit models of society—they encapsulate histories and bear legal, economic and moral implications that can create new relationships between individuals, groups, and objects. These goals are, however, mostly silenced or disguised, constituting policies as presumably a set of technical solutions that are unrelated to morality, politics, or ideology (Ong 2006: 3). The use of seemingly objective, neutral language endows policies with an instrumental appearance aiming to promote efficiency, thereby concealing their operation as a vehicle of power (ibid.: 8, 11).

Assisted reproduction and adoption are sensitive issues, both heavily loaded with personal meaning and as such, are crucial sites of governance and regulation. Societies interfere with reproduction, primarily through sanctioned norms of behavior, but also by means of formal policies. Recent technological and pharmaceutical developments that have transferred key aspects of human reproduction to the medical domain have opened up new channels for state intervention in this personal sphere. Some countries shape the use of assisted reproduction technologies (ARTs) by policies that exclude ART services almost fully from public health care schemes, thus placing these expensive treatments beyond the reach of large populations. Other states police these technologies by setting exclusionary eligibility criteria that render whole categories of people—e.g., unmarried, homosexual, mentally impaired individuals and couples—un-entitled. A third type of policy restricts application indirectly by keeping ART solely in the public sector, where available clinics cannot fully provide for the existing demand (Pashigian, 2009). Additionally, many states prescribe limitations on the range of permitted treatments and combinations thereof (e.g., prohibiting the use of donor gametes in IVF procedures).

Child adoption is as closely state-monitored in industrialized societies. Here, the intervention is legitimized primarily in terms of the child's best interest and entails varying degrees of scrutiny of the adoption applicants' lives. Though being regulated by formal statutes and laws since the late 19th century and becoming fully formalized during the second half of the 20th century, adoption has been shown to be still deeply steeped with ambivalence in the public eye (Miall 1996). A consistent gap that was also found between people's positive statements regarding adoption, and actual adoption practices, may suggest that this route to family formation is often perceived as a last resort for infertile couples or—increasingly—as the feasible option for marginalized groups like single individuals, and homosexual individuals or couples (Fisher 2003; Miller 1992). The media tendency, observed in many countries, to highlight adoption-related difficulties and to overlook "happy stories" (Wegar, cited in March & Miall 2000), alongside the growing emphasis on genetics as the basis of one's identity and inventory of future therapies (Lebner, cited in March & Miall 2000) both reflect and enhance this view. Adopted children thus emerge in the public domain as more prone to mental and physical developmental problems (Miall 1996; Fisher 2003; Bharadwaj 2003). These concerns are especially heightened in cases of inter-country adoption (ICA), wherein the children's mostly poorer countries of origin further nurture such fears (Lovelock 2000). Still, despite the concerns, adoption is practiced in all industrialized countries, as specified below.

ART policies in Israel

Israel's ART policy is an international exception in terms of its inclusiveness. Fertility treatments are state funded and offered to women of all family statuses and sexual orientations up to the age of 45—51 if using a donor egg. The state covers treatment for the first two live births with the present partner. This policy means that each partner may have children from previous relationships and may end up with more than two "IVF children," given Israel's high frequency of multiple births following fertility treatments. In practice, even these policy limitations can be bypassed rather easily. In line with this situation, Israel has the world's highest number of IVF clinics per capita and the largest number of treatment cycles per woman (Collins 2002). As the subject of ART policies and practice in Israel is presented more extensively in the introduction to this volume, we focus this chapter's background section on the subject of adoption. We start with a cross-country comparative overview which will then ground our comparative analysis.

Adoption: International perspectives

Countries vary in their regulation and practice of adoption. A brief summary of main adoption principles in several industrialized countries will provide an illustrative framework for our subsequent analysis of the Israeli policy.

Table 8   Selected adoption guidelines: International profiles[1]

	Single Persons	Same sex	Age requirements	Additional requirements	Estimated costs and reimbursement *excluding travel expenses*
Sweden	V	V	25+ (younger, if adopting a related child)		$20,000 State subsidy of $5,000
Norway	No	No	Usually <45y difference from child	-good health - stable financial situation -police clearance	
Denmark	V	No	Usually <40y difference from child		Roughly $14,000 State grant: $7,600
U.K. [2]	V	Can adopt individually, not as a couple	21y+	Medical examination; Police record doesn't necessarily exclude	$70,000[3] State support is provided in cases some cases [4]
Germany	V	Not as a couple but one member may adopt alone	25y+ (general preference for age difference <40		Several thousands
Netherlands	No	Only adoption of a child born in the Netherlands	Age difference <41	-Health assessment -judicial/police records -sureties for adoption costs agree to provide child's medical care	$25,000
Ontario, Canada [5]	V	V		Be Ontario resident Home study	State subsidy in some cases of children with special needs
U.S.A.	V				Up to $40,000 but, federal and state tax credits, state reimbursement for costs, employer benefits, Adoption Loans and Grants[6]

As shown in Table 8, quite a few industrialized countries allow single persons to adopt a child; some allow same sex pairs to adopt as a couple; some set no upper age limit to adoptive parents. Additional requirements, like medical reports, financial status or police clearance also vary. In all countries adoption entails substantial expenses, but most states provide some financial assistance. Countries also vary in the proportion of domestic vs. inter-country adoptions. In the U.K., for instance, overseas adoptions comprise a mere 1 to 6 percent of adoptions while in Germany and Norway the comparable figures are 34 percent and 81 percent respectively (General Register Office for Scotland 2004). Some countries appear to proactively support adoption. For instance, in Canada, the federal umbrella organization for adoption (The Adoption Council of Canada) has as its patron the Governor General of Canada, who is the country's Head of State, thus granting the organization the status of vice-regal office. In the same spirit, Canada's National Statistical Agency consistently merges "child birth or adoption" into a single statistical category (Statistics Canada 2006).

Whether reflective or constitutive of local variations, countries also differ significantly in their total rates of adoption, with a range as broad as 11.2 adoptions per 1,000 births in Norway, to 5.2 in Canada and 0.4 in the U.K. (see table 9).

Table 9 Intercountry adoptions per 1,000 live births: 1998 and 1989. Selected receiving countries.

Country	No. of adoptions 1997*/1998	No. of births (1,000) 1998	Adoptions per 1,000 births 1997*/1998	Adoptions per 1,000 birth 1989
Norway	643	57	11.2	11.0
Sweden	928	86	10.8	9.4
Denmark	624	63	9.9	8.5
Switzerland	733*	80	9.2*	6.2
France	3,777	713	5.3	3.0
Canada	1,799	344	5.2*	2.7
Netherlands	825	179	4.6	3.7
U.S.A.	15,774	3.788	4.2	2.0
Italy	2,019*	512	3.9*	3.8
Germany	1,819	749	2.4	1.6
Finland	181	57	3.2	2.0
Australia	245	245	1.0	1.4
U.K.	258	689	0.4	N/A

asterisked rates are for 1997
Table source: Selman 2002

Adoption policy in Israel

The cursory outlines of Israel's ART policy, and international adoption policies, provide instructive background for the description and subsequent analysis of Israel's adoption policy. Though available, adoption in Israel entails much bureaucratic hassle and extensive waiting periods. ICA is also licensed but entails high expenditure that is not reimbursed. The following sections critically locate Israel's policy within the international adoption landscape, and compare it with the local ART regulations.

As elsewhere in the industrialized world, demand for adoption in Israel outstrips the number of "available" local babies. Increased use of contraceptives, the normalization of single motherhood and the financial provisions allocated to them coincide with rising rates of infertility to generate a chronic shortage. This is particularly true in regard to healthy newborns. Over 400 Israeli couples wait for a baby at any given time, but only 50 (local) healthy young babies (up to two years of age) will be handed out for adoption every year.

In contradistinction to the local world record of IVF consumption, Israel ranks low on adoption in comparison with industrialized countries. In 2005, Israel had 115 domestic adoptions (of babies and older children, including ones with developmental problems) and 193 ICAs (National Council for the Child 2006),[7] mostly from Russia and the Ukraine (Zwebner 2003). This is measured against the country's 143,913 live births in 2005 (Central Bureau of Statistics 2005).

Israel's ICA ratio is 1.34 per 1,000 births (193/143,913 x 1,000 = 1.34). When all adoptions are included the figure rises but is still modest at 2.14; just over two children are adopted for every 1,000 babies being born. This figure is roughly 5 to 6 times lower than in Norway or Sweden. Whereas these figures are not in themselves exceptional—the U.K. for instance has a lower adoption rate—they acquire greater significance in the light of the extensive state support of ART. It is this gap that we try to address in the present chapter.

Domestic adoption in Israel is regulated by the Ministry of Law and Justice, sometimes in consultation with the Ministry of Labor and Welfare.[8] The concerted work of these state bureaus makes the adoption of a young healthy Israeli child a tightly regulated procedure. Applicants must fulfill numerous strict requirements. They must be legally married for at least 3 years, without any children (a couple may adopt up to 2 children), be no more than 43 years older than the adopted child, and have at least 12 years of schooling. The couple must have a regular source of income and earn at least the national average income. They must also have a reasonable place of residence wherein the child will be offered a room of its own. Additionally, the couple is assessed for their spousal, familial, and social functioning and for their projected ability to cope with adoption-related complexities. Adoptive parents must be of the same religion as the child's birth religion.[9] Unofficially, a senior practitioner in the field has told us that the state consistently prioritizes religious over secular applicants. To this list of requirements—visibly on the tighter side when compared to other countries in table 8—one should add a waiting period of 5 to 6 years on the average. Couples are offered babies on a "first come, first offered" basis. Of great significance here is the law's license—in fact encouragement—of couples to carry on with fertility treatments during the years of waiting in the adoption line.

A shorter waiting time—two years on average—is required for the adoption of an Israeli baby who is affected by a health, development, or drug addiction problem. Fifty such babies are placed with adoptive families in Israel every year.

A third route leads to the adoption of an older (Israeli born) child—aged 2 to 10 years—with some special needs. The special feature of this option is that siblings are mostly placed together in one family.

Single individuals are allowed to adopt only those children who could not be placed with an adoptive couple. The state's rationale here is that it is better for the child to grow up with a single parent, often supported by an extended family, than to remain in institutional care. Possibly implied in the prescription is, however, a notion that less desirable children would in some sense match somewhat marginalized families. A recent proposal to amend the adoption law by allowing same sex partners to adopt their partner's child has not been ratified so far (Political Council for GLBT Rights in Israel 2003). All adoptive parents are required to undergo a preparatory program, designed to fit their specific circumstances.

In section 33 of Israel's 1981 Adoption Law, ICA was prohibited and up to a year imprisonment prescribed for law breakers. However, the shortage of Israeli babies offered for adoption became so severe, waiting periods so long and applicant requirements so restrictive, that many Israelis seeking adoption eventually resorted to illegal ICA. For several years, improvised arrangements were carried out informally, occasionally resulting in financial losses and child trafficking (Kislinger n.d.). Two high profile cases around 1990 became especially publicized. In 1988, Bruna Caroline, who had been adopted in Brazil two years earlier, was returned to her birth mother after an Israeli court was convinced that the baby had been kidnapped from her birth mother. Five years later, in 1993, Sapirit Friedman, an Israeli celebrity, was arrested in Brazil for charges of child trafficking when she went there to adopt a baby. These cases, as well as the growing pressure and the signing of the Hague Convention, eventually prompted amendment of the Israeli adoption law. As of January 1998, ICA is allowed when conducted through government-licensed non-governmental organizations (NGOs). At present, twenty such NGOs operate in Israel (ibid.). Other forms of ICA remain criminal offenses.

The state presents strict requirements for the operation of NGOs (e.g., licensing operation only for a specific county and retaining the right to suspend or cancel an NGO's license under certain circumstances). At the applicants' end, however, eligibility criteria for ICA are much more relaxed than for domestic adoption. Applicants are required to undergo a psychologist's assessment of their ability to adopt, and later may be requested to present additional documents required by the adoptee's country of origin. Notably, on the part of the State of Israel, no additional requirements apply.

Though the law prohibits any payment for adoption, it does allow the attending agencies to charge applicants for related costs of up to $20,000 (U.S.). To these one should add concomitant costs like travel expenses or loss of work days. The total sum is privately covered without any state assistance. Our inquiry revealed one single source of financial support: an interest-free loan of up to $5,000 to be repaid over a 30-month period that is offered by a special NGO (Child Welfare Information Gateway 2004). In a country where the gross monthly salary was just under $1,700 in 2006 (Central Bureau of Statistics 2007), the basic adoption-related expenditure thus equaled one's entire annual income, placing ICA beyond the reach of many childless people, let alone single individuals. By law, NGOs are required to subsidize a few applicants who cannot afford the full costs. However, our investigation has not revealed any evidence of such subsidized or cost free placements. As of 2000, the State's comptroller report criticized state authorities for not having defined clear criteria for handling adoption requests on the part of applicants of lesser financial means (Knesset-Research and Information Center 2003). CA procedures are also highly intricate bureaucratically.

Having said that, people who do embark on the ICA route normally end up with a healthy baby within 6 to 12 months. Between the years 1998 and 2003, about 1,000 children were adopted by Israelis (Knesset Research and Information Center 2003), mostly from Russia and the Ukraine (Ministry of Labor and Welfare n.d.a).[10]

All adoption registries are confidential but adopted children may view their files at the age of 18. Inappropriate disclosure of adoptive parents' or adoptee's identity is a criminal offense.

In the Revised Adoption Law of 1998, Israel's policies regarding both local and inter-country adoption define the adoptee's best interest as their guiding principle. The law attributes to this guideline the thorough investigation of applicants' family backgrounds, their legal and medical records and psychological fitness. It also prescribes a 6-month probation period following placement (of an Israeli or foreign baby) to obtain the Ministry of Interior Affairs' final approval. Applicants must wait at least 18 months between adoptions, unless the adoptees are related to each other. The state retains the right to remove an adopted child from the parents if this is found to be in the child's best interest.

Once they adopt a child—aged up to 10 years—parents are entitled in principle to all maternity-related provisions, including birth allowance and a 12-week paid parental leave. An adoptive mother who decides to quit her job is entitled to Dismissal Compensation Payment like any other mother, as long as she resigned within 9 months following adoption. The maximum qualifying age of the child for this clause is 13. Maternity tax exemptions also apply equally to adoptive mothers. Though they have been guaranteed by law only as late as 1994, these provisions had been unanimously supported by otherwise bitterly divided Knesset members of all parties (Sered 2000: 27).

If the adoption entails religion conversion of the baby—normally required in ICA where most babies are not of a Jewish origin—the parents would have to approach a conversion center. If they are not married, they would be encouraged, though not forced, to marry. If the adoptee is an older boy and his circumcision would involve a surgeon's fee, the state would cover these costs. At the end of the process, the adoptee is considered Jewish. However, according to the religious law, converted girls are not allowed to marry a Cohen.[11] This dictate may be applied at the discretion of the involved parties. While the conversion court does not normally enforce an observant lifestyle on the adoptive family, the requirement is nevertheless presented, thus placing many adoptive parents who are secular in an allegedly uncomfortable situation.

The conversion requirement is but one way in which the state tacitly places adoptive parents at disadvantage. A more systematic comparison with fertility treatment provisions reveals a consistent disparity. Probably the most striking contrast is between the practically universal admission of any woman to fertility treatments and the tight eligibility criteria for domestic adoption. As mentioned, these go beyond one's health to place applicants' familial, social, and financial lives under State inspection, from the time of initial application to the 6-month post-placement probation period. A second substantial difference is financial. Domestic adoption is indeed free of charge. However, as mentioned, this option is scarce and entails, in addition to the strict requirements, an extensive waiting period and an age limit, which many applicants exceed, owing to long years spent in fertility treatments. Many adoption applicants must therefore resort to ICA and privately cover the $20,000 initial fees, further expanded by traveling expenditure and missed work days. Unlike fertility treatments, which qualify women to sick leave of up to 80 work days a year, absence from work for adoption-related reasons is not equally subsidized. Adoptive mothers are also not as protected from being fired during the pre-adoption period as women undergoing fertility treatment.

At the ideological level, the difference in ensuring the child's best interest is significant. In ART policy, which shapes the state's proactive intervention in the very creation of a baby, this aspect of assisted family formation is never mentioned or even implied in any part of the document. In contradistinction, in adoption the child's best interest is construed as the guiding principle and the grounds for the pedantic applicant scrutiny. On the other hand, or actually following the same spirit, the state provides adoptive parents with psychological and some technical support in the first stages following adoption, which it does not offer to families created by ART.

Analysis and discussion

Our main interest is in the differences between ART and adoption policies. In order to explore these differences systematically, we divide the ensuing analysis into three sets of comparisons. We start by comparing the two types of adoption: inter-country vs. domestic adoption, then move on to compare ART and ICA, followed by a comparison of ART with domestic adoption.

Inter-country vs. domestic adoption. The differences between domestic and inter-country adoption in Israel seem particularly sharp. As noted, in domestic adoption, applicants must satisfy a long list of requirements. They have to be heterosexual, married (in fact, happily married), young, well-educated, financially stable, and preferably (informally) also religious. In other words, they must fully conform to the traditional middle class family model. No such requirements bind people seeking adoption abroad, who must undergo a psychologist's assessment, but would then depend on the adoption agency and the child's country of origin for any additional investigation.

Now, if adoption is guided, as claimed, by the child's best interest, the difference in criteria raises questions regarding the well being of foreign children. If a child needs a traditional family in order to develop and flourish, as required in domestic adoption, how can the state be so "lenient" in matters of ICA?

An initial explanation of Israel's domestic adoption policy could apply a demand/supply model: the demand for healthy Israeli babies exceeds the number of children offered for adoption to such an extent that the state can implement a highly selective policy, namely, privilege these homes in which adoptees will presumably be best off, i.e., homes of normative middle class couples. In this respect, Israel's domestic adoption policy tacitly establishes the middle class family as the optimal habitat for child growth and development, thus disclosing clear middle class hegemony.

While this interpretation seems obviously valid, it still appears partial in the light of the country's "liberal" admission to ICA. The policy's openness to the creation of practically any family formation suggests that the state views adoptive commitment as solid and stable also beyond the typical middle class: evidently, older and less "established" couples or even individuals are considered capable of handling the challenges of inter-country adoption. This openness leads to the possibility that a crucial factor contributing to the difference between the two types of adoption is the Jewishness of the adoptees, with its concomitant symbolic significance of Jewish blood ties, and the "natural family." As we consider this symbolic complex to be of formative import to the scrutinized policies, we now turn to a brief description of its main components.

In Jewish tradition the "natural family" is viewed as obviously "good." This view is not an exclusively Jewish idea, as observed in many studies that have found adoption to be considered inferior to "natural kinship" (e.g., Bartholet 1993; March & Miall 2000; Fisher 2003). However, within this broad framework, the particular significance bestowed on the "natural family" varies culturally and historically and as such renders adoption policies an encapsulation of cultural codes and historical transformations within a society.

In Israel, the preference for the "natural family" is anchored in Jewish law. However, traditional perceptions of this issue are not monolithic. At a certain level, Jewish sources (the Bible and Talmud) do praise adoption through favorable examples: Abraham adopted his servant Eliezer; Mordecai raised his orphaned cousin Esther; the Talmudic sage Abaye used to attribute wise observations to his foster mother (Gold 1988: 1). At the same time, the transferring of the biological parents' rights and duties in their entirety to another couple or individual, as pertinent to contemporary adoption, is alien to Judaic law, which anchors a person's identity in bloodlines. The birth mother's Jewishness determines the child's religious identity. When the mother is Jewish, the father's "tribal status" (Cohen, Levi, or ordinary Israel) is transferred on to his son. Contemporary modes of adoption obviously interfere with this tradition.

Perceptions of the "natural family" go beyond individual families to effect the definition of collectivities. Collective identity is shaped from within and from without (e.g., Barth 1969). Jewish collective definition has been largely dictated from the outside during centuries of exile. Quite often, "natural" components were central in these definitions, climaxing in the Nazi pedantic tracing of Jewish ancestry. Jewishness was thus constituted as inborn and sometimes even imposed on dismayed members.

From within, the centrality of the "natural" element in the collective definition has varied historically. In biblical times and into the 2nd century B.C.E., the Jewish collectivity was founded on tribal myths but also expanded via exogamy. The biblical stories of Moses's Midianite wife Zipporah, of Ruth the Moabite who became King David's grandmother, and King Solomon's Hittite mother and his foreign wives are all paradigmatic examples. More generally, the biblical prohibition on marrying non-Jews did not apply to female captives, many of whom were taken as Israel's wives. The "natural" myth of the Biblical tribes was thus mitigated by territorial expansion and political alliances (Leach 1969). In addition to fusion by exogamy, the myth has also been supplemented by some cases of large scale conversion. In the Babylonian Talmud, Rabbi Johannan praised conversion ("The Holy One, blessed be He, dispersed the people of Israel among the nations in order that they might acquire proselytes" [Pesachim 87b]). In the pre-Christian Roman Empire, Jewish proselytizing had reached its peak, and during the 7th century C.E. the Khazars gradually endorsed Judaism as the state religion (Brook 2005; Shepard 1998). However, since the Middle Ages, most Jewish communities have been segregated in ghettos. Intermarriage with non-Jews, let alone mass conversions, was placed beyond the possible. The Jewish family was charged with virtually full responsibility for the collectivity's continuity while the community and nation assumed an image of a mythical natural family (Katz 1971).

In contemporary Israel, "nature," though occasionally challenged, has remained central in the definition of the collectivity. The biblical ancestors' myth of the "natural family" pervades daily parlance, and family metaphors (e.g., "the patriarchs and the matriarchs" [*ha'avot veha'imahot*], "the children of Israel" [*bnei Israel*], "the tribes of Israel"

[*Shivtey Israel*]) are being taught in schools and are commonly used, connoting blood relations as constitutive of the Jewish collectivity (see introduction, this volume). Often, the mythical "natural" component is used as a unifying vehicle of Israeli Jewish identity.

Beyond parlance, the "natural" family is ritualized in the blending of historical family myths with nation building. A prominent example is the major holiday of Passover, wherein Jewish Israelis celebrate in families the mythical flee of the "Children of Israel" (*Bnei Israel)* from Egypt, which has become fused with present day sovereignty. Indeed, the basic Jewish Israeli claim on the land is phrased in the familial Biblical idiom of *Eretz Avotenu*—"Land of our Ancestors."

The "natural family" element also imbues the local discourse of social integration. Unlike in other immigration countries, where parameters like voting, mastering the language or economic mobility are tokens of integration, in Israel such indices are considered significant but (at least until the 1990s) secondary to the "ultimate" sign of absorption: inter-ethnic marriage and the creation of blood ties through "natural" offspring. Occasionally, economic and even social gaps would be presented as secondary to endogamy, which is highlighted as the guarantee for "the continuity of the Jewish people" (Ritterband 1995).

A fresh rephrasing of the "nature" argument has been provided by recent genetic findings that have identified typical Jewish genetic formations (e.g., Hammer et al. 1997; Thomas et al. 2002) and claims that all Jews have descended from a small number of women (probably nine). Notably, in contrast to the extensive publicizing of these studies, other findings which showed genetic resemblance between Jews and Palestinians (Arnaiz-Villena et al. 2001; Oppenheim et al. 2000) and thereby undermined the "natural" identity thesis and the consequent religious/political monopolist claim on the land, were sidelined and never picked up as a basis for political change.

To sum up, in present day Israel, the Jewish "natural family" encapsulates a mythological descent from ancestors and thus "the people" to whom the land has been promised. Historically, it is perceived as an embodiment of a remote common origin and a history of persecution that legitimizes the return to this land. In daily experience, living "natural" families are the site of reproduction, regenerating the precarious "natural" Jewish identity. We take this religious-ideological and political notion of the Jewish collectivity as the explanatory context for both the centrality of the "natural family" in Israel (discussed in numerous chapters in this volume), and for the marginalization of adoption. At the same time, the above illustrations of the historicity and constructedness of "natural" kinship and of the relationship among myth, religious law, and daily practice points to some tension between the religious-ideological definition of the Jewish Israeli collectivity as "natural," and the lived reality that destabilizes it. This tension will be the vantage point for the ensuing assessment of the observed differences between ART and the two types of adoption.

ART-ICA. As described, we found great similarity in the "liberal" admission to both these veins of child pursuit, primarily in the "liberal" eligibility criteria that admit practically any applicant. Consequently, both options can equally result in the founding of either traditional or completely unconventional families. The similarity stops, however, in the financial sphere, with ART being fully state funded and ICA being entirely private. The difference becomes particularly striking when we recall that the $20,000 (U.S.) "cost of an IVF baby" (Stern et al. 1995), covered in its entirety by the state, is identical to the charges of ICA agencies in which the state does not participate at all. In comparison to its ART policy, Israel's policy of ICA thus emerges as ambivalent: accommodating, though financially disengaged. The reluctant side, namely the lack of state investment, lends itself to a simple explanation: ICA is not fully funded in any country, and Israel is not any different in its budgetary constraints. However, this reluctance may also be underpinned by the traditional Jewish association of the "natural family" with the collectivity, thus prescribing a preference for ART over adoption. Within this framework, the acceptance of non-Jewish children into the collectivity thus acquires a strong symbolic significance.

Having said that, in its tolerant eligibility criteria and in enabling a relatively simple conversion process for adoptees, the state does manifest openness towards ICA. We understand the state policy as an attempt to reconcile the effort of sustaining a "Jewish state" with contemporary "cracks" due to politics of survival.

The legalization of ICA came into effect in 1998. By that time, Israel had already signed the Hague Convention (in 1991) and had "absorbed" two distinct waves of immigration that indirectly challenged the "natural" basis of its Jewish identity. The "Jewishness" of the Ethiopian immigrants of the 1990s was for years a matter of doubt and negotiation, thus becoming a vivid demonstration of the constructed "nature" of Jewish collective identity. The second wave consisted of roughly a million immigrants from the Former Soviet Union, which included many newcomers of mixed religious origin, as well as Christians who joined Jewish partners, parents or children. A minority of these Christians converted, but the majority went on leading a Christian life in Israel. Church attendance and Christian burial thus gained unprecedented visibility in Israel during the 1990s. In terms of the definition of the Jewish state, both the Christians and recent converts embodied the erosion of the "natural" basis of the country's "Jewishness." The growing number of legal and illegal foreign workers has also challenged the state's Jewish definition. Thus, in the wake of the 1990s, Israel has been somewhat pluralized, almost inadvertently, despite its immigration policy, as if eroded by the pragmatics of its own survival.

At that historical point, the idea of raising a non-Jewish baby from Eastern Europe seemed so familiar it could hardly be rejected. Moreover, the general exchange with Eastern Europe had become so routinized and ICA had become so established throughout the industrialized world that prohibition would have been practically irrelevant. Against this international background, and given the shortage of local babies, the state was almost forced to respond to adoption seekers' needs by legalizing ICA. However, it did so very cautiously: In sealing all public resources to ICA, it signaled reluctance and decreased the likelihood of public debate; and by mandating a strictly Orthodox conversion of adoptees it appeased the religious bodies and more generally, re-endorsed the existing religious-political status quo.

ART-domestic adoption. Unlike the certain similarity between ART and ICA, the rift between ART and domestic adoption policies is conspicuous. First, the state establishes a clear hierarchy between these two modes of family formation by encouraging domestic adoption applicants to continue fertility treatments during the waiting years. Through this recommendation, policy makers construct adoption as a last resort, to be undertaken only when all routes to the "natural family" have failed. This privileging of "natural" relatedness is scattered throughout the adoption policy. For instance, when applicants are "naturally" related to the adoptee, the state waives the requirements for minimum age and married status; and when a child's biological parents are not alive, the state grants her or his grandparents special adoption-related rights. It also privileges birth mothers by allowing withdrawal from pre-birth consent to adoption.[12]

A second major difference is established through the dissimilar admission criteria. The same state apparatuses that screen domestic adoption applicants so conservatively actively support the creation of the most unconventional families through ART. Older women, single women, and lesbian couples are all invited to found families via IVF and gamete donation under state auspices. Even post-divorce embryo transfer (Birenbaum-Carmeli 2007) and post-mortem sperm aspiration from an unmarried man (Hasson 2007) have been approved by Israeli Courts. Hypothetically, a woman of 51, who would be totally excluded from domestic adoption (and completely unsupported financially if opting for ICA), would receive immediate, free treatment if she chose to undergo IVF with a donor egg. How should we understand this difference?

Our explanation revolves around both the centrality of the "natural family" in current definitions of the Jewish collectivity and its precariousness.

Starting with Israel's "liberal" ART policy that accommodates all applicants and treatment combinations, we view this openness as materializing the notion of "natural" ties as solid enough to support any family formation. According to this logic, extensive ART services represent the state's attempt to hold on to the natural family basis, or at least to its guise.

If the "natural" family is indeed the stronghold—possibly the last viable resort—of the "natural" Jewish bond, and if, as such, it is perceived as crucial to the Jewishness of the state and its concomitant geopolitical claims, then the naturalness of the family acquires a ritual, symbolic import, tied up not only in the definition but also in the survival of the collectivity, as a strategic vehicle supporting a challenged collectivity (see Seeman, this volume). It is in order to serve this purpose that "the natural family" needs to be so sharply distinguished from any social alternative.

Within this framework, domestic adoption, i.e., the adoption of Jewish children, blurs the demarcation between "natural" and social family alliances by evoking some all-Jewish "natural" relatedness between parents and their adopted child. If natural relatedness is at the heart of the collectivity's definition, then this vagueness poses a symbolic threat to the distinctiveness of the "natural family" and therefore needs to be construed as weaker, i.e., requiring every possible guarantee to "survive" as a family.

According to this line of thought, the implied weakness of domestic adoption families is not a matter of a weaker parent-child bond. In fact, being based on an act of choice, these families might well be perceived as stronger. Rather, the weakness lies in the symbolic threat and consequent marginalization of the adoptive family vs. the "natural" definition of the collectivity. It is in order to curb the symbolic threat represented by social relatedness that Israel's domestic adoption policy is so highly restrictive. (Similar preferences for a "natural" appearance were expressed by recipients of sperm donation who would not disclose the third party contribution and who preferred physically similar donors [see Carmeli and Birenbaum-Carmeli 2000;

Birenbaum-Carmeli and Carmeli 2002a, 2002b].) The tight state scrutiny of adoption applicants, the introduction of mutual suspicion into adoptive family relations, the denial of financial assistance to ICA, and conversely, the encouragement of "natural" families, including partially- or seemingly- natural families created by gamete donation all point in this direction: the attempt to sustain the singular significance of "natural" bonds as a vehicle of collective definition in contemporary Israel.

Israel's ART as well as adoption policies have served in this chapter as "cultural texts," which enhance a particular ideology and related groups and marginalize others. Whereas the view of biological relatedness as superior to social alternatives is not exclusive to Israel, the observed discrepancy in eligibility, financial provisions, and bureaucracy between fertility treatments and adoption tells the story of a collectivity trying to define itself in terms of blood relatedness in the name of familial and national bio-survival. Within this perspective, reproductive technologies themselves could be turned into a symbol, representing Jewish scientific ingenuity, determination, and commitment to national regeneration—a symbol charged with an intensity that adoption, so it seems, will continue to be equally denied.

Notes

1. All material on the particular countries was obtained from the U.S Department of State (2006).
2. British Association for Adopting and Fostering (n.d.a).
3. British Association for Adopting and Fostering (n.d.b).
4. Office of Public Sector Information (2005).
5. On the web site of the Ontario Ministry of Children and Youth Services (n.d.), the following declaration is made: "If you are 18 years of age and over and a resident of Ontario, you may apply to adopt."
6. Child Welfare Information Gateway (2004).
7. Also cited in the Knesset Committee on Work, Welfare and Health (2002: 4).
8. The latter also provides various types of support to birth mothers (See Ministry of Labor and Welfare n.d.a.). This subject is, however, beyond the scope of the present chapter.
9. Among Muslim Israelis formal adoption is rarely opted for, whereas various modes of informal intra-familial fostering are more popular. However, being mostly informal, these arrangements are not state monitored.
10. Notably, there have not been any significant concerns regarding the social origin of foreign babies, as, for instance Indians were claimed to have expressed (Bharadwaj 2003).

11. A Cohen is a traditional Jewish priest. Today, the title bears little meaning for most Jews. However, it still retains some symbolic significance and in orthodox circles has considerable practically implications.

12. When the State severs birth parents' rights and removes a child from their home in the name of her or his best interest, the emphasis is on the exceptionality and the gravity of the circumstances that had justified such a sanction. As such it reaffirms yet again the primacy of "natural" kinship.

References

Andersen, A.N., Gianaroli, L. and Nygren, K.G. 2004. "Assisted Reproductive Technology in Europe, 2000. Results Generated from European Registers by ESHRE." *Human Reproduction* 19, no. 3 (March): 490–503.

Arnaiz-Villena A, Elaiwa N, Silvera C, Rostom A, Moscoso J, Gómez-Casado E, Allende L, Varela P, Martínez-Laso J. 2001. "The Origin of Palestinians and their Genetic Relatedness with other Mediterranean Populations." *Human Immunology* 62, no. 9 (September): 889–900.

Barkai, H. 1998. *The Evolution of Israel's Social Security System: Structure, Time Pattern and Macroeconomic Impact.* Aldershot: Ashgate.

Barth, Fredrik, ed. 1969. *Ethnic Groups and Boundaries.* Boston: Little, Brown.

Bartholet, E. 1993. *Family Bonds: Adoption and the Practice of Parenting.* New York: Houghton Mifflin.

Bentley, Gillian R., and Nicholas Mascie-Taylor, eds. 2000. *Infertility in the Modern World: Present and Future Prospects.* Cambridge: Cambridge University Press.

Bharadwaj, Aditya. 2003. "Why Adoption is not an Option in India: The Visibility of Infertility, the Secrecy of Donor Insemination, and other Cultural Complexities." *Social Science and Medicine* 56: 1867–80.

Birenbaum-Carmeli, D.1997. "Pioneering Procreation: Israel's First Test-Tube Baby." *Science as Culture*6: 525–40.

———. 2003. "Contextualising a Medical Breakthrough: An Overview of the Case of IVF."*Health Care for Women International*24, no. 7: 591–607.

———. 2004a.'Cheaper than a Newcomer': On the Political Economy of IVF in Israel." *The Sociology of Health and Illness* 26, no. 7: 897–924.

———. 2004b. The Prevalence of Jews as Subjects in Genetic Research: Explanation and Potential Implications." *American Journal of Medical Genetics* 130A, no. 1: 76–83.

———. 2007. "Contested Surrogacy and the Gender Order: An Israeli Case Study." *Journal of Middle East Women Studies* 3, no. 3: 21–44.

Birenbaum-Carmeli Daphna and Yoram S. Carmeli. 2002a. "Hegemony and Homogeneity: Donor Preferences of Recipients of Donor Insemination." *The Journal of Material Culture* 7, no. 1: 73–94.

———. 2002b. "Physiognomy, Familism and Consumerism: Preferences among Jewish-Israeli Recipients of Donor Insemination." *Social Science & Medicine* 54, no. 3: 363–76.

Birenbaum-Carmeli, D., Y. S. Carmeli, and R. Cohen. 2000. "Press Coverage of the First IVF in Israel and Canada." *International Journal of Sociology and Social Policy*20, no. 7: 1–38.

Birenbaum-Carmeli, D. Yoram S. Carmeli and H. Yavetz. 2000. "Secrecy among Israeli Recipients of Donor Insemination." *Politics and the Life Sciences* 19, no. 1: 69–76.

British Association for Adoption and Fostering. n.d.a. "Adoption: Who Can Adopt?" (accessed November 4, 2007. <http://www.baaf.org.uk/info/firstq/adoption.shtml#whocan>

British Association for Adoption and Fostering. n.d.b. "Inter-Agency Fees: 1 April 2006—31 March 2007." <http://www.baaf.org.uk/info/financial/iafees2006.pdf> (accessed 4 November 2007).

Brook, Kevin Alan. 2005. "Khazars and Judaism." In *The Encyclopedia of Judaism*, 2nd ed., vol. 2, eds. Jacob Neusner, Alan J. Avery-Peck and William Scott Green. Leiden, Netherlands: Brill Academic Publishers.

Carmeli, Yoram S. and Birenbaum-Carmeli, D. 2000. "Ritualizing the 'Natural Family': Secrecy in Israeli Donor Insemination." *Science as Culture* 9, no. 3: 301–25.

Central Bureau of Statistics. 2005. "Live Births: Selected Findings." http://www1.cbs.gov.il/reader/cw_usr_view_SHTML?ID=630 (accessed June 30, 2007).

Central Bureau of Statistics. 2007. "Table: Average Employee Monthly Salary". http://www.cbs.gov.il/yarhon/k4_h.htm (accessed November 13, 2007).

Child Welfare Information Gateway. 2004. "Costs of Adopting: Factsheet for Families." http://www.childwelfare.gov/pubs/s_cost/s_costb.cfm (accessed June 30, 2007).

Chinitz, D., Shalev, C., Galai, N., and Israeli A. 1998. "Israel's Basket of Health Services: the Importance of Being Explicitly Implicit." *British Medical Journal*317: 1005–7.

Collins, J. 2002. "An International Survey of the Health Economics of IVF and ICSI." *Human Reproduction Update*8, no. 3: 265–77.

Doron, A. and R.M. Kramer. 1991. *The Welfare State in Israel: The Evolution of Social Security Policy and Practice*. Boulder. Colorado: Westview Press.

Douglas, M. 1970 [1966]. Purity and Danger: *An Analysis of the Concepts of Pollution and Taboo*. London: Routledge & Kegan Paul.

Ekstein J. and H. Katzenstein. 2001. "The Dor Yeshorim Story: Community-based Carrier Screening for Tay-Sachs Disease." *Advances in Genetics* 44: 297–310.

Fisher, A.P. 2003. "Still 'Not Quite as Good as Having your Own?' Toward a Sociology of Adoption." *Annual Review of Sociology* 29: 335–61.

Fogiel-Bijaoui, S. 1999. "Families in Israel: Between Familism and Post-modernism." In *Sex, Gender, Politics: Women in Israel* [Hebrew], ed. A. Friedman. Tel Aviv: Hakibbutz Hameuchad.

General Register Office for Scotland. 2004. "Adoption Statistics." http://www.gro-scotland.gov.uk/press/news2004/03adopt-press.html (accessed November 4, 2007).

Glickman, A. 2003. "Marriage on the Verge of the 21st Century" [Hebrew]. *Deot Ba'am* no. 7.

Gold, M. 1988. *And Hannah Wept: Infertility, Adoption and the Jewish Couple.* Philadelphia: The Jewish Publication Society.

Hammer MF, Skorecki K, Selig S, Blazer S, Rappaport B, Bradman R, Bradman N, Warburton PJ, Ismajlowicz M. 1997. "Y Chromosomes of Jewish Priests." *Nature* 385: 32.

Haraway, Donna. 1997. *Modest_Witness@Second_Millennium.FemaleMan_ Meets_ OncoMouse: Feminism and Technoscience.* New York: Routledge.

Hasson, N. 2007. "Dead Soldier's Parents Allowed to Use his Sperm to Fertilize a Woman He Had Not Known." *Ha'aretz,* January 15.

Ifrah, A. ed. 1999. *"Women's Health in Israel 1999: A Data Book"* [Hebrew]. Hadassah, the Women's Zionist Organization of America, The Israel Women's Network, Israel Centre for Disease Control and Hadassah-Israel.

Jones, C. A. 2005. "Cost-effectiveness of the Single Embryo Transfer." Presentation given at the Reproductive Disruption Conference, Ann Arbour, Michigan.

Kahn, S.M. 1998. "Putting Jewish Wombs to Work: Israelis Confront New Reproductive Technologies." *Lilith,* 23, no. 2: 30–31.

Kahn, S.M. 1998. "Rabbis and Reproduction: The Uses of New Reproductive Technologies among Ultraorthodox Jews in Israel." Working Paper No. 3, HRIJW.

———. 2000. "Reproducing Jews: A Cultural Account of Assisted Conception in Israel." Durham and London: Duke University Press.

———. 2004. "Eggs and Wombs: The Origin of Jewishness." In *Kinship and Family: An Anthropological Reader,*eds. R. Parkin and L. Stone. Oxford: Blackwell.

———. 2005. "Are Genes Jewish? Conceptual Ambiguities in the New Genetic Age." Paper given at the Reproductive Disruption Conference, Ann Arbour, Michigan.

Katz, J. 1971. *Tradition and Crisis: Jewish Society at the End of the Middle Ages.* New York: Schoken Books.

Kislinger, Lara. N.D. "Inter-Country Adoption: A Brief Background and Case Study." http://www.adoptionpolicy.org/pdf/backgroundCS.pdf (accessed November 4, 2007).

Knesset Committee on Work, Welfare and Health. 2002. "Child Welfare Services (Adoption Services)" [Hebrew]. http://www.knesset.gov.il/ mmm/data/docs/m00231.rtf (accessed November 12, 2007).

Knesset Research and Information Center. 2003. "Inter-Country Adoption Background Report" [Hebrew]. http://www.knesset.gov.il/MMM/data/ docs/m00526.doc (accessed November 7, 2007).

Leach, E. 1969. "The Legitimacy of Solomon." In *Genesis as Myth and Other Essays,* ed. E. Leach. London: Jonathan Cape.

Lovelock. K. 2000. "Intercountry Adoption as a Migratory Practice: A Comparative Analysis of Intercountry Adoption and Immigration Policy and Practice in the United States, Canada and New Zealand in the Post WWII Period." *International Migration Review*34, no. 3: 907–949.

March, K., & Miall, C. 2000. "Adoption as a Family Form." *Family Relations*49, no. 4: 359–62.

Miall, C.E. 1996. "The Social Construction of Adoption: Clinical and Community Perspectives." *Family Relations*45, no. 3: 309–217.

Miller, N. 1992. *Single Parents by Choice: A Growing Trend in Family Life*. New York: Plenum Press.

Ministry of Health. 1999. *Health Status in Israel—1999*. Ramat Gan: Israel Centre for Disease Control.

———. 2005. *IVF Treatments: Absolute Numbers, Percentages, Medical Facilities and Equipment Licensing*. Jerusalem: Division and Department of Health Information.

Ministry of Labor and Welfare. n.d.a. "Inter-Country Adoption Statistics" [Hebrew].   http://www.molsa.gov.il/NR/rdonlyres/FB594336–596D-435B-87C7-CD4FB273CD24/3575/ישראליקוחצומיאמסינותנ.doc (accessed November 13, 2007).

Ministry of Labor and Welfare. n.d.b. "Single Pregnant Women" [Hebrew]. <http://www.molsa.gov.il/MisradHarevacha/Females/PregnantNotMarried/> (accessed 15 November, 2007).

Nachman, Michal. 2005. "'Ze Intimi': Reflections on Israeli Egg Donation in Israel." Paper given at the Reproductive Disruption Conference, Ann Arbour, Michigan.

National Council for the Child. 2006. "Children in Israel—2006." *Annual Statistical Bulletin* 3, no. 28. http://children.org.il/UploadPic/2006.doc (accessed on November 12, 2007).

Office of Public Sector Information. 2005. "The Adoption Support Services Regulations 2005". http://www.opsi.gov.uk/si/si2005/20050691.htm#8 (accessed November 4, 2007).

Ong, Aihwa. 2006. *Neoliberalism as Exception: Mutations in Citizenship and Sovereignty*. Durham and London: Duke University Press.

Ontario Ministry of Child and Youth Services. N.D. "Who Can Adopt in Ontario." http://www.children.gov.on.ca/mcys/english/programs/child/adoption/index.asp#who_can_adopt (accessed December 23, 2007).

Oppenheim A, Nebel A, Filon D, Thomas MG, Weiss DA, Weale M, and Faerman M. 2000. "High-resolution Y Chromosome Haplotypes of Israeli and Palestinian Arabs Reveal Geographic Substructure and Substantial Overlap with Haplotypes of Jews." *Human Genetics* 107, no. 6: 630–41.

Pashigian, Melissa J. 2009. "Inappropriate Relations: The Ban on Surrogacy with In Vitro Fertilization and the Limits of State Renovation in Contemporary Vietnam." In *Assisting Reproduction, Testing Genes: Global Encounters with New Biotechnologies*, eds. Daphna Birenbaum-Carmeli and Marcia C. Inhorn. Oxford and New York: Berghahn Books.

Perets, Y. and Katz, R. 1981. "The Family in Israel: Change and Continuity" [Hebrew]. In *Families in Israel*, eds. R. Bar-Yosef and L. Shamgar-Handelman. Jerusalem: Academon.

Political Council for GLBT Rights in Israel. 2003. "Political Parties' Agenda" [Hebrew]. http://www.geocities.com/pcgri/chapter7.html (accessed November 13, 2007).

Portugese, J. 1998. *Fertility Policy in Israel: The Politics of Religion, Gender and Nation*. Westport, Connecticut: Praeger.

Ritterband, Paul. 1995. "Modern Times and Jewish Assimilation". In *The Americanization of the Jews*, eds. Robert M. Seltzer and Norman J. Cohen. New York: New York University Press.

Rose N. and Carlos Novas. 2005. "Biological Citizenship." In *Global Assemblages: Technology, Politics and Ethics as Anthropological Problems*, eds. Aihwa Ong and Stephen Collier. Oxford: Blackwell.

Roberts, E. Forthcoming. "The Traffic Between Women: Female Alliance and Familial Egg Donation in Ecuador." In *Assisting Reproduction, Testing Genes: Global Encounters with New Biotechnologies*, eds. Daphna Birenbaum-Carmeli and Marcia C. Inhorn. Oxford and New York: Berghahn Books.

Rosenzweig, F. 1971 [1930]. *The Star of Redemption*. London: Routledge and Kegan Paul.

Safir, M. P. 1986. "Religion, Tradition and Public Policy Give Family First Priority." In *Calling the Equality Bluff*, eds. B. Swirski. and M. P. Safir. New York: Pergamon.

Schenker, J.G. 2003. "Ethical Aspects of Advanced Reproductive Technologies." *Annals New York Academy of Science* 997: 11–21. <http://www.nyas.org/pdfs/v997_11.pdf>. (accessed on November 25, 2007).

Selman, P. 2002. "Intercountry Adoption in the New Millennium: the 'Quiet Migration' Revisited." *Population Research and Policy Review* 21: 205–25.

Sered, S. 2000. *What Makes Women Sick: Maternity, Modesty and Militarism in Israeli Society*. Hanover and London: Brandeis University Press.

Shalev, C., & B. Lev. 1999. "Public Funding for IVF in Israel—Ethical Aspects."Working paper.

Shepard, Jonathan. 1998. "The Khazars' Formal Adoption of Judaism and Byzantium's Northern Policy." *Oxford Slavonic Papers, New Series*31: 11–34.

Shokeid, M. 1999. "The Emergence of Supernatural Explanations for Male Barenness among Morroccan Immigrants." In *The Predicament of Homecoming*, eds. S. Deshen and M. Shokeid. Ithaca: Cornell University Press.

Shore, C. & Wright, S. 1997. "Policy: A New Field of Anthropology." In *Anthropology of Policy: Critical Perspectives on Governance and Power*, eds. C. Shore and S. Wright. London: Routledge.

Shtal, A. 1999. *Family and Childrearing in Oriental Judaism*. Jerusalem: Academon Press.

Statistics Canada. 2006. "General Social Survey: Navigating Family Transitions." http://www.statcan.ca/Daily/English/070613/d070613b.htm (accessed November 4, 2007).

Stern Z., N. Laufer, R. Levy, D. Ben-Shushan, S. Mor-Yosef. 1995. "Cost Analysis of In Vitro Fertilization." *Israel Journal of Medical Science*31: 492–96.

Stolley, Kathy S. 1993. "Statistics on Adoption in the United States." *The Future of Children*3, no. 1 (Adoption): 26–42.

Struewing, J. P., P. Hartge, S. Wachholder, S. M. Baker, M. Berlin, M. McAdams, M. M. Timmerman, L. C. Brody, and M. A. Tucker. 1997. "The Risk of Cancer Associated with Specific Mutations of BRCA1 and BRCA2 among Ashkenazi Jews." *The New England Journal of Medicine* 15, 336, no. 20 :1401–08.

Swirski, S. 1976. "Community and the Meaning of the Modern State: The Case of Israel." *The Jewish Journal of Sociology* 18: 123–40.

Swirski, S., E. Konor-Attias, B. Swirski, and Y. Yecheskel. 2001. *Women in the Labor Force of the Israeli Welfare State* [Hebrew]. Tel Aviv: Adva Centre.

Teman, Elly. 2006. "The Birth of a Mother: Mythologies of Surrogate Motherhood in Israel" (PhD dissertation, Department of Sociology and Social Anthropology, Hebrew University of Jerusalem).

Thomas, Mark G., Michael E. Weale, Abigail L. Jones, Martin Richards, Karl Skorecki, Antonio Torroni, Rosaria Scozzari, Fiona Gratrix, Ayele Tarekegn, James F. Wilson, Cristian Capelli, Neil Bradman, and David B. Goldstein. 2002. "Founding Mothers of Jewish Communities: Geographically Separated Jewish Groups were Independently Founded by Very Few Female Ancestors." *American Journal of Human Genetics* 70: 1411–20.

U.S Department of State. 2006. "Intercountry Adoption." http://travel.state. gov/family/adoption/intercountry/intercountry_473.html (accessed 30 June, 2007).

Wolpe, P.R. 1997. "If I am Only My Genes, What am I? Genetic Essentialism and a Jewish Response." *Kennedy Institute of Ethics Journal* 7: 213–30.

Zwebner, Sarah. 2003. Inter-Country Adoption: Background Material for a Knesset Discussion." Ministry of Social Affairs and Social Services. http://www.knesset.gov.il/mmm/data/docs/m00526.doc (accessed on November 7, 2007).

Part II

Gene:
Reproductive Technologies and the Quest for the Perfect Child

Chapter 6

Genetic Testing and Screening in Religious Groups: Perspectives of Jewish *Haredi* Communities[1]

Barbara Prainsack and Gil Sigal

Introduction

Genetic testing and screening in Israel

The uptake of genetic testing varies greatly between occidental nations. Some countries, such as Germany (e.g., see German National Ethics Council 2003) are somewhat reluctant to engage with the full array of genetic possibilities, while other societies are more inclined to exploit genetic knowledge (see also Wertz 1994–1995; The Nuffield Council on Bioethics 2006; Hashiloni-Dolev 2007).

In Israel, genetic testing and screening[2] is used in various contexts. Similarly to most countries, its use extends to prenatal and neonatal diagnosis, genetic counseling services, HLA for tissue typing, paternity testing, and use in criminal forensics (identification of victims, their remains, or crime perpetrators). Genetic testing is relatively widely and intensely embraced in Israel as well as in Jewish communities in the Diaspora (Green et al 2006; Nuffield Council on Bioethics 2006). Furthermore, voices of non-governmental organizations (NGOs) and disability rights groups expressing skepticism towards genetic testing are virtually absent in Israel (Raz 2004, 2005;

Hashiloni-Dolev 2007; Lori 2003), rendering it a relatively unusual case within the range of the world's wealthy nations.

Medical genetics and genetic counseling is a recognized sub-specialty in Israel; the 2001 Genetic Information Law[3] grants its practitioners exclusive authorization to provide genetic counseling. Currently, fourteen clinical genetic centers serve a population of seven million (Efron 2007), implementing a broad range of partly subsidized screening policies for various population sectors (Zlotogora and Leventhal 2000; Gross 2002; Zlotogora and Chemke 1995; Broide et al. 1993; Shahrabani-Gargir et al. 1998). Current population screening programs include Fragile X, Cystic Fibrosis, Gaucher and Canavan disease, Bloom syndrome, Fanconi anemia types B and A, Familial Dysautonomia, Mucolipidosis type IV, and recently also for Usher syndrome type I, Glycogen storage disease type I, Nieman-Pick type A, SMA, Alfa-1 Antitripsin, and several others (Hashiloni-Dolev 2007).

Most genetic screening programs revolve around reproduction; at the core of those are screening policies aiming at the detection of embryos affected by one of the aforementioned conditions. Women or couples could decide to abort such affected embryos (abortions require an approval by a medical committee in Israel), or, in case embryos have been diagnosed *ex-utero* (in the course of pre-implantation genetic diagnosis [PGD]), they could choose non-affected embryo(s) for implantation. Many genetic tests are not covered by national health insurance; many patients are willing to pay significant amounts of money for these services. There is large societal consensus on the benefits of a wide array of perinatal genetic tests (Hashiloni-Dolev 2007; Kahn 2000).

One explanation for a favourable attitude towards genetics in this population rests on the high prevalence of genetic diseases resulting from high rate of endogamy within Ashkenazi-Jewish communities.[4] Besides this "technical" explanation, the utilization of science and technology in general, and genetics in particular, in the context of procreation is seen by most as entirely compatible with Jewish values; many also regard it as part of the ethos of Jewish societies. This ethos, which emphasizes reproduction as a religious obligation, is also shared by the non-Orthodox Jewish majority in Israel—a majority that makes relatively intense use of perinatal genetic testing and screening (Hashiloni-Dolev 2007; Sher et al. 2003).

It has been argued that the Zionist heritage of the country accounts for the generally relatively positive view of science and technology, which also includes medical technologies (Efron 2007). In addition, it has also been argued that the relatively positive attitude towards genetic testing in Israel must also be seen within a larger cultural context where physical health and fitness are defined according to relatively narrow criteria, and this context can lead to a narrow contemporary understanding of what a "healthy" newborn should be (Weiss 2002; Hashiloni-Dolev 2007).

Haredi Jews and reproductive/genetic technologies

It has been recognized that for a variety of reasons the population of *Haredi* (sometimes also referred to as "ultra-Orthodox") Jews in Israel represents a special case with regard to their increased use of genetic tests. The group of *Haredim* (pl. of *Haredi* ["fearful," or "anxious"]; more adequately translated as "trembling in the awe of God" [see Isaiah 66: 2, 5]) is comprised of Jews who believe that *Halachah* (Jewish Law) should be observed literally and who reject any progressive interpretation of it. Jewish Law encompasses every practice of daily life, and the *Haredim* feel that it should be strictly adhered to.[5] The founders of today's *Haredi* movements are seen as those who resisted attempts to "reform" Judaism in 18th century Europe.

Apart from these generalized observations, it is difficult to define what constitutes *Haredi* Judaism. Therefore, it might be more helpful to list a number of characteristics applying to most *Haredi* Jews in order to understand what distinguishes *Haredim* from other Jewish groups in Israel. To begin with, most *Haredim* live in tightly knit communities separated from the non-*Haredi* world. The lives of many *Haredi* Jews revolve around Torah study (for males), prayer, and family and community involvement. Much attention is devoted to the religious and moral education of new generations, and to the promotion of modesty in behaviour and clothing. The *Haredi* understanding of modesty necessitates the separation of genders in most settings outside of the family. Also within the family and among married partners, matters of love, sexuality, and procreation are framed by *Halachah*, and are not discussed in the same manner as among most non-Orthodox Jews. Young *Haredim* are exempt from military service in Israel as long as they commit to *Yeshiva* studies. The use of modern technology, such as cell phones, Internet, and other mass media, is usually restricted to business or controlled use; emphasis is placed on disabling the features of modern life which could expose the *Haredi* individual to morally compromising contents and materials.[6] In respect to the use of technology, a general rule is that whatever fosters the observance of commandments and does not conflict with other commandments or *Halachic* prohibitions will be accepted in *Haredi* communities (see also Berger 2005). Likewise, the use of medical technologies is guided by this rationale.[7] Due to the great importance vested in reproduction—it is seen by many as one of the most important commandments of the Torah—the use of medical technologies to facilitate reproduction is generally regarded very positively by *Halachic* authorities. (Again, as long as there is no conflict of the particularities of their use with other *Halachic* provisions.)

With regard to genetic testing, there are a number of possible *Halachic* complications. The avoidance of human suffering (such as the birth of a child with a life-threatening genetic disorder) is generally seen as desirable goal. However, "traditional" genetic prenatal testing is not deemed acceptable for most *Haredim* because of the religious prohibition on abortion unless the life and/or health of the potential mother are in danger. In addition, premarital genetic testing (testing the carrier status of individuals for particular genetic disorders) is most often not feasible because of the possible detrimental impact on family members in a society where arranged marriages are the norm. Knowing that a member of a particular family is a carrier for a severe inheritable genetic disorder could stigmatize the entire family and therefore decrease marriage prospects for all unmarried members of the family (see Prainsack and Siegal 2006). These beforementioned characteristics constitute the infrastructure that explains the establishment and warm acceptance of the Dor Yeshorim (DY) genetic screening initiative, the focus of our research.

What has not received much scholarly attention so far are the perspectives of the addressees of the DY initiative (and other projects targeting the *Haredi* population). Therefore, our study aims to explore the attitudes of *Haredi* men and women towards genetic testing in general and DY in particular. As (to the best of our knowledge) this is the first empirical study on this topic, we lack data that would embed our findings in a comparative context; further research in this field would be highly desirable.

Kehilah ("community"), family, and the concept of "genetic couplehood"

In previous work (Prainsack and Siegal 2006) on the topic of genetic testing in the *Haredi* context we argued that the embrace of premarital genetic testing in these communities is rooted in distinct conceptions of risks and benefits, and of what constitutes permissible intervention. We reasoned that the particular ways of performing genetic tests in the *Haredi* population create a unique understanding of genetic responsibility which bypasses the level of the individual. We coined the term "genetic couplehood" to describe a genetic identity which is seen as a "joint fate" of a couple as opposed to the awareness of genetic "risks" and "advantages" at the level of the single individual.

In the following section, we will outline the core characteristics of the concept of genetic couplehood in the context of the Dor Yeshorim preconception genetic testing initiative.

The Dor Yeshorim premarital genetic testing initiative

Founded in the early 1980s, DY today operates in Orthodox Jewish communities in Israel, the United States, and some European countries (such as the U.K.). Since its founding, DY has tested more than 200,000 men and women. Over the years, DY's panel of genetic tests has become a standard step in the matching process (*Shiduch*) within these communities (Ekstein and Katzenstein 2001; Broide et al. 1993; Zlotogora and Leventhal 2000; Cowley et al. 1990; Bach et al. 2001). Most importantly, the birth rate of afflicted children has dropped to near zero in screened couples.

DY has been set up as a *preconception* (in this case, premarital) genetic testing program designed to discourage the marriage of carrier couples who would face a high risk (25 percent in the case of autosomal recessive genetic diseases such as Tay-Sachs[8]) of any of their children being affected by a particular genetic disease. DY targets young adults in *Haredi* communities, where blood samples are taken in religious high schools and *Yeshivas* (parents give informed consent in the place of minors). All tested individuals receive an identification number and are encouraged to call DY and check their "genetic compatibility" with their potential spouse at the time of a proposed match. DY tests for carrier status on a set of genetic diseases consisting of autosomal-recessive and fatal or severely debilitating conditions.[9] The founder of the DY initiative, Brooklyn-based Rabbi Joseph Ekstein, has determined the criteria for incorporating new screened-for diseases to include only recessive diseases with significant morbidity and/or mortality, where premarital genetic knowledge would prevent an undesired match but not preclude procreation altogether. Therefore, DY does not, for example, test for a disease such as Fragile X syndrome where the carrier mother would present the same 50 percent chance of transmission with all her potential spouses. As it is unusual for *Haredi* couples to go through a "dating" period prior to marriage, participating families and communities see the dissolution of marriage plans in case of "genetic incompatibility" as an acceptable option.

As we emphasized elsewhere (Prainsack and Siegal 2006), DY does not aim to create an individual health care delivery interaction. It intends to avoid a patient/consumer-provider relationship with its inherent legal and ethical responsibilities and liabilities. At the time of the test, neither the tested individuals nor their families receive information about the results, in order to prevent stigmatization, discrimination, and the burden of "useless" genetic knowledge for carriers. As carrier status becomes relevant only when two carriers of the same recessive disease plan to marry, it is only then that DY provides counseling, and only in cases in which both potential partners are carriers for the same genetic disease. (Put differently, tested individuals are not informed of what genetic conditions they are carriers for, unless a potential couple are *both* carriers for *the same* autosomal recessive genetic condition.) The counseling itself is free, provided anonymously, and only over the phone. Due to the fact that DY is usually consulted very early in the process of arranging a potential marriage, virtually all marriage plans of "genetically in-compatible" individuals are cancelled. (Also, DY requires individuals to declare that they are not already engaged prior to requesting a genetic compatibility check.) Instead, the young man and the young woman (and/or their families) orient themselves towards other pos-sible partners with whom the risk of carrying the same genetic dis-ease is statistically very low. Stigmatization of "carrier families" is usually successfully avoided due to the discretion of involved par-ties, as well as due to the early timing of the DY consultation in the matchmaking process. Most importantly, DY adheres to strict confi-dentiality and prevents any information leak, even to the degree of not sharing carrier status with tested individuals.

DY does not keep records on the fate of "incompatible couples." Given the religious objection to abortions and the obligation to pro-create in the Jewish religion, however, the community considers avoiding the union in the first place as a sound choice. Couples who are determined to marry despite double carrier status for the same genetic disease are likely to face significant resistance from their families and allegedly also from their Rabbis (see Chen 2001; DY rejects the claim that such rabbinical stances are practiced).

Indeed, despite the absence of binding measures, compliance with DY's policies in *Haredi* communities is very high. (As DY does not target the non-*Haredi* sector, where marriages are not arranged, "tra-ditional" preconception carrier testing instead of the DY method is used in large parts of the modern-Orthodox as well as the "secular"[10] sectors.) Resistant at first, prominent rabbis of *Haredi* communities have eventually (and gradually) endorsed DY premarital genetic testing by issuing public and personal religious rulings. Opponents of the program are mainly found in the modern-Orthodox sector of the Jewish community, including Rabbi Tendler from Yeshiva University in New York City. His criticism is leveled against the applicability of premarital genetic testing in communities where arranged marriages are uncommon, and against withholding information on the carrier status of tested individuals (Rosen 2003).

In addition to DY's effectiveness in preventing the stigmatization of "carrier families," its success is of course conditioned by the aforementioned *Haredi* rejection of abortion in all cases where the life or health of the potential mother is not in danger. Attempts to preclude a need for abortion are therefore viewed favorably. In addition, ensuring that the offspring of a couple will be healthy (and thereby supposedly reducing suffering for all parties involved) is seen not as a selfish objective but rather as part of the fulfilment of the Biblical commandment to "go forth and multiply." No conflicting religious rulings prohibit attempts to assure this commandment's successful, disease-free completion. As we argued elsewhere (Prainsack and Siegal 2006: 26):

> In Judaism, the betterment of God's creation entails the lasting commitment of every generation to actively seek to improve their conditions of life, to fight existing imperfections such as maladies (. . .) and to fulfil the Biblical commandment: "Conquer the land and subdue it." The concept of using genetic testing and genetic matching programs to avoid the affliction of newborns with diseases has suffused Jewish culture for many years.

Hence, premarital (preconception) interventions are commonly regarded as legitimate tools to improve the chances of having genetically healthy[11] offspring.

Risk as a relational category

Relating to discussions of the geneticization/somaticization of identities in the genomic and post-genomic era (Brown and Webster 2004; Collins et al. 2003; Franklin 2000; Conrad and Gabe 1999; Petersen 1999; Rabinow 1999; Lippman 1991), in our 2006 paper we argued that DY fosters the establishment of an interesting alternative to "somatic selfhood" (Rose 2001: 18). In the context of DY, genetic responsibility is not primarily tied to the individual but to the couple. In cases of conventional carrier screening in non-*Haredi* populations, we can assume that the tested subjects usually have established senses of their "genetic selves" prior to taking the genetic tests, and also confront risks for diseases in the framework of these programs individually (see Novas and Rose 2000; Lemke 2002). Thus, even though the genetic makeup of a person may become *relevant* only in connection with his or her partner carrying the same autosomal-recessive disorder, the person is usually still constructed as an independent "genetic individual" due to his or her knowledge of individual carrier status. Strong exposure to media and public conceptions accentuating genetics as a "personal future diary," or of genes being "responsible" for one's fitness, health, and attractiveness also add to the formation of this "genetic self."

In conventional preconception testing programs, genetic "risk" is inscribed in the individual. If, for example, a woman gets tested to find out whether she is a carrier for an autosomal-recessive genetic disorder that renders her at risk to pass on this "faulty gene" to her offspring, risk is defined in individual terms. Furthermore, individuals who, after undergoing a genetic test, are established as belonging to a "risk group" cannot entirely get rid of this status; they may be able, however, to alleviate it by making "responsible" decisions (such as deciding to undergo mastectomy, or deciding to undergo prenatal testing when two carriers of the same autosomal recessive genetic disorder procreate together). Despite her efforts to engage in "responsible" behavior and reduce "her risks," however, the person in question will always remain part of the genetically determined "risk group." In the context of DY, on the other hand, genetic risk is conceived as absent if the potential match is found out to be "compatible." Individuals are never told their individual carrier status. The "rational" thing to do in the case of an "unadvisable match" (again, without the concerned individuals being informed about the condition[s] for which they are both carriers) is consequently not to look for options to uphold the marriage plans but rather to enter an "advisable" matching situation, where there is no presence of genetic risk. The medical and societal imperative to control and manage one's health and procreate in a responsible manner (see Atkin and Ahmad 1998: 448) rests upon the individual as much as it rests upon the joint shoulders of a prospective couple. Here, risk is a relational concept; consideration of one's "genetic body" is only manifest and relevant once it is seen in conjunction with another individual. As we have argued (Prainsack and Siegal 2006), in the framework of DY, the "medicalization of spouse selection," as Raz and Atar (2004) termed it, turns into a medicalization *through* spouse selection. In *Haredi* communities, where "genetic screening [. . .] is somewhat de-medicalized and linked to marriage arrangements, rather than prenatal care" (Rapp 1999: 170; see also Sher et al. 2003), the "geneticization" of a person's identity is not likely to arise independently of the field of matchmaking and reproduction. Individuals conceive of themselves as inseparable parts of a couple/family and a community for whose sake they live and procreate "well."

In summary, DY's genetic panel has become the "gold standard" in *Haredi* communities within only one decade. This astonishing phenomenon can be explained by several particular features of these communities such as a strong focus on communal values, strong intercommunity bonding and solidarity, the embrace of reproductive technology, and the power of religious authorities.

While we and others have studied the operation and rationales of DY (Prainsack & Siegal 2006), knowledge and attitudes of the target group of DY, *Haredi* Jews, towards genetic testing (especially premarital genetic testing) have not received considerable scholarly attention so far. What accounts for the (virtually) comprehensive uptake of DY testing in *Haredi* communities?

In order to shed light on this question, we carried out a (self-administered) survey of 182 Israeli first- and second-year law students from the *Haredi* sector. Our findings, which will be presented and discussed in the following section, show that a) with the exception of DY, both knowledge about, and the uptake of, genetic testing services in the studied group is relatively limited; b) DY is perceived primarily not as a medical but as a social institution embedded in the process of matchmaking; and c) DY is perceived by the majority of our respondents as a beneficial institution which should be improved further. This overall very positive evaluation of DY by our respondents could be interpreted as corresponding with dominant values within their communities, such as a focus on the well being of the family and the community (*kehilah*) rather than of the individual. These prevalent values might have served as a reference point for many (if not all) of our interviewees. As we will argue in the conclusion, however, this should not be interpreted as a denial of individuality but rather as a situation in which the individual is not typically conceived and conceptualized as independent of his or her familial and community relations.

Experiences and attitudes towards genetic testing among Haredi Jews

We composed a questionnaire containing closed and open questions on experiences with and attitudes towards genetic testing in general and towards DY in particular. The questionnaire (in

Hebrew) was distributed to *Haredi* first- and second-year law students. As it is relatively unusual for members of *Haredi* communities to devote large portions of their time to the study of secular subjects, these law students study in a unique academic setting which meets the religious requirements of *Haredi* Jews. (For example, males and females study on separate weekdays; lecturers are of the same gender as their students; and formal dress codes are enforced.) The program is situated at the Ono Academic College near Tel Aviv.

Questionnaires were distributed in class after a brief explanation of the purpose of the study and its technicalities (mainly, the protection of anonymity). Answers to closed and quantifiable questions were analyzed using SAS software (version 9.1). Answers to open questions were grouped and coded accordingly.

The demographic parameters within the group of our respondents can be described as follows (see table 10): The majority (62 percent[12]) of our respondents were male. Respondents were between 19 and 67 years old (median 27); 57 percent were married, 41 percent were unmarried, and 2 percent were divorced. Fifty-two percent already had children (1 to 10 children; median 3.3).

Eighty-seven percent of our respondents were born in Israel; 3 percent in Morocco, 3 percent in France, and 1 percent were born in Tunisia and Switzerland respectively. Forty percent of our respondents had Israel-born parents; 30 percent had parents born in Morocco, Lebanon, Iraq, Iran, Yemen, or Tunisia; and 20 percent had parents from Eastern or Western Europe (Ashkenazi). Parents of the remaining 10 percent were born in other countries.

Table 10 Demographic Parameters (in %)

Age: 19–67 [median 27]						
Male	Female	married	unmarried	divorced	children	no children
62	38	57	41	2	52	48
						[1-10; mean 3.3]
born in	Israel	Morocco	France		Tunisia	Switzerland
	87	3	3		1	1
Parents' birth place	Israel	The Levant	Eastern & Western Europe [Ashkenazi]		other countries	
	40	30	20		10	

Compared with the general Jewish population in Israel, and with *Haredi* Jews in Israel in particular, Israel-born individuals are overrepresented among our respondents (87 percent in our sample compared to about 68 percent of the total population in Israel, and about 44 percent of *Haredi* Jews in Israel), while immigrants from Europe and the Americas are underrepresented (4 percent of our respondents compared to about 22 percent of the total Jewish population in Israel, and about 17 percent of *Haredi* Jews in Israel [see Israeli Central Bureau of Statistics 2005]; the proportions might vary according to different age groups; however, age-based data for comparison could not be obtained).

i. Knowledge and practices

When asked whether they had any knowledge about any genetic condition, only 8 percent answered that they were aware of such a problem, whereas 90 percent said that they were not (See table 11). When asked to name organizations providing genetic testing services, 42 percent of our respondents mentioned only DY. Another 8 percent were familiar with DY as well as other programs. Fifty-one percent did not indicate any organization providing genetic services.

Seventy percent said that neither they nor any of their family members had ever been referred to genetic counseling; 27 percent said that they (or their family members) had been referred; and 3 percent did not respond to this item.

Forty percent of our respondents reported that either they (27 percent) or a close family member (13 percent) had undergone genetic testing. The main reasons for performing genetic tests had been pre-marital/Dor Yeshorim testing (27 percent, equal to 67 percent of those who had a genetic test) and genetic tests during pregnancy (6 percent, equal to 16 percent of those who had a genetic test). Fifty-seven percent said that they, or their family members, had never had a genetic test, and 3 percent did not answer. Very few respondents provided reasons for not performing recommended genetic tests: only 5 percent of our respondents did so. Among the reasons given were religious convictions (3 cases, equalling 2 percent), and tests being too costly (2 cases, equalling 1 percent).

When asked specifically whether they knew DY, 59 percent of our respondents answered in the affirmative.[13] When respondents were asked to write down, in their own words, what DY was, the majority (44 percent, equal to 74 percent who said that they were familiar with DY) wrote words to the effect that DY belongs in the realm of genetics for the purpose of matching couples. Five percent (equal to 8 percent of those who were familiar with DY) said that DY's mission was to detect diseases in general; 10 percent (equal to 17 percent of those who knew DY) provided miscellaneous answers. Forty-one percent left the space for answers blank, and one answer was illegible.

Consequently, although we lack concrete comparative data regarding familiarity with genetic testing institutions in general and DY in particular, we can conclude that knowledge with regard to both seems to be relatively low. Nevertheless, those who knew DY saw it as relatively positive: When asked what respondents would change in DY's form of activity if they could, and why they would do so, 29 percent provided an answer: 10 percent (equal to 34 percent of those who answered this question) said that it should have more publicity; 7 percent (equal to 23 percent of those who provided answers) said that it should produce faster results; 3 percent (10 percent of those who answered) said it should cost less.

Table 11 Knowledge and Practices (in %)

Familiar only with DY	42
Familiar with DY and other programmes	8
Did not indicate any organization that provides genetic services	51
They or their family members were referred to genetic counselling	27
Neither they nor one of their family members were were ever referred to genetic counselling	70
Have had a genetic test	40
themselves	27
immediate family members	13
Main reasons for performing genetic tests:	
premarital/Dor Yeshorim testing	27
genetic tests during pregnancy	6
They (or their family members) never had a genetic test	57
Familiarity with DY:	
Familiarity with DY	59
Description of DY's role:	
DY belongs in the realm of genetics for the purpose of matching couples	44
DY's mission is to detect diseases in general	5
various answers	10

Percentages might not add up to 100 due to rounding

ii. Attitudes

Respondents were given four statements and asked to indicate their agreement or disagreement on a 4-point scale (1 = "strongly agree", 4 = "strongly disagree," and an additional option was "don't know") regarding genetic testing in general and DY in particular.

Eighty-five percent agreed, or strongly agreed, with the statement that "extending the use of genetic testing is a positive thing" (64 percent strongly), while only 4 percent disagreed (2 percent strongly). Seven percent said that they did not know, and 4 percent did not answer.

In the same vein, the vast majority of our respondents rejected (62 percent; 34 percent strongly) the statement that "DY is a project which limits self-determination and free choice"; only 9 percent agreed (3 percent strongly). Twenty-three percent said that they did not know, and 7 percent refrained from answering.

Most did not accept the claim that "genetic tests are an instance of wrongful interference with creation": Seventy-six percent disagreed (36 percent strongly), while only 9 percent agreed (3 percent strongly). Nine percent did not know, and 6 percent did not provide an answer.

More than half (53 percent) agreed that "DY has a positive impact on my community" (34 percent agreed strongly), while 5 percent said that it did not (2 percent strongly). However, a considerable number of respondents (32 percent) said that they did not know, and 9 percent chose not to answer.

Table 12 Attitudes towards genetic testing in general and DY in particular (in %)

Statement	strongly agree	agree	disagree	strongly disagree	don't know	no answer
(a) Extending the use of genetic testing is a positive thing	64	21	2	2	7	4
(b) DY is a project which limits self-determination and free choice	3	6	28	34	23	7
(c) Genetic tests are an instance of wrongful interference with creation	3	6	40	36	9	6
(d) DY has a positive impact on my community	34	19	3	2	32	9

Percentages might not add up to 100 due to rounding

Discussion and concluding remarks

The diverse embrace of novel medical technologies by different societies reflects particular concepts of benefits, risks, and responsibilities. It is also a result of varying levels of the public's level of
education, awareness, concerns, and existing incentives/disincen-
tives (see Prainsack and Hashiloni-Dolev 2009). The high uptake of
perinatal tests in Jewish populations has been noticed before, and
the DY program operating within *Haredi* communities represents a
special case.

The intuition that Jewish Orthodoxy is inversely related to usage
of novel technology seems accurate at first. However, DY successfully displays a way to surmount such hesitancy once the underlying
paradigms of a specific cultural and religious group are identified and
mitigated (Bowen et al. 2003). In DY's operation, the following te-
nets were incorporated: strict confidentiality (to protect families and
individuals from stigmatization and negatively influencing their marriage prospects); diminished reliance on prenatal diagnosis and painful agony surrounding abortions; and a social compact allowing the
relinquishing of personal information (carrier status) for the benefit
of future couplehood and reproduction of the prospective couple.

Our survey of potential and actual participants in DY's premarital genetic screening program provides several interesting (although
preliminary) insights into this unique and under-recognized and
often-stereotyped population.

As expected, we found relatively poor knowledge with respect
to genetics in general and to genetic services in particular: When
asked to list organizations providing genetic testing, 42 percent of
our respondents mentioned only DY, while only 8 percent were familiar with DY and other genetic testing services. This means that
despite their high level of education, only half of our respondents
listed *any* organization providing genetic testing services. Although
there is no data which would allow a direct comparison, we assume
that this result stands in contrast to the non-Orthodox population
in Israel, which seems to be very well aware of its availability and
potential uses (see Hashiloni-Dolev 2007). While the relatively poor
knowledge of genetic testing services in the group we studied can
possibly be explained by the general lack of medical knowledge
about genetic testing, the high level of familiarity with DY and its
function within the group we studied could be explained by the
way DY is viewed and appropriated by its addressees: It is organized
and seen less as a medical service provider but rather as a beneficial social institution that complements (and perfects) the process of

matchmaking and helps to avoid pain and suffering. Undergoing DY genetic testing requires very little "technical" knowledge but rather ample trust. Making a socially responsible decision is the requirement, and the genetic discourse is just the backdrop. Consequently, knowledge about DY seems to be regarded as social rather than genetic knowledge.

The majority of our respondents (57 percent) were unaware of any "genetic" test they or their family members have performed, which is a very high figure if one takes into account the entire array of possible genetic tests in modern medicine. The fact that in our surveyed population 57 percent were married and 52 percent already had children renders them very likely to have been exposed to offers for genetic tests for conditions such as Tay-Sachs or Down Syndrome (see, for example, Sher et al. 2003). Respondents who said that either they or their family members had undergone genetic testing associated it primarily with DY or perinatal tests, again accentuating the perceived role of genetics mainly for reproduction. Indeed, this may add to our understanding of why 85 percent of our respondents thought that extending genetic tests was a positive thing. Evidence from other studies suggests that other societies hold stronger reservations, usually considering possible negative effects of extended genetic testing such as genetic discrimination in employment or insurance (see, for example, Catz et al. 2005). Similarly, most of our respondents rejected the "playing God" notion in respect to genetics, a notion that is not part of the Jewish ethos (Barilan and Siegal 2005). In our survey, the majority regarded DY as a positive development benefiting their communities.

The points of criticism expressed by our respondents were constructive—they pertain to various operational elements of DY (the need for more publicity, lower costs, and faster results). No objections to DY's overall rationale and/or justifications were articulated. This acceptance is a direct demonstration of DY's remarkable acceptance within the *Haredi* community, having become an inherent part in the matchmaking process for the majority of *Haredi* couples-to-be.

A possible interpretation regarding the high uptake in *Haredi* communities could be that individuals take part mainly due to social pressure. The results of our study, however, lend themselves to the interpretation that the positive attitude towards DY stems from a positive perception of the impact of genetic testing in improving the chances of disease-free procreation. In this light, DY is primarily seen as a social and not a medical institution.

Nevertheless, a large portion of our respondents (30 percent) did not answer the question about whether DY limits self-determination and free choice, while an additional 10 percent thought that it does limit those two capacities. Forty-one percent did not know or did not answer the question on whether DY has a positive impact on their community. It could be argued that the relatively high percentage of respondents in this category is due to problems with understanding the question. This, however, is relatively unlikely to apply to the particular group of respondents in our study. Law students are familiar with terms and concepts of individual freedom, self-determination, and personal choice, even if they live in a community that emphasizes communal values and solidarity. Therefore, the relatively large percentage of non-responses to this question could also be a reflection of a significant portion within the *Haredi* community questioning the dominant "social order" in the community, which in turn could be a result of the selection bias of our survey: Our respondents, although they are *Haredi* Jews, study in an academic program towards a law degree, which is unusual in the sense that they do not devote their entire time to Torah studies or family duties and are exposed to Western legal norms such as autonomy, liberalism, and human rights. If this assessment is plausible, it may point to possible fragmentation of the community we have discussed. On the other hand, it may also be considered as indicating that other segments of *Haredi* population hold even more positive views of DY than the participants in our survey. As we currently have no possible way to validate either explanation on the basis of the material available to us, we call for further research on this aspect.

Another limitation of our survey is an overrepresentation of respondents from one geographical area: Thirty percent of our respondents were non-Ashkenazi Jews (that is, in the case of our respondents, of North African, Lebanese, Iraqi, or Iranian origin). This could be relevant for the interpretation of our results in the sense that diseases targeted by DY are commonly considered to be more prevalent in Ashkenazi Jews. In addition, Ashkenazi Jews are regarded as the most technology-driven subpopulation within the *Haredi* communities, and overall they participate more readily in health promotion initiatives. Further studies will be necessary to determine whether our results can be generalized to the *Haredi* population.

The current study, however, also draws attention to a bias of the prevalent individual-based bioethical approach which conceptualizes humans primarily (and sometimes only) as individuals whose individual autonomy needs to be protected (Beauchamp and Childress 1979; for the implications of this view on public health genetics, see Dabrock 2006). Following this line of reasoning, it can be the case in some instances that another value outweighs individual autonomy and leads to its (justified) infringement; this argument cannot escape, however, a conflictual and antagonistic depiction of individual vs. common interests. What we encounter in this study of attitudes among *Haredi* communities, on the other hand, is the inconceivability of any individual interest detached from the wellbeing of the person embedded in his or her "couplehood," family, and community. Therefore, what is seen as positive for those entities is perceived by the person as positive for him or herself. Without being deterministic of all actions and convictions, the values of the community are adopted by people into their own individual life choices.

Notes

1. The description and analysis of the "Dor Yeshorim" initiative in the first part of this chapter draws heavily upon a previous article published in *BioSocieties* (see Prainsack & Siegal 2006). The authors are grateful to the editors and publishers of *BioSocieties* for their kind permission to include parts of the article in this chapter. In addition, we thank Yoram Carmeli, Daphna Birenbaum-Carmeli, and Shiri Shkedi for very helpful comments on this manuscript.

2. Our use of the terms "genetic testing" and "genetic screening" is in accordance with the UNESCO *International Declaration on Human Genetic Data* (2003). Art. 2xii of this declaration defines genetic testing as a "diagnostic procedure to detect the presence or absence of, or change in, a particular gene or chromosome, including an indirect test for a gene product or other specific betabolite that is primarily indicative of a specific genetic change." Genetic screening, on the other hand, is defined as (Art. xiii) "large-scale systematic genetic testing offered in a programme to a population or subsection thereof intended to detect genetic characteristics in asymptomatic people" (see also Chadwick et al. 1998: 257). We attempted to harmonize our terminology, but nevertheless, "testing" and "screening" are widely used interchangeably.

3. An English translation of the law is available at the website of the Israeli Ministry of Justice: <http://www.justice.gov.il/NR/rdonlyres/46993742-CA48–41D6-A785–21CA8A0E2B52/0/**GeneticInformation**LawEdited_050901.doc>.

4. The high incidence of genetically inheritable diseases among this group is said to be due to two phenomena: first, the "founder effect," which is understood as the loss of genetic variation because of endogamy, and second, so-called "genetic drift," the inter-generational change of gene frequencies due to chance, instead of natural selection. Ashkenazi Jews, who make up more than 80 percent of world Jewry, are believed to descend from about 1,500 Jewish families dating back to the 14th century.

5. Non-Orthodox Jews might contend that the *Haredi* interpretation of commandments and prohibitions is more extensive than in other Jewish streams and therefore overrules these competing interpretations.

6. Efron (2007: 251, note 20) points out that as concerns communication and other high technology, "[i]n the past, Ultra-orthodox rabbis were rarely exercised about apparent conflicts between contemporary science and ancient books, relying on well-established traditions of interpretation to harmonize between the laboratory and the yeshiva. Lately, however, this seems to be changing."

7. There are a variety of guide books and overviews of *Halachic* issues related to the use of assisted reproduction and genetic testing (see, for example, Broyde 1999; Rosner & Schulman 2005), although individuals seeking guidance are always required to consult with their local *Halachic* authorities (a process often abbreviated as CYLAH, "Consult Your Local Authority on *Halachah*").

8. An autosomal recessive disorder means two copies of an abnormal gene must be present in order for the disease or trait to develop. Tay-Sachs disease has lethal neuro-degenerative effects due to ongoing accumulation of a lipid called GM2 ganglioside in nervous system cells, which causes progressive damage. The destructive process begins in the fetus early in pregnancy, although the disease is clinically apparent when the child is several months old. Children with classical Tay-Sachs usually die by the age of five as no treatment is available apart from supportive measures.

9. This applies to Tay-Sachs disease, cystic fibrosis, Gaucher's disease type I, Canavan's disease, familial dysautonomia, Bloom syndrome, Fanconi's anemia, glycogen storage disease type 1A, mucolipidosis type IV, and Niemann-Pick disease type A. Recently, DY in Israel also added Connexin 26 on demand by the proposed couple, a disease which leads to hearing loss but does not meet the criteria for "severe and debilitating conditions."

10. The term "secular" (*chiloni*) refers to lifestyle rather than religious conviction; many individuals in the "secular" sector believe in God and attend religious services at special times of the year.

11. On varying understandings of the term "genetically healthy" in this context, see Hashiloni-Dolev 2007.

12. Numbers might not always add up to 100 percent due to rounding.

13. This means that while "only" 42 percent spontaneously thought of DY when asked what organization providing genetic testing they knew, 59 percent said that they knew DY when explicitly asked about this organization.

References

Atkin, K., and W.I.U. Ahmad. 1998. "Genetic Screening and Haemoglobinopathies: Ethics, Politics and Practice." *Social Science & Medicine* 46, no.3: 445–58.

Bach, G., J. Tomczak, N. Risch, and J. Ekstein. 2001. "Tay-Sachs Screening in the Jewish Ashkenazi Population: DNA Testing is the Preferred Procedure." *American Journal of Medical Genetics* 99: 70–75.

Barilan, Y.M. and G. Siegal. 2005. "The Stem Cell Debate: A Jewish Perspective on Human Dignity, Human Creativity, and Inter-Religious Dialogues." In *Crossing Borders: Cultural, Political and Religious Differences Concerning Stem Cell Research*, eds. W. Bender, A. Manzei, and C. Hauskeller. Münster: Agenda Verlag.

Berger, Y. 2005. *Judaism, Science, and Moral Responsibility*. Lanham, MD: Rowman & Littlefield Publishers.

Beauchamp, T.L. and J.F. Childress. 2001. *Principles of Biomedical Ethics*, 5th ed. Oxford: Oxford University Press.

Bowen, D.J., R. Singal, E. Eng, S. Crystal, and W. Burke. 2003. "Jewish Identity and Intentions to Obtain Breast Cancer Screening." *Cultural Diversity and Ethnic Minority Psychology* 9, no.1: 79–87.

Broide, E., M. Zeigler, J. Ekstein, and G. Bach. 1993. "Screening for Carriers of Tay-Sachs Disease in the Ultraorthodox Ashkenazi Jewish Community in Israel." *American Journal of Medical Genetics* 47, no. 2: 213–215.

Brown, N. and A. Webster. 2004. *New Medical Technologies and Society—Reordering Life*. Cambridge, UK: Polity Press.

Broyde, M.J. 1999. *Assisted Reproduction and Jewish Law*. Cincinnati, Ohio: University of Cincinnati.

Catz, D.S., N.S. Green, J.N. Tobin, M.A. Lloyd-Puryear, P. Kyler, A. Umemoto, J. Cernoch, R. Brown, and F. Wolman. 2005. "Attitudes about Genetics in Underserved, Culturally Diverse Populations." *Community Genetics* 8, no. 3: 161–72.

Chadwick, R., H. Ten Have, J. Husted, M. Levitt, T. McGleenan, D. Shickle, and U. Wiesing. 1998. "Genetic Screening and Ethics: European Perspectives." *Journal of Medicine and Philosophy* 23, no. 3: 255–273.

Chen, S. 2001. "The Rabbi Said: 'Marriage is Forbidden (without genetic test)'" [Hebrew]. *Yediot Aharonot*, 19 August.

Collins, F.S., E.D.Green, A.E. Guttmacher, and M.S. Gyer. 2003. "A Vision for the Future of Genomics Research." *Nature* 422 (April): 835–47.

Conrad, P and J. Gabe. 1999. "Sociological Perspectives on the New Genetics: An Overview." *Sociology of Health and Illness* 21: 505–16.

Cowley, G., E. Leonard, G. Cerio, and D. Glick. 1990. "Made to Order Babies." *Newsweek* 114, no. 27: 94–95.

Dabrock, P. 2006. "Public Health Genetics and Social Justice." *Community Genetics* 9: 34–39.

Efron, N.J. 2007. *Judaism and Science: A Historical Introduction*. Westport: Greenwood Press.

Ekstein, J. and H. Katzenstein. 2001. "The Dor Yeshorim Story: Community-based Carrier Screening for Tay-Sachs Disease." *Advances in Genetics* 44: 297–310.

Franklin, S. 2000. "Life Itself: Global Nature and the New Genetic Imaginary." In *Global Nature, Global Culture*, eds. Sarah Franklin, Celia Lury, and Jackie Stacey. London: Sage Publications.

German National Ethics Council ("Nationaler Ethikrat"). 2003. "Genetic Diagnosis Before and During Pregnancy." http://www.ethikrat.org/_english/publications/Stn_PID_engl.pdf (accessed 4 January, 2008)

Green, N.S., Dolan, S.M., and Murray, T.H. 2006. "Newborn Screening: Complexities in Universal Genetic Testing." *American Journal of Public Health* 96: 955–59.

Gross, M.L. 2002. "Ethics, Policy, and Rare Genetic Disorders: The Case of Gaucher Disease in Israel." *Theoretical Medicine and Bioethics* 23, no. 2: 151–70.

Hashiloni-Dolev, Y. 2007. *A Life (Un)Worthy of Living: Reproductive Genetics in Israel and Germany*. Dordrecht, NL: Springer/Kluwer.

Israeli Central Bureau of Statistics. 2005. <http://www1.cbs.gov.il/reader/cw_usr_view_Folder?ID=141>. (accessed 4 January, 2008).

Kahn, S.M. 2000. *Reproducing Jews. A Cultural Account of Assisted Conception in Israel*. Durham, NC: Duke University Press.

Lemke, T. 2002. "Genetic Testing, Eugenics and Risk." *Critical Public Health* 12, no. 3: 283–90.

Lippman, A. 1991. "Prenatal Genetic Testing and Screening: Constructing Needs and Reinforcing Inequities." *American Journal of Law and Medicine* 1: 15–50.

Lori, A. 2003. "What Did Daddy Mean?" [Hebrew]. *Ha´aretz*, April 16.

Novas, C. and N. Rose. 2000. "Genetic Risk and the Birth of the Somatic Individual." *Economy and Society* 29, no. 4: 485–513.

Petersen, A. 1999. "Counseling the Genetically 'at risk': The Poetics and Politics of 'Nondirectiveness'." *Health, Risk and Society* 3, no. 1: 253–265.

Prainsack, B. and G. Siegal. 2006. "The Rise of Genetic Couplehood? A Comparative View of Premarital Genetic Testing." *BioSocieties* 1: 17–36.

Prainsack, B. and Y. Hashiloni-Dolev. 2009. "Religion and Nationhood." In *Handbook of Genetics and Society: Mapping the Genomic Era*, eds. P. Atkinson, P. Glasner, and M. Lock. London: Routledge. 404–421.

Rabinow, P. 1999. *French DNA: Trouble in Purgatory*. Chicago: University of Chicago Press.

Rapp, R. 1999. *Testing Women, Testing the Fetus: The Social Impact of Amniocentesis in America*. London: Routledge.

Raz, A. 2004. "'Important to Test, Important to Support': Attitudes Toward Disability Rights and Prenatal Diagnosis among Leaders of Support Groups for Genetic Disorders in Israel." *Social Science & Medicine* 59, no. 9: 1857–66.

Raz, A.E. 2005. "Disability Rights, Prenatal Diagnosis and Eugenics: A Cross-Cultural View." *Journal of Genetic Counseling* 14, no. 3: 183–87.

Raz, A. and M. Atar. 2004. "Upright Generations of the Future: Tradition and Medicalization in Community Genetics." *Journal of Contemporary Ethnography* 33, no. 3: 296–322.

Rose, N. 2001. "The Politics of Life Itself." *Theory, Culture & Society* 18: 1–30.

Rosen, C. 2003. "Eugenics—Sacred and Profane." *The New Atlantis* 2: 79–89.

Rosner, F. 1997. "Judaism, Genetic Screening, and Genetic Therapy." (accessed December 28, 2007. <http://www.mssm.edu/msjournal/65/16_Rosner.pdf>.

Rosner, F., and R. Schulman. 2005. *Medicine and Jewish Law*, vol. 3. Brooklyn, New York: Yashar Books.

Shahrabani, L., R. Shomrat, Y. Yaron, A. Orr-Urtreger, J. Groden, and C. Legum. 1998. "High Frequency of a Common Bloom Syndrome Ashkenazi Mutation among Jews of Polish Origin." *Genetic Testing* 2, no. 4: 293–96.

Sher, C., O. Romano-Zelekha, M.S. Green, and T. Shohat. 2003. "Factors Affecting Performance of Prenatal Genetic Testing by Israeli Jewish Women." *American Journal of Medical Genetics* 120A: 418–22.

Shohat, M. 2000. "The Future of Genetics: Where Are We Going in the Next Forty Years?" *Israel Medical Association Journal* 2: 690–91.

The Nuffield Council on Bioethics. 2006. *Genetic Screening: Ethical Issues.* <http://www.nuffieldbioethics.org/fileLibrary/pdf/genetic_screening. pdf> and <http://www.nuffieldbioethics.org/fileLibrary/pdf/Genetic _Screening_-_a_Supplement_to_the_1993_Report_(2006).pdf> (accessed December 28, 2007).

UNESCO. 2003. *International Declaration on Human Genetic Data* (General Conference, 32nd session, Paris: 32 C/29 Add.2, October 8, 2003). http:// unesdoc.unesco.org/images/0013/001331/133171E.pdf (accessed January 4, 2008).

Weiss, M. 2002. *The Chosen Body: The Politics of the Body in Israeli Society.* Stanford: University Press.

Wertz, D.C. and Fletcher, J.C. 1994–1995. *Genetics Approaches to Ethics: A Survey in 37 Nations.* Waltham, MA: Shriver Center.

Zlotogora, J. and A. Leventhal. 2000. "Screening for Genetic Disorders among Jews: How Should the Tay-Sachs Screening be Continued?" *Israel Medical Association Journal* 2, no. 9: 665–67.

Zlotogora, J. and G. Bach. 2003. "The Possibility of a Selection Process in the Ashkenazi Jewish Population" (Letter to the Editor). *American Journal of Human Genetics* 73: 438–40.

Zlotogora, J. and J. Chemke. 1995. "Medical Genetics in Israel." *European Journal of Human Genetics* 3, no. 3: 147–54.

Chapter 7

ULTRASONIC CHALLENGES TO PRO-NATALISM

Tsipy Ivry

Introduction

Israel, so many scholars claim, is a pro-natal state. But what does that mean in terms of the public imagery of pregnancy? That *failing* to conceive is pictured as an unbearable tragedy might come as no surprise, but what about a normal healthy pregnancy? One could hypothesize that since such a pregnancy is the height of the pro-natal fantasy, then it should be depicted in the most positive of terms. How then, can one interpret the following scene in which terror is so tightly intertwined into the very fabric of the social imagery of gestation?

The scene I am referring to took place in the summer of 2003, when I was sitting together with an audience of 500 pregnant women and their partners in a lecture about obstetrical ultrasound. The lecture was given by Professor Bloch (not his real name), the distinguished head of a maternity ward in one of the largest medical centers in Israel. It was part of a "pregnancy study day"—one of many consumer-oriented events organized throughout the country by hospitals in order to attract pregnant women to give birth in their institution. As became quite obvious during the course of his lecture, Bloch was trying to literally *entertain* the audience with short videos of ultrasonic fetal images to which he matched unpredictable soundtracks to construct humorous "clips" with fetuses starring as the main protagonists. In the same spirit he started his lecture with a joke. "Let me tell you a joke: Why do pregnant women have two eyes?" asked Professor Bloch. Answer: "One eye is to observe the ultrasound screen, and the other eye is to look at the doctor to see if everything [i.e., the fetus] is OK." The audience smiled faintly.

I find this joke to be a powerful assemblage of gender stereotypes and ideas about gestation. To begin with, it implies that (even) the eyes have a different function in women, and are part of the project of medically monitored pregnancy. Otherwise, the joke implies that if women were not reproducers, they could suffice with one eye. Second, the joke depicts the woman as an external spectator of her own pregnancy, who is totally dependent on her authoritative ob-gyn, but this might not be surprising in the context of any medicalized regime of pregnancy. However, what about the anxiety? The joke depicts a grotesque image of a woman split by anxiety in the course of a non-eventual ultrasound scan of her non-eventual pregnancy. In fact it is not merely an image of an anxious woman who is dependent on medical "assurance," but the embodiment of fear in a woman's body.

Delving into the literature written by Euro-American scholars about the images produced by obstetrical ultrasound, one becomes further perplexed, for it is precisely the technology of obstetrical ultrasound that has been associated in these societies with maternal-fetal bonding—a sphere of meaning that prescribes quite a different range of emotions to pregnant women (a range that is also much more congruent with a pro-natal regime).

It is with the intent of interpreting such "jokes" and more "serious" public representations of pregnancy through ultrasonography that I was looking for a comparative analysis of public images of obstetrical ultrasound in other similarly medicalized settings. The only scene I found that involves public images of obstetrical ultrasound that can parallel the emotional intensity reflected in the above joke is that of the *Silent Scream* discussed at length in the works of Rosalind Pollack-Petchesky (1987), Fay Ginsburg (1989), and Janelle S. Taylor (1992). *The Silent Scream* is a video widely used in anti-abortion campaigns in America. It depicts an abortion being performed during the twelfth week of gestation, as viewed via the screen of an ultrasound. The voiceover of the video, however, explains that this is how the abortion is experienced by the fetus itself, the "unborn child." These scholars have worked to deconstruct the rhetorical and visual techniques through which the "silent scream" attempts to "convert" women out of abortion (Ginsburg 1989: 104): They exposed the use of an elaborate combination of blurry images (presented as "truth" as viewed from an authoritative biomedical technological device) and interpreted by a voiceover that attempts to "fix" its meaning (Taylor 1992: 70) and "speak for" the fetus. The climax towards which the "silent scream" propels its audience comes when "the ultrasound appears to show (and the narrator points out lest we not see it) the mouth of the fetus opening in what the narrator tells us is a 'silent scream' of fear and pain" (Taylor 1992: 79).

Whereas the political statement *The Silent Scream* wants to make about abortion in the U.S. personifies the fetus as a sacred, vulnerable, helpless *person* who is silently screaming for help before catastrophe hits, Bloch's joke depicts the parallel image of a terrified woman, silently screaming through her eyes, similarly helpless and awaiting catastrophe (in the form of a fetal health problem or a pregnancy complication), even though positioned, as it seems, on the opposite side of the abortion debate. All this happens in the context of an ordinary ultrasound scan. As Taylor and others have shown in the American context, though the potential of ultrasound to enhance prenatal bonding with the fetus is almost taken for granted in medical and public spheres, at the same time ultrasound remains a tool of prenatal diagnosis. According to Taylor (1998), Draper (working in England) (2002) and others, however, the diagnostic aspects together with their possible implications on the state of mind of pregnant women and their partners, are greatly ameliorated as the scan is communicated to them in terms of "reassurance" that the fetus is healthy.

In contrast, in Bloch's straightforward description of a terrified woman, whose sight is split by anxiety, terror is explicit to the extent that it becomes grotesque. It echoes the way Israeli pregnant women are often conceptualized by their ob-gyns, by their partners, and by themselves as "hysterical," a notion I encountered throughout my field work. That Bloch felt it was legitimate to tell such a joke in a hall filled with pregnant women further attests that the association between pregnancy and anxiety is considered common knowledge and thus openly acknowledged in the Israeli public sphere.

Clearly Bloch's joke raises a host of issues that touch upon the discursive construction and practical implications of Israeli gender stereotypes and the relations between women and biomedical technologies, a thorough discussion of which goes beyond the scope of this chapter. Rather, I will focus on exploring the local meanings that obstetrical ultrasound assumes as it is talked about by experts and others in the public sphere, and look for the particular cultural paradigms of pregnancy as well as the political, national, and international circumstances in which such meanings come into being. Underlying my endeavor, however, is an attempt to challenge the widely accepted assumption about Israeli pro-natalism, or at least to complicate our understanding of it by paying heed to the multiple layers of the technological, political, and cosmological contributions to the terrorization of pregnancy—a pattern seemingly incongruent with pro-natal regimes. Before I proceed to discuss these inconsistencies through a specific segment of my ethnography, it is useful to situate the technology of obstetrical ultrasound within the broader context of the technologization of reproduction in Israeli society.

Hyper-tech reproduction and the pro-natal state

That NRTs (new reproductive technologies) have been enthusiastically embraced in Israel by both medical experts and large parts of the Israeli public has been used in the social scientific literature as one piece of evidence for the pro-natalist attitudes of Israeli policy makers. This line of arguments points out impressive figures—Israel's highest rate of IVF treatments per capita (Kahn 2000); the generous funding of fertility treatments by the state (Birenbaum-Carmeli 2004); the overwhelming tendency of Israeli couples to refer to fertility treatments not so much as a last resort but more as a first priority; and the institutionalization of surrogacy through the surrogacy law of 1996 (Teman, this volume; see also 2001, 2003, 2010)—as illustrations to an Israeli pro-natal regime.

Thus by using evidence from technologies of assisted conception, social scientists often associate the technologization of reproduction with an Israeli "cult of fertility" (an expression coined by Hazelton 1977), and continue to reason that such reproductive policies and behaviors are devised against a conspicuous public discourse about Israel—a Jewish state surrounded by Arab countries and involved in almost continuous armed conflict—and its "demographic threat."

My analysis in no way denies the predominance of such discourse, nor the overwhelming popularity of assisted conception in Israel (though I return to re-examine assisted conception in the epilogue of this chapter). Rather, I wish to complicate our ideas of pro-natalism. For the picture might change radically once one shifts the focus onto a different set of technologies that predominate in the way that the Israeli state manages pregnancy from the moment conception has taken place—that is prenatal diagnosis (PND).

In 1978, the Israeli government enacted a "program for the prevention of inborn abnormalities." The services offered under the plan were, and still are, free of charge. Clearly, the initiators of the plan were trying to minimize the birth of children with congenital abnormalities that occur in high rates among Jews of various ethnic origins. Thus, in the beginning the plan dealt with lethal diseases such as Tay-Sachs. However, soon the range of diseases being screened for was perceptibly widened (Weiss 2002: 80).[1]

Since the initiation of "the program," an increasing number of prenatal tests have been included in the "health basket" covered by the National Health Insurance, including those for genetic conditions that are not lethal, as well as for various chromosomal conditions that are not particularly frequent in Jews, such as Down's Syndrome.

Moreover, prenatal testing is "backed up" by the Israeli abortion law, which seems relatively liberal for a "pro-natal" state. The Israeli abortion law accommodates selective reproduction using an elaborate formulation of vague definitions. The law permits the abortion of defective fetuses without specifying kinds of defects or setting a maximum time threshold beyond which abortion is forbidden (Amir 1995). Neither of these points were ever a matter of either public or parliamentary debate, even in those rare instances when abortion debates in the Israeli Parliament momentarily managed to capture public attention.[2] When, in the mid 1980s, several ultra-religious parties, who are a potent electoral force, tried to change the abortion law, this was in order to erase the "economic article" (that permitted abortion due to financial hardships of the mother), and not to prevent "the murder of fetuses."

Adding to this picture is that virtually no criticism has been voiced by disability movements in Israel against the social meaning of prenatal diagnosis. The most vocal among these is an organization of military veterans who have been wounded in combat, who do not affiliate themselves with other disabled people, nor show any commitment to the rights of the non-military disabled.[3] Thus "the proliferation of publicly circulating representations of disability as a form of diversity" that Rapp and Ginsburg (2001: 534) point out in the context of post-industrial societies is only starting to emerge in very limited segments of Israeli Jewish society—namely the ultra-religious and religious circles (who are formally opposed to abortions for religious reasons)—and is still fairly unfamiliar among the non-religious population.

In this context it might not come as a surprise that although *The Silent Scream* has immigrated to Israel and been translated to Hebrew by an Israeli anti-abortion organization called Efrat, it has not gained any significant visual presence in the Israeli public sphere. The anti-abortion activists Taylor describes as "waving grisly 'war pictures' and wailing 'Mommy, don't kill me!!'" (Taylor 1992: 79) are still an unheard of phenomenon in the Israeli public sphere.

Within such a moral economy, obstetrical ultrasound has been incorporated into prenatal care together with other screening tests and diagnostic technologies. Currently the standard health basket includes three ultrasound scans in the course of a "low risk" pregnancy: a first trimester scan to negate the possibility of an ectopic pregnancy; a second trimester scan that is performed with a "check list" of the inner and outer fetal organs that have to be screened for deformations and indications of abnormality; and a third trimester scan that focuses on evaluating fetal weight towards birth. However, a growing number of patients from a variety of socio-economic backgrounds do not suffice with the "cheaper" scans covered by the health funds, but consume additional scans from doctors who have established reputations as ultrasound experts. An example of this is a scan performed in the twelfth week of gestation, during which the "nuchel-translucency"—the width of the back of the fetus' neck—is measured as one more indicator of Down's Syndrome. Moreover, more doctors today offer "bargains" that include the three diagnostic scans at "affordable rates."

The Israeli prenatal experts I spoke with claimed that their detection rates of fetal abnormalities are higher than those reported by their Euro-American counterparts, although they use similar technologies. Among many parameters, such high detection rates may have to do with the fact that Israeli ultrasound experts continue to look for fetal abnormalities up to birth. Thus, whereas in many places in the industrial world the law limits abortions to a certain gestational age, the Israeli legal and social context provides experts with a wider scope of practice, since even minor abnormalities detected in the latest stages of gestation may still have a practical solution sanctioned by law—abortion.

At the same time, the growing number of lawsuits in gynecology places considerable pressure on prenatal experts and pushes them to practice defensively. As the Yarkoni case cited below shows, the expectation that ultrasound experts will diagnose rare abnormalities with this technology plays a significant role in the construction of such pressure.

In 1998, in a landmark ruling, a court for the first time convicted an ob-gyn of negligence, though he had acted in accordance with the guidelines laid down by the Ministry of Health. The plaintiff was a woman by the name of Yarkoni who had undergone all the prenatal tests in the health basket as recommended by her ob-gyn, none of which had given any indication of fetal health problems. The baby she then gave birth to proved to have Dandy-Walker syndrome, an extremely rare genetic syndrome that causes mental retardation and paralysis. The plaintiff sued her doctor and her health fund for having failed to inform her of the additional testing she could have opted for, i.e., an extended ultrasound scan by privately paid experts that might have diagnosed the condition, in which case she would have had an abortion (Davies 1999). As stated above, the court found the ob-gyn guilty. The precedent of the Yarkoni case shows clearly that the plaintiff and her lawyer understood obstetrical ultrasound as a powerful prenatal diagnostic technology that can detect rare abnormalities. Moreover, the Yarkoni case has placed medico-legal considerations right at the heart of gynecological practice. At present, a woman visiting an ob-gyn for an initial prenatal visit may be presented with an integrated list of about thirty or more prenatal tests, some of which are subsidized by her health fund (under specific conditions), others being expensive tests that she can pursue in government hospitals or private clinics. Some ob-gyns may ask her to sign a declaration that she has been made aware of the existence of all these tests.

Given the pressure posed by the risk of a lawsuit, it might come as no surprise that a number of ultrasound experts that I spoke with explained to me that they are always on guard to detect fetal anomalies in any pregnancy regardless of its categorization as low-risk or high-risk, and up until the last stages of gestation. A senior ob-gyn close to retirement who claimed that pregnancy at any age is like a "dangerous gamble" (given the chance of bearing a child with an anomaly), or a prominent ultrasound expert in his mid-forties who told me explicitly that for him the category of a "low-risk pregnancy" simply does not exist (he treats all pregnancies as high-risk), are only too examples of the broadening of the concept of "risk" in Israeli prenatal care. Most importantly, all these professionals understood their risk-oriented style of practice as designed according to the best interests of their pregnant patients (Ivry 2010). Moreover, their attitudes echoed the insistence of the majority of my non-religious pregnant informants to undergo as much testing as possible in order to minimize the risk of bearing a child with an abnormality (see also Remennick 2006; Sher et al. 2003).[4]

Thus, within a general absence of public debates about prenatal diagnosis and selective abortions (Hashiloni-Dolev 2006a, 2006b, 2007), a growing reliance on ultrasound to indicate fetal anomalies, and the simultaneous pressure of lawsuits, a local industry of ultrasound scans is flourishing in Israel as part of the broader embrace of prenatal diagnostic testing.

Exploring pregnancy

The data presented in this chapter is part of a larger comparative study that explores conceptions of pregnancy in Japan and in Israel

(Ivry 2006, 2007, 2010). In that study I attempted to understand the experiential, medical, and social meanings of pregnancy in these two countries through the perspectives of a variety of human experiences and sets of medical knowledge about pregnancy. I used a combination of anthropological methods that Marcus (1995) calls "multi-sited-ethnography": I conducted participant observations in prenatal clinics, maternity and birth-education courses, and clinics that perform prenatal tests—among them ultrasound scans and amniocentesis—as well as more than one hundred in-depth interviews with Japanese and Israeli ob-gyns and pregnant women. Interviews were conducted in Japanese and Hebrew respectively. In addition I collected pregnancy guides, medical forms, and medical literature.

In this chapter, however, I will focus on a specific segment of my Israeli data: the study days that medical centers and hospitals organize throughout the country for pregnant women. I chose this set of observations for the light they help shed on the range of meanings that ultrasound can acquire in public. However, concerns that have arisen from observing Israeli women and men experiencing ultrasound scans (Ivry 2008), and insights from my observations of other reproductive technologies as well as those that arise from in-depth interviews with Israeli women and ob-gyns, all feed into the concerns of this chapter.

During my years of fieldwork (1996–2003) "pregnancy events" proliferated throughout Israel, their major target being to attract women to give birth in the medical institutions that organize them. This increase can be seen as the reaction of medical institutions to the "threat" of ideas of "natural birth." Institutions of conventional medicine are reacting to the slightly rising rates of home births by making active attempts to re-hospitalize birth on the patients' terms, utilizing "pregnancy events" as opportunities to explain and advertise their progressive approaches to childbearing. Interestingly, such childbirth-oriented events very often took to discussing the management of pregnancy, although most of the women in the audience were approaching its very last stages. For our matter it should be borne in mind that the lectures about obstetrical ultrasound discussed here were given in the course of pregnancy days to pregnant women who had already undergone an array of prenatal tests, ultrasound included: women who were towards the end of term and who came to inquire about birthing facilities.

The pregnancy events documented here are advertised in daily newspapers and childrearing magazines in Hebrew under titles that associate them with pleasure and indulgence: "Pregnancy and Fun Fair," "A Friday Coffee," or "Pregnancy Fair" are examples of titles under which such events are advertised. The advertisements invite women to hear lectures from the best obstetrical experts and to enjoy a nice breakfast free of charge. According to the organizers, hundreds of pregnant women participate in each event. My impression (though I have no way of corroborating this statistically) is that the participants were from secular as well as modern orthodox backgrounds, and came from a wide range of socio-economic strata and various levels of education. Women from ultra-religious communities clearly do not attend the pregnancy events discussed here, and the study days they are exposed to are significantly different in their content. The paradigms for thinking about reproduction in ultra-religious communities in Israel deserve analysis in and of themselves and are beyond the scope of this study.[5]

The pregnancy events that I attended took place in various geographical locations throughout Israel. Some were held in hospitals and some in large community centers. "Pregnancy events" are always joint enterprises of medical establishments and certain commercial companies who market their pregnancy and childrearing products at these events. Cosmetic ointments to lubricate the stretched skin of a pregnant belly, pregnancy work-out videos, maternity outfits, childrearing magazines, baby carriers, water filters and even amulets to protect pregnant women and future babies from the evil eye are only part of a long list of commodities that are offered for sale in such events. As they stroll among the stands, pregnant women and their companions are offered food and drink and given presents of all kinds.

At the core of such "fun days," however, is a series of lectures by prominent medical practitioners who are well-known experts in their own fields and/or hold senior positions as heads of maternity wards in distinguished medical centers. Lecturers explore a range of topics in obstetrical medicine from different medical perspectives: "pain management in labor," "the pros and cons of cesarean births," and "alternative methods of pain relief" are examples of subjects that are often taken up. That organizers make a point of including lectures on obstetrical ultrasound—lectures that stand out as somewhat indirectly related to the main topic—says something about the general importance attached to ultrasound, and also about the expectation that the audience will welcome lectures of this sort. Often using absorbing *PowerPoint* presentations, lecturers do their best to entertain their audience with jokes and humorous pictures inserted into these serious presentations.[6]

Since 1999 I have observed ten events throughout the country that lasted an average of three to five hours. I tape-recorded all the lectures presented on pregnancy days and also took notes of what happened in the exhibition halls. Throughout, in presenting data I have changed the names and identifying features of all informants.

Though I focus on the ways in which ultrasound is talked about and presented in the public sphere, the images that emerge often echo the uses of ultrasound in the privacy of the clinic, as well as broader patterns of use of prenatal diagnosis by the Israeli public. However, as the only pregnancy activities that are explicitly defined and designed as large scale events, pregnancy study days offer especially condensed and powerful perspectives from which to explore the local meanings of pregnancy as it is articulated by a specific technology.

In what follows, and as my analytical point of departure, I will treat Israeli pregnancy events as social constructs that speak about culturally specific reproductive relations and as embedded within local reproductive politics (cf. Ginsburg and Rapp 1991, 1995). That such "fun" days can host horrific ultrasonic shows is a phenomenon that deserves interpretation.

The ultrasound picture show

It was a sunny Friday morning in November 2002. After a short walk through the lanes of the medical center following the signs "To the pregnant women's day," I finally reached the tidy plaza of a well-maintained building surrounded by greenery. Since I had come one hour ahead of schedule, the plaza was still almost empty, but hospital workers were already arranging a buffet in the hall and the organizers were busily moving around the assembly room. When I came into the assembly room, I found Ms. Shein, an elegant woman in her mid-thirties, standing and looking at the huge placard that was hanging from the ceiling covering the wall behind the lecturers' lectern. The placard featured the plump face of a blue-eyed baby about eight months old with the words, "Seeing the unborn" [*lir'ot et hanolad*] written above the picture in thick black letters. As I learned later, Ms. Shein worked in the office of public relations at the medical center and was thus in charge of the organization of pregnancy events for the general public. She defines herself as a feminist and told me, "I organize these pregnancy days for the benefit of pregnant women. I want them to feel good and have a nice morning. But I also think it is most important to see to it that they get correct and up-to-date medical information." Lectures about obstetrical ultrasound play a double role in this venture: Ms. Shein described them as both "fun" and "informative." As she and other organizers of pregnancy events often told me, it goes without saying that a "pregnancy day" should include a lecture given by an ultrasound specialist.

An hour later, the assembly room had filled up with about 300 pregnant women and about 20 male partners. Ms. Shein warmly invited all the participants to be seated and welcomed them on behalf of the medical staff. Then she introduced the first lecturer as follows:

> Undoubtedly, one of the exciting moments in pregnancy is viewing the fetus in ultrasound. Ultrasound screening, which entered wider use during the late 1970s, has changed the face of gynecology and obstetrics and brought about a real revolution. Let me introduce Professor Cohen, who is the head of our Ultrasound unit . . . and is currently heading the disability clinic in our hospital.

Observing the women in the audience moving uneasily in their seats, I felt that the idea of pregnancy as exciting quickly subsided when they realized that the "head of the ultrasound unit," who was to be giving the ultrasound lecture, was also the head of the "disability clinic."

Immediately on taking his place behind the lectern, Professor Cohen responded to the introduction by "assuring" the audience that "I did my best not to show you many disabilities today, only one or two examples; anyway it is unpleasant." "So don't show us any," a woman in the audience called out. Professor Cohen continued:

> We, the experts, we the ultrasound people, began observing fetuses in the womb about twenty-five years ago, and with time we learned many things that even our embryology books still don't tell us. The things that we see in the womb are not in the books even today: all kinds of indications that changed the face of medicine. Ask your ob-gyns what is the most significant thing that has happened generally in gynecology during the last two decades, and undoubtedly they will say, "The first thing that happened is that obstetrical ultrasound came into use. . . ."
>
> Anyone who worked in birthing rooms twenty years ago knows the huge difference in diagnosing now, in ways that I now wonder how we did it then. For example, identifying twins during labor using X-ray. I remember an X-ray of twins in the birthing room, and they were identical twins, and not only identical, they were Siamese, and during the delivery, it was simply horrible what happened there, how they got out all completely torn apart.

> Nowadays you [Cohen used the Hebrew second person singular male] do ultrasound, you identify it during the first trimester of pregnancy and I will show you the pictures. This is what makes all the difference. Nowadays we are wiser because we can see the unborn.

This proud meta-narrative of biotechnological progress (achieved by an expert collective designated as "we") serves as the starting point for the narration of obstetrical ultrasound. However, I argue that neither progress itself nor its aim can be understood without the notion of reproductive catastrophe. Catastrophe is both the foil against which one is encouraged to measure progress, and the reason why such progress is necessary in the first place. The horrifying example described above of what can happen in a world without obstetrical ultrasound (evidence of progress) is only one example of a pattern repeating itself throughout this and other lectures.

I heard Professor Cohen giving this same lecture three times during three different pregnancy events. What particularly struck me was his apparent assumption that it is legitimate to tell such horror stories to pregnant women, even though he was fully aware of the intimidating effect they were bound to have. However, that such representations "go public" also suggests that they are based, at least to some degree, on shared understandings by doctors and patients. In fact, it tells us much about how far terrorization can reach, undisturbed. Otherwise, it is hard to explain why Ms. Shein made sure that Professor Cohen's lecture always came first on the schedule, and why the woman mentioned earlier voiced the only protest I heard against this lecture.

Cohen's lectures were saturated with ultrasound pictures of deformed fetuses that he had integrated into the thematic flow of the lecture. These alternated between pictures of human-like fetuses doing human-like things (that are supposed to make the audience laugh) and images of anomalous fetuses. An illustrative example is when Cohen shows the audience ultrasound pictures of fetal male and female sexual organs, leading to a brief, humorous account of a fetus he had screened masturbating for 15 seconds. The audience laughs, but he then immediately follows this by telling them that this particular fetus died in the 28th week of gestation because of a heart problem. "Maybe he died from this [masturbation, T.I.]," adds Cohen laughing, as he proceeds to show a series of pictures of fetuses with deformed sexual organs, discussing each deformation at length. Another example is when he shows the audience "how nicely you can see small details like the fingers and the toes," but then proceeds to show pictures of fetuses with six fingers.

Since for each and every 'normal' organ he discussed Cohen showed pictures of the same organ deformed (with no notification of how rarely these deformities occur), the overall impression of the lecture was that a myriad of deformations and abnormalities occur all the time and that each and every organ may be subject to deformity and abnormality. A partial list of disabilities and fetal deformations that were discussed in detail and shown on the big screen includes cleft lip, hernia, distorted sexual organs, extra fingers, fetuses with two heads (a form of Siamism) and more. It should be borne in mind that the visibility of deformed fetuses in Cohen's *PowerPoint* presentation stands in sharp contrast with the relative absence of people with deformities in the Israeli public sphere (either because the public sphere is largely still physically inaccessible to people with disabilities in spite of recent attempts to improve access, because their status and rights are still subject of debate within the legal system, or because a multitude of implicit and explicit symbolic mechanisms reinforce their distance from the collective of "the fit").[7]

Returning to Cohen's lecture, along with the numerous deformations and abnormalities, the audience also learns about new tests that can be performed to detect them (with the clear implication that abortion of these fetuses is an acceptable solution to the problem). Although some of these tests are irrelevant for many of the women in the audience who are approaching birth, the expert does not spare any efforts to recommend them to the women "for the next pregnancy." At the same time, he makes sure to warn the audience that undergoing multiple screening throughout gestation can never bring absolute "assurance" to the patient. He explains that although for the detection of some abnormalities it is recommended to undergo a first trimester vaginal ultrasound screening, the patient must bear in mind that vital organs, like the heart and the brain, have not completely developed, and that therefore to detect problems in the latter it is recommended to undergo an additional screening in the 20th week during the second trimester. Yet, even this cannot provide assurance, as he explained:

> The subject of dwarfism, well this is something you can miss in earlier screening, . . . and even in later screening, because sometimes shortened limbs become apparent only in later weeks, and sometimes they are discovered only when fetal weight estimation is done in the 30th week, so take it into consideration.

While numerous tests are brought to the awareness of the audience and offered for consumption, at the same time people are told that the apparent limitations of these tests "should be taken into consideration." But it is the following statement that, I think, delivers the knock-out blow to the idea of obstetrical ultrasonography as "assurance." Cohen shows the audience a clear fetal profile and says:

> Look how beautifully you can see, you can really see the tongue, those of you who have especially good sight can recognize the lens of the eye. Look how nice. If we can see a lens it says that the fetus has an eye but it does not say that he can see because we cannot see the nerves of sight.

It is notable, first, that Professor Cohen's fascination clearly is not with the fetus, but rather with the ability of ultrasonic devices to display detailed images of fetuses. Secondly, whereas the narrative of abnormality detection relies on the "panoptic" illusion of ultrasound's enhanced vision, it becomes clear that not all disabilities are visually observable. The destruction of "assurance" also destroys the pleasure that might come from seeing even the most "beautiful pictures" that ultrasonography can provide, not to speak of the idea of the "psychological benefits" of maternal–fetal bonding discussed by Taylor (1998).

Finally, when speaking of "beautiful pictures" such as those shown on three-dimensional ultrasound scans, Cohen says:

> Look at these faces; here is a fetus that lay down his head and went to sleep "on" the womb; look at the lips and the nostrils, really very nice pictures, but you should bear in mind that three-dimensional ultrasound is a gimmick and see it the way it is—it does not always have an additional diagnostic value.

To conclude this example, I suggest that Cohen's lecture illustrates how far the idea of reproductive catastrophe can go in public discourse. His lecture powerfully illustrates a meta-message saying that no assurance can be ever given about fetal health and prospects of living, until well after birth. Cohen understands women and encourages them to understand themselves as being in the process of carrying a potential fetal catastrophe. In this sense the lecture echoes Professor Bloch's joke about pregnant women having two eyes. Ultrasound is presented as a diagnostic tool that can help prevent fetal anomalies as one type of reproductive catastrophe. Presented under such an overarching meta-message all alternative interpretations of the images of deformed fetuses are repressed. Deformed fetuses are presented in the context of being warned against rather than nurtured, cared for, corrected or "saved." Thus in its potential to generate terror and anxiety, Cohen's lecture parallels *The Silent Scream*. However, while *The Silent Scream* attempts to generate terror to scare women away from abortion, Professor Cohen's ultrasonic picture show is likely to work the opposite effect, i.e., frighten women away from pregnancy.

Significantly, Professor Navon's lecture, focusing on issues of nutrition during pregnancy, was always scheduled after Professor Cohen's. In the three events at this medical center that I attended, Navon opened his lecture by saying:

> There is a division of roles between me and Professor Cohen: He frightens you a little and then I calm you down. Usually it works well. We are graduates of the Shabak [Israel's General Security Service or secret police]. He "shakes" [a euphemism for the physical torture the Shabak uses when interrogating detainees] and then I come and put things in order. Because he is the one who finds the disabilities and I am the one who maybe is trying to prevent them, he gets his share of problems, but I will try to give you the more optimistic approach.

Here Navon was proposing an alternative, a preventive approach to pregnancy. Using the Shabak euphemism was his way of breaking the tension his predecessor had generated by trying to make the audience laugh, in which he succeeded. His borrowing of metaphors from conflict-saturated life-worlds of physical violence in Israel is one more technique that I came across in several pregnancy events, particularly when lecturers tried to alleviate tensions, or simply to entertain the audience.

Trying to suggest an alternative to the fatalistic view of pregnancy conveyed by Professor Cohen's lecture, Professor Navon focused on the description of a new nutritional supplement, a "cocktail-pill" for pregnant women, which he is helping to develop. However, relatively little information was given to the women about how to "take charge" of their health while pregnant by consuming the ideal calorific intake or through balancing different nutrients in a meal.

Moreover, the order of the lectures of these two medical experts (Cohen's always coming first), together with Navon's cautious way of presenting his professional endeavor as "maybe preventing" fetal disabilities, suggests an implicit hierarchy between the knowledge systems that focus on "nutrition/prevention" and "detection/diagnosis" respectively. This hierarchy is also reflected in the audience's differential reactions to the two lectures. Whereas the women and their partners sit quietly throughout Cohen's lecture, once the topic shifts to more preventive issues, people tend to pay less attention, whisper to each other, joke, and even leave the room to indulge in the buffet on offer outside the lecture hall. The kinds of foods and drinks that are offered at such buffets include sweets, fried food, and coffee—precisely the sort of foods that preventive discourses emphasizing nutrition as a factor in fetal health tend to warn against (Markens, Browner, and Press 1997; Browner and Press 1997). Thus, while Navon was enthusiastically urging the women to "contribute to the future health of the fetus by taking care of your diets now," coffee was being served to the women in the hallway and consumed by them uninterruptedly.

Of course the disabled fetus is not the only fetal image present in the public sphere. One can find the image of the personified fetus—one that at the outset might seem quite similar to the one reported by scholars working in America—in the public discourse about ultrasound. Except that, once again, the meaning of this image seems to undergo a considerable shift. This brings us back to the word "gimmick" that Cohen and other ob-gyns whom I interviewed used when they referred to the strategy of "humanizing" the fetus for its parents during ultrasound scans. For example, in a lecture given on 14 July 2003 at a pregnancy day that took place in a medical center in the south of Israel, Dr. Gil showed his audience a series of ultrasound pictures of fetuses in different positions and gave them "humanizing" titles. One fetus holding her fist against her face he called "the boxer," another, who was suckling his thumb, was presented as "the sucker," and another, who was caught moving his hands and legs as if he was driving a car, was called "the driver"; he also showed a picture of a fetus making the gesture of "the finger," as well as one of twin fetuses kicking each other's heads while "playing soccer." Towards the end of his presentation, however, Dr. Gil told the audience about a pair of twins whose ultrasound picture showed how their umbilical cords had become tightly wound around each other while in the womb. He said that these twins had been saved due to this prognosis and the subsequent recommendation to deliver them in a cesarean section, and then showed the wound umbilical cords just after the birth. This presentation was an example of a more light-hearted sort of discourse of obstetrical ultrasound. Yet even this relatively optimistic presentation included at least some examples of possible reproductive catastrophe pre-empted by technology. When Dr. Gil finished his presentation and the next lecturer was being announced, I overheard the couple sitting next to me saying to each other "What bullshit!" Having watched them out of the corner of my eye intimately hugging, and the husband massaging his wife and stroking her belly throughout the presentation, I had expected them to enjoy it: this couple looked as if they were "connected" or "bonded" to each other and to the unborn baby in a way that reminded me of the idealized American discourse of maternal–fetal bonding described in Taylor's work. However, as they told me later, both husband and wife thought that this "baby talk" before birth was totally out of place. "Is he trying to make idiots of us?" asked the husband.

The responses of this couple to Dr. Gil's attempt to "humanize the fetus" echoed the insistence of my ob-gyn informants that, as a 46-year-old ultrasound expert I call Dr. Shalev said, "There is a mutual understanding between the patients and the doctors that this blah blah of "Hey look, the baby is waving goodbye to you" is a joke. Both parties know what ultrasound is for." After all, as Alan Dundes reminds us, "[P]eople joke about only what is most serious" (Dundes 1987: viii). And pregnancy, as one might expect, is a most serious business in pro-natal states.

Terrorized pregnancies in Israeli-Jewish culture

In her account of the public fetus in American culture, Janelle S. Taylor points out that whereas fetal images have come to deploy the fetus as "endangered childhood in need of protection" (Taylor 1992: 67), there is nevertheless a whole set of significations of fear and horror that are repressed in the American public sphere: significations such as "the possibility of a deformed baby, or indeed the unknown future itself as evoked by such an image—not to mention by the political climate of the moral horror of abortion which the public deployment of such images has helped to create" (Taylor 1992: 77). In the Israeli ethnography presented here, it is precisely the deformed fetus as well as other reproductive misfortunes that are powerfully made explicit. Those, however, are not even the most dramatic examples. Rather, I decided to focus on ultrasound shows, first and foremost for their being public representations forged by authoritative experts, but also since they are particularly condensed examples of a much broader pattern that cuts through the social spheres in which I conducted my fieldwork: namely the terrorization of pregnancy through narratives that couple humor and horror, narratives that assume and evoke anxiety while simultaneously suggesting (doubtful) practical ways to mitigate it. Elsewhere, I call this structured system of narratives and practices "the politics of threatened life" where "life" stands typically for the pregnant woman and "threat" for the fetus, and elaborate on *how* this politics works within an Israeli local mode of biomedical care complete with its own theories about fetal development and imagined relations between women and fetuses (Ivry 2009). Here, I focus my analysis on excavating the cultural and cosmological paradigms of thinking that go beyond pregnancy and the modern medicine that underpins such local forms of terrorized pregnancies, while considering their implications for our understanding of pro-natalism.

To give a sense of how broad is the terrorization of pregnancy I encountered throughout my fieldwork, it is useful to locate it in the everyday experiences of pregnant women. The pregnancy accounts of Israeli women revealed that once pregnancy was announced, women became the target of reproductive horror stories. Relatives and far acquaintances made a point to call them (sometimes even while they were abroad) to tell about women friends who had received a positive diagnosis of fetal anomaly and terminated the pregnancy, had had a pregnancy complication, a still birth, a difficult birth or a caesarian. These stories often ended with unsolicited advice about the necessity to undergo a certain test or the importance of medical monitoring of the birth. At the same time, women who followed up on these messages and became enthusiastic consumers of prenatal diagnosis were often narrated by their partners and medical care-takers as "hysterical" and subjected to cynicism.

Moreover, taking a broader look away from prenatal care reveals that the implicit assumptions behind folk practices of pregnancy common among Israeli Jews provide an especially fertile ground for pregnancy anxieties. More specifically, there is evidence to claim that a notion of pregnancy as a tentative state of being prevails in large parts of the Israeli-Jewish society. One illustrative example is the custom of delaying the preparations for a new baby. While it is customary for many American "expectant mothers" to celebrate baby showers—events that "carry tremendous emotional importance for the nascent mother" (Davis-Floyd 1992: 36)—during the seventh month of pregnancy, many Israeli mothers-to-be would prefer that baby clothes, cribs, and other maternity ware will be brought to the house only after the baby has been born. They adhere, to varying degrees, to a custom that draws on Jewish folk traditions predating the constitution of the State. This strategy is reflected in much broader marketing trends for maternity products.

Chain stores in Israel selling baby's furniture and clothing invite expecting couples to choose whatever they need for their future baby prior to birth, that is, to make a "birth order" without paying for it immediately. What is particular to Israel is that the order can be made without the couple having to take it home. The store keeps their order on hold until the baby has been born. Israeli would-be parents (particularly first-time ones) are expected to be completely disorganized in expecting the new baby. This marketing strategy echoes Jewish folk beliefs and practices devised to protect pregnancies against the evil eye.[8] That it proves so successful suggests that this strategy is tuned in to a broad and common perception of pregnancy that in fact acknowledges it as a fertile enterprise only retrospectively—after a healthy baby has been born.

Whereas Barbara Kaz-Rothman (1986, 1989) sees PND at the heart of the process through which pregnancies are being transformed into tentative states, the above examples suggest that in the Israeli Jewish case the understanding of pregnancy as tentative predates modern medicine and the advent of prenatal diagnosis in particular. Rather, as I see it, the rise of prenatal diagnosis in the 1980s has only worked to corroborate the notion of pregnancy as tentative—an idea that was already prevalent in the cosmologies of many Israeli Jews, professional and non-professional alike.

When pregnancy is seen and experienced as tentative, ultrasonography takes on a different set of meanings. Israeli fetuses are represented as separate from their mothers and carry the authority of visual knowledge in the same way that Taylor (1992) and Pollack Petchesky (1987) pointed out for their American counterparts. But this authority is used to convey different meanings: Rather than a personified fetus entitled to fetal rights, Israeli fetal images may strive towards individuality and personification, but always threaten to collapse at any moment into either deformation or into a joke. To be sure, the image of the deformed fetus is often narrated as if it were the embodiment of reproductive catastrophe: precisely the kind technology promises to prevent from erupting. Thus, while more inclusive interpretations of the disabled body are silenced, images of deformed fetuses are presented in public discourse as if they were warning signs situated at all the dangerous turning points along the road.

In fact, considering the seemingly less frightening, "humorous" presentations of fetuses, one realizes that these too belong to the same paradigmatic system of thinking that sees pregnancy as threatened by catastrophe almost by definition, and thus constructs mechanisms to lower the stress pregnancy causes. In this vein, the "funny" fetus and the deformed fetus are the implicit and explicit versions of the same concern that supposedly unites all the agents taking part in reproduction.

Moreover, as Dundes (1987: vii-viii) has taught us, humor and horror have much in common: Not only are they mutually constituted in the sense that "where there is anxiety, there is humor," but they also tend to suggest a similar range of scripts for action. At the outset both produce distance from the horrified/ridiculed object. In the specific case of pregnancy this means distance between the pregnant woman and her fetus.

It is notable that, while the representation of the American fetus as separate helps anti-abortionists in their attempt to adorn it with individual rights, the Israeli fetus reminds us that in a different socio-cultural setting separateness can also facilitate the distance required to keep it a potential candidate for abortion.

Thus in the Israeli discourse, worst case scenarios loom large. What is significant about them is that they are typically understood and represented as arbitrary, basically unpredictable, and as very realistic possibilities about which the patient can do little or nothing to prevent them from happening. The most significant feature that the ethnography demonstrates, I think, is that such representations may "go public": It is considered legitimate to show images of deformed fetuses to pregnant women towards the end of term with an explicit message that fetuses with such abnormalities should be detected and aborted. Thus, that pregnant women might be split by anxiety is only logical when the constant message is that catastrophe awaits each one of them around the corner.

It is notable that, in both the Israeli and the American public spheres, the "implicit logic" has it that women may be terrorized while pregnant for "legitimate" reasons: Israeli medical experts may feel that it is legitimate to horrify women with images of deformed fetuses so that they keep alert and help to gate-keep their own family and society against the birth of deformed fetuses.[9] American anti-abortion activists may feel that it is legitimate to horrify women so that they continue keeping and protecting their "unborn children." Finally, in both cases the terrorization of pregnant women attempts to silence women's voices, experiences, and powers of reasoning, together with any alternative interpretations of how the fetal images could be read. The silencing effect of terror powerfully emerged from the accounts that doctors, male partners and women themselves gave me of the time they spent once a medical practitioner had suggested the possibility of a fetal anomaly, while struggling with a decision whether to undergo an invasive test that endangers maternal and fetal health. Doctors told me how patients get "completely blocked out," male partners spoke of how it becomes "impossible to communicate with her," and women kept telling how they "could not afford to take chances." These accounts, I think, radically differ from the "moral pioneering" that Rapp (1999) describes among American women. After all, terror tends not to leave space for lengthy moral indecision; rather, it calls for emergency defense actions.

What I find most remarkable in the Israeli context, however, is that the terrorization of pregnancy has come to predominate the public narrations of pregnancy in the context of a state that claims to be, and is widely acknowledged as being, "pro-natal." Such incongruence between powerful ultrasonic images and other cultural practices and ideas of pregnancy as a potential catastrophe, and the pro-natalistic desire to bear more children, I suggest, should be used to challenge, re-examine and complicate the assumptions of pronatalism that seem to prevail in much of the social critique about fertility in Israel. Terrorizing women in the context of the criminalization of abortions is a well known pattern of pro-natal states. But how can we explain the terrorization of pregnancy itself in the context of "pro-natalism"?

Pro-natalism and the key scenario of catastrophe

I suggest that to understand the worst-case-scenario-oriented thinking so prevalent in the ethnography, one must explore broader Jewish-Israeli key scenarios of catastrophe that are very much present in the thinking of Israeli professionals as well as lay ideas about reproduction that go far beyond pregnancy and birth to the core of the collective national identity of Jewish Israelis. From such a vantage point, the tentative pregnancy is a specific articulation of a key scheme of thinking that is continuously perpetuated in segments of public discourse in Israel in areas beyond reproduction: a thinking that generates the self, both as an individual and part of a collective, as threatened by catastrophe.

In fact, the idea that terrible catastrophes—either physical, spiritual or both—are around the corner predominates in parts of the collective Jewish memory and reestablishes itself through the commemoration of key events in Jewish history. In Jewish canonical narratives that pre-date the constitution of the State of Israel, the threat of extinction is usually countered by a miraculous redemption/salvation brought about by God and thus the relief from the threat is commemorated. Examples include the enslavement of the Israelites by Pharaoh followed by their exodus from Egypt, which is celebrated at Passover; a temporary relief in the bitter struggles for national and spiritual independence from Hellenistic rule that is celebrated in Hanukah; and the inversion of the magisterial verdict to extinguish all Jews in the Persian Empire that is celebrated in Purim.

It is beyond the scope of this chapter to provide a full historical and cultural account of the evolution and diversity of Jewish narratives of existential threats. However, it is clear that when Zionism absorbed this scheme of thinking into Israeli state narratives, it transformed it in significant ways. In fact, towards the beginning of the 20th century, the Zionist movement put forward the constitution of a Jewish state as the most recent form of redemption from the age-old threat of Jewish extinction. The role of the state as redeemer appeared to be vindicated soon after the Holocaust, as refugees sought sanctuary in the Jewish state. Since the constitution of the State of Israel, the notion of redemption took on alternative trajectories, one of which has been the military as a symbolic substitute for the redemptive power of God.

However, with the rise in the late 1970s of public and scholarly criticism of the military and the militarization of Israeli society—only to intensify during the first and second Intifada—the "threat/redemption" formula appears to have jettisoned the latter part of the scenario, where catastrophe now looms large as a lone key scenario, powerfully transforming the world view of those who have difficulty believing in divine redemption into one of pessimism. As Gerald Cromer (2006) points out, the *threat* of terror transcends terror events themselves and becomes a key notion to think with, an index case against which claimants, regardless of their political positions, weigh other unrelated issues.

Returning to pregnancy, it seems to me that the hovering presence of reproductive misfortune has to do with the readiness of Israeli Jews to think with the key scenario of "threat": to imagine that the worst is about to happen and to adopt the emotional posture familiar to many, if not all, Israelis: distancing oneself from what is understood to embody the threat and of defending oneself against it (i.e., undergo invasive testing, and abort fetuses with minor anomalies).

The above is true to a considerably lesser degree for Jewish ultra-Orthodox women. Although initial findings from a series of in-depth interviews with ultra-Orthodox women that Elly Teman and myself have conducted show that these women might be very anxious about the health of their fetuses as well as other complications of pregnancy and birth, they consume prenatal diagnosis cautiously and speak about their faith in God, who will provide them with the mental and physical resources to deal with whatever ordeal they have been destined to take on (Teman and Ivry n.d.). Their narratives echo the attitudes of their communities, which purposely set themselves apart from state ideology, and in turn adhere to the traditional narratives of Judaism that include divine redemption. Yet, ultra-Orthodox women, it should be borne in mind, are not exempt from anxiety while pregnant.

I do not mean to claim, of course, that all Israeli-Jewish nonreligious pregnancies are haunted, nor that any given pregnancy is experienced as haunted in each and every moment. In fact, I spoke to a considerable number of women who tried their best to create a cozy and friendly world in which to carry their pregnancies as cheerfully as they possibly could, while trying to establish certain degrees of connection with their fetuses especially during the last trimester of pregnancy. Such women were actively blocking the streaming information about reproductive misfortunes often by keeping their encounters with the medical system to what they perceived as minimum. Such constructions, however, quickly collapsed when a woman found herself unwillingly facing threatening predictions delivered by medical practitioners in the course of one of the medical checkups to which she did show up. Thus, what I argue is not that all pregnancies are haunted in each and every moment, but rather that thinking through the powerful threat paradigm makes Israeli experiences of pregnancy considerably more vulnerable to terrorization.

Returning to the horror picture show from the vantage point of the threat/redemption scheme, it seems that the ultrasound experts quoted in the ethnography were trying to situate themselves and their technologies at the redemption side of the scheme. At the same time, in a narrative process that parallels the weakening of the notion of redemption, they again and again reminded their audience that no assurance could be given.

Similarly, the "demographic threat" analyzed by scholars as part of their discussion of pro-natalism can now be seen as the recent re-formulation by the Jewish state of quite an ancient narrative. Paradoxically, while the threat of losing the Jewish majority within the borders of the State of Israel is often presented as an important component in the rationale of the "Israeli cult of fertility" and its recent technologization, it becomes clear that the scheme of thinking in terms of threat also has opposite effects. In other words, the predominance of the narrative of this existential threat simultaneously encourages and discourages fertility. State officials would use it as a reminder of how important the bearing of children is for assuring the continued existence of the (Jewish) State of Israel. Yet when catastrophe becomes a key scenario to think with for medical professionals, pregnant women, and their partners, pregnancies become more easily "haunted," and post-diagnostic abortions become a reasonable defensive act against it. It is precisely within the tensions generated by the paradigm of threat that women and doctors manage pregnancies and make procreative decisions.

Thus, rather than a regime that simply opts to "encourage" the birth of more children, the analysis here suggests that Israeli pro-natalism be understood as a complex system of tensions around the bearing of children, complete with its moral economy and order of priorities. It is not only that Israeli pro-natalism is torn between concerns with the number of children born and with their "quality." To fully understand the meaning of these tensions one should bear in mind the overarching Jewish-Israeli key scenario of catastrophe as it is replayed in the public images of pregnancy. Ultrasonic images are but one example of how this set of tensions can be played out, and what its consequences could be. In fact, once pro-natalism is understood as a set of tensions, one can reread the Israeli politics of high-tech reproduction.

Epilogue: Rereading reproductive technologies and pro-natalism

Statistics suggest that Israeli neonates are nowadays more likely to die or become affected due to premature birth than by inborn genetic or chromosomal anomalies. Paradoxically, fertility treatments contribute greatly to the heightened rates of neonatal mortality and morbidity.

In Israel as in fertility clinics elsewhere, usually more than one embryo is returned to the womb in order to maximize the chances of impregnation in a single treatment cycle. However, while in many European countries the regulations fix the number of returned embryos at two, in Israel the regulations allow greater "freedom."[10] In practice, in many cases more than three embryos are returned. According to medical statistics, the more embryos implanted in the womb, the shorter the pregnancy, the lower the neonatal weight at birth, and the higher mortality and morbidity rates. The logic behind the Israeli regulations is that enabling more embryos to attempt implantation will produce the maximum rate of success in fertilization per treatment cycle. The logic behind such regulations seems to be one of a pro-natal state fighting to increase birth rates at all costs. However, through a vicious circle, the obsession with quantity again brings forth a dilemma over quality.

Being aware of the distributions of morbidity and mortality rates among neonates, Israeli ob-gyns are not interested in creating pregnancies with more than two fetuses. However, they rely on the legitimate possibility of aborting "residual" fetuses if fertilization becomes "too" successful, bringing about great dramas concerning the decision of whether and which embryos to "thin out." Thus, while practicing a most pro-natal technology, Israeli experts and laypersons are caught within the set of tensions characteristic of the Israeli version of pro-natalism—a structure that perpetually leads them to face dilemmas and experience contradictions: in this case, between the attempts to increase fertility as much as possible on the one hand, and to maintain "fetal quality control" on the other. Here is another example to how within a local pro-natal regime tinted with an omnipresent threat of reproductive misfortunes, technologies that are so closely associated with pro-natalism can have confusing consequences on fertility.

Notes

1. After offering amniocentesis free of charge to women over the age of 35 for many years, Israeli medical health funds have recently extended this offer to women over the age of 31.
2. For a discussion of abortion debates in the Israeli Parliament, see Sered (2000).
3. The privileged status of "IDF disabled persons" in the eyes of decision makers is reflected in the special benefits granted to them in Israeli law. Note how the predominance of military symbols differentiates disabled persons according to their relationship to the nation-state through participation in the military, and silences other categories (such as their ability to live a meaningful life, enrich human experience, etc.) that are voiced in the U.S. This is not to say that there are no other disability movements in existence in Israel, but that acting within the above set of binary categories (IDF/non-IDF disabled person) it is difficult for them to elicit attention in the public sphere. In 2002 a group of disabled persons went on a "strike of the disabled" and did get a fair amount of public attention through the media; however, their public concerns focused on financial government budget issues and much less on changing Israeli social perceptions of disabled persons or deconstructing the binary categorization code.
4. Elsewhere I analyze and discuss a range of pregnancy experiences based on the accounts of Israeli pregnant women and show how they develop strategies to maintain different degrees of cautious distance from their fetuses in order to cope with the possibility that an abnormality will be detected in them (Ivry 2010).
5. Elly Teman and I address these issues in our present study on ultra-Orthodox women and their encounters with prenatal diagnosis (Teman and Ivry n.d).
6. The effort to entertain the audience reached a climax when, in the course of an event that took place in June 2002, an IVF specialist treated the audience to a pantomime performance animating scenes of pregnancy and birth.
7. For a discussion of the state of people with disabilities in the socio-cultural context of Israeli society see Weiss (2002: 88–91).
8. As Sered observes (2000), Jews continually used amulets to protect them from the evil eye (in spite of the fact that many rabbis condemned this practice as idol worship). Pregnancy and birth are only particular

cases of this. In her book, Sered includes a long list of amulets and incantations that were used specifically to protect pregnancy and birth from the evil eye and bad ghosts.

9. Or as the editors of this volume reformulated: The experts see it as their obligation to warn the women against deformed fetuses in order to help them "gate keep" their families and society from such reproductive misfortunes, and so do most women.

10. In a 1998 working paper of the Israeli Association of Gynecologists and Obstetricians, the number of returned embryos for women under 35 was three. However, for women over 35 and for those who had undergone three unsuccessful IVF treatments the number is unspecified. An update of this working paper, from 2004, has tightened up the considerations: It recommends that up to two embryos will be returned in the first three cycles. After specifying three more cases in which more embryos can be returned—three unsuccessful treatment cycles with two returned embryos, women over 35 who underwent two unsuccessful treatment cycles with two returned embryos, and the first cycle of a woman over 41—the paper states that the number of returned embryos will not be more than four in any case.

References

Amir, Delila. 1995. "Responsible, Committed and Wise: The Establishment of Israeli Femininity in Committees to Terminate Pregnancy" [Hebrew]. *Teoria VeBikoret* 7: 247–54.

Birenbaum-Carmeli, Daphna. 2004. "'Cheaper than a Newcomer': On the Social Production of IVF Policy in Israel." *Sociology of Health and Illness* 26, no. 7: 897–924.

Cromer, Gerald. 2006. "Analogies to Terror: The Constriction of Social Problems in Israel During the Intifada Al Aqsa." *Terrorism and Political Violence* 18, no. 3: 389–98.

Draper, Jan. 2002. "'It Was a Real Good Show': The Ultrasound Scan, Fathers and the Power of Visual Knowledge." *Sociology of Health and Illness* 24, no. 6: 771–95.

Davis-Floyd, Robbie. 1992. *Birth as an American Rite of Passage.* Berkeley: University of California Press.

Davies, Jonathan. 1999. *Medicolegal Case Law in Obstetrics and Gynecology* [Hebrew]. Jerusalem: Avi Law Books.

Dundes, Alan. 1987. *Cracking Jokes: Studies of Sick Humor Cycles & Stereotypes.* Berkeley: Ten Speed Press.

Ginsburg, Faye D. 1989. *Contested Lives: The Abortion Debate in an American Community.* Berkeley: University of California Press.

Ginsburg, Faye and Rayna Rapp. 1991. "The Politics of Reproduction." *Annual Review of Anthropology* 20: 311–43.

Ginsburg, Faye and Rayna Rapp, eds. 1995. *Conceiving the New World Order: The Global Politics of Reproduction.* Berkeley: University of California Press.

Hashiloni-Dolev, Yael. 2006a. "Between Mothers, Fetuses and Society: Re-productive Genetics in the Israeli-Jewish Context." *Nashim: A Journal of Jewish Women's Studies and Gender Issues* 12: 129–50.

———. 2006b. "Genetic Counseling for Sex Chromosome Anomalies (SCAs) in Israel and Germany: Assessing Medical Risks According to the Importance of Fertility in Two Cultures." *Medical Anthropology Quarterly* 20, no. 4: 469–86.

———. 2007. *What is a Life (un)Worthy of Living? Reproductive Genetics in Germany and Israel.* Dordrecht: Springer-Kluwer.

Hazleton, Lesley. 1977. *Israeli Women: The Reality Behind the Myths.* New York: Simon and Schuster.

Ivry, Tsipy. 2006. "At the Back Stage of Prenatal Care: Japanese Ob-gyns Negotiating Prenatal Diagnosis." *Medical Anthropology Quarterly* 20, no. 4: 441–68.

———. 2007. "Embodied Responsibilities: Pregnancy in the Eyes of Japanese Ob-gyns." *Sociology of Health and Illness* 29, no. 2: 251–74.

———. 2008. "We are Pregnant: Israeli Men and the Paradoxes of Sharing." In *Reconceiving theSecond Sex: Men, Masculinity, and Reproduction,* eds. Marcia C. Inhorn, Tine Tjørnhøj-Thomsen, Helene Goldberg, and Maruska la Cour Mosegaard. Oxford: Berghahn Books.

———. 2008. *Embodying Culture: Pregnancy in Japan and Israel.* New Brunswick: Rutgers University Press.

———. 2009. "The Ultrasonic Picture Show and the Politics of Threatened Life." *Medical Anthropology Quarterly* 23, no. 3: 189–211.

Kahn, Susan Martha. 1999. *Reproducing Jews: A Cultural Account of Assisted Conception in Israel.* Durham: Duke University Press.

Marcus, George E. 1995. "Ethnography in/of the World System: The Emergence of Multi-Sited Ethnography." *Annual Review of* Anthropology 24: 95–117.

Markens, Susan, Carol H. Browner, and Nancy Press. 1997. Feeding the Fetus: On Interrogating the Notion of Maternal-Fetal Conflict. *Feminist Studies* 23, no. 2: 351–72.

Petchesky-Pollack, Rosalind. 1987. "Fetal Images: The Power of Visual Culture in the Politics of Reproduction. *Feminist Studies* 13, no. 2: 263–92.

Rapp, Rayna. 1999. *Testing Women, Testing the Fetus: The Social Impact of Amniocentesis in America.* New York: Routledge.

Rapp, Rayna and Faye D. Ginsburg. 2001. "Enabling Disability: Rewriting Kinship, Reimaging Citizenship." *Public Culture* 13, no. 3: 533–56.

Remennick, Larisa. 2006. "The Quest for the Perfect Baby: Why do Israeli Women Seek Prenatal Genetic Testing?" *Sociology of Health and Illness* 28, no. 1: 21–53.

Rothman, Barbara Katz. 1986. *The Tentative Pregnancy: How Amniocentesis Changes the Experience of Motherhood.* New York: Norton.

———. 1989. *Recreating Motherhood: Ideology and Technology in a Patriarchal Society.* New York: Norton.

Sered, Susan. 2000. *What Makes Women Sick? Maternity, Modesty, and Militarism in Israeli Society.* Hanover: Brandeis University Press.

Sher, Carron, Orly Romano-Zelekha, Manfred S. Greed, and Tamy Shohat. 2003. "Factors Affecting Performance of Prenatal Genetic Testing by Israeli Jewish Women." *American Journal of Medical Genetics* 120A: 418–22.

Taylor, Janelle S. 1992. "The Public Fetus and the Family Car: From Abortion Politics to a Volvo Advertisement." *Public Culture* 4, no. 2: 67–80.

———. 1998. Images of Contradiction: Obstetrical Ultrasound in American Culture. In *Reproducing Reproduction: Kinship, Power, and Technological Innovation*, ed. Sarah Franklin, and Helena Ragone. Philadelphia: University of Pennsylvania Press.

Teman, Elly. 2001. Technological Fragmentation and Women's Empowerment: Surrogate Motherhood in Israel. *Women's Studies Quarterly* 29, nos. 3–4: 11–34.

———. 2003. "The Medicalization of "Nature" in the "Artificial Body": Surrogate Motherhood in Israel." *Medical Anthropology Quarterly* 17, no. 1: 78–98.

———. Birthing a Mother: The Surrogate Body and the Pregnant Self. Berkeley: University of California Press.

Teman, Elly and Tsipy Ivry. n.d. "Ultra-Orthodox Women and Prenatal Testing: God Sent Ordeals and their Discontent."

Weiss, Meira. 2002. *The Chosen Body: The Politics of the Body in Israeli Society*. Stanford, CA: Stanford University Press.

Chapter 8

ABORTION COMMITTEES AS AGENTS OF EUGENICS: MEDICAL AND PUBLIC VIEWS ON SELECTIVE ABORTION FOLLOWING MILD OR LIKELY FETAL PATHOLOGY

Nitzan Rimon-Zarfaty and Aviad Raz

Introduction

The Israeli penal law concerning the interruption of pregnancy (1977) authorizes hospital committees to assess parents' requests for selective abortion. Applications for abortion due to "genetic defects" counted for 15 to 20 percent of all applications submitted to hospital "abortion committees" from 1990 to 2007 (Israeli ministry of health 2008). However, the law does not provide any definition of these "genetic defects" in terms of severity and/or likelihood of expression. Rather, the legal phrasing—kept unchanged since 1977—allows an abortion on the basis of any medical diagnosis for which the fetus "may suffer from physical or mental defect." These definitions remain open to interpretation, negotiation, and boundary-work by parents and committee members. The multi-faceted discussion of these cases involves medical views as well as public discourse, which this chapter seeks to unveil.

Previous research has focused on the role of abortion committees as agents of the Israeli nation-state that subject women to rituals of moral education that reflect the stigma of abortion in a pro-natalist collectivity haunted by the "demographic war" (Amir and Binyamin 1992a, 1992b). However, in the case of applications due to fetal diagnosis, the conventional role of the committee as an agent of moral socialization becomes irrelevant, presumably since the woman does not take the blame for wanting an abortion. The focus of our analysis therefore shifts, in the context of fetal diagnosis and requested abortion, to questions of eugenics: for example, whether parents and committee members in Israel tend to select abortion in relatively mild cases, in cases where the probability of expressing the phenotype is low, as well as in late-stage pregnancies. We focus on this phenomenon, which has not been empirically studied before, in order to explore its cultural, sociological, and bioethical meanings.

Since the term "eugenics" carries loaded and ambiguous meanings (Paul 1994; Mahowald 2003) it is important that we clarify how we use it. "Eugenics" would be regarded today by many scientists as the idea of improving the gene pool of a population. This could be done through selective breeding or genetic enhancement (so-called "positive" eugenics) and/or by preventing the birth of undesirable offspring or preventing them from reproducing (so-called "negative" eugenics). When abortions are selected due to genetic defects in the embryo this would be widely regarded as negative eugenics. Of note, from the perspective of population genetics, such abortions are not, strictly speaking, negative eugenics, because preventing the birth of embryos with genetic defects does not obliterate deleterious genes or even necessarily reduce their prevalence in the population. "Real" negative eugenics, scientifically speaking, would be to prevent all carriers from reproducing. Notwithstanding the importance of such objective definitions, our use of "eugenic abortions" here follows the social construction of this phenomenon by the public (Raz 2009). It is also important to emphasize that this research deals with committee deliberations regarding selective abortion due to mild or likely embryopathies. It does not deal with cases in which the embryopathies are "clear-cut" or "severe" by medical definition. Focusing on those borderline cases enables us to examine the normative boundaries, as well as the negotiation of those boundaries, as they are reflected through committee deliberations. We use the term "mild or likely" embryopathies to denote medical conditions in which affected individuals usually have normal intelligence, normal life span and a reasonable quality of life. Evidently, there is no consensus over the definition of what makes life "worth living"—which is exactly our point. Examples of relatively mild or likely genetic embryopathies include: (i) Gaucher disease, a disease with several severity degrees that cannot be predicted by genetic testing. The mildest form (which is also the common one) is expressed by symptoms similar to anemia. The genetic test for Gaucher, which is a relatively prevalent disease in the Jewish population, is being offered by most of the genetic institutes in Israel; (ii) congenital deafness, which can be tested for in some of the genetic institutes in Israel as part of the standard battery of tests offered to the public, and constitutes another controversial case in which the disease is relatively mild as well as often treatable; (iii) dwarfism, where in milder forms of achondroplasia, for example, affected individuals usually have normal intelligence and a normal life span. However, affected children have a number of medical complications that can affect their development.

Interviews with committee members (physicians and social workers), as well as with geneticists who serve as committee advisors, are used in order to describe and analyze exemplary cases and recurrent themes reflecting the opinions of respondents. We conclude the chapter with an international comparison in order to highlight the characteristics of the Israeli case, and then discuss the possible links between the discourses of health professionals, parents, and the media.

Setting the theoretical scene

The socio-anthropological interest in selective abortion following genetic diagnosis is multi-faceted. The prevalence and popularity of prenatal diagnosis have been discussed, following Foucault (1976, 1977, 1991), as reflecting a growing governmentality of bio-power and medicalization. In this view, pregnancy and reproduction join an increasing range of human "problems" that are defined as genetic in origin, a phenomenon termed "geneticization" (Conrad 1997, 1999; Lippman 1992; Nye 2003; Sawicki 1999). Others have examined the public images and popular discourses around the "new genetics," including motifs of essentialism, reductionism, and determinism and their implications for moral issues such as parental responsibility (Nelkin and Lindee 1995; Lock 1998). Another major focus has been to examine the profession of genetic counseling and its associated ethical and social dilemmas (Bosk 1992; Wertz 1998). Sociologists and anthropologists studying prenatal diagnosis have also asked how the culture-bound and value-laden concepts of the "severity" and "mildness" of the embryopathy are constructed and negotiated (Franklin 2003; Rothman 1998; Rapp 1999; Rapp and Ginsburg 2001).

Prenatal diagnosis is meant to provide individuals with non-directive and understandable medical information while respecting personal and cultural differences (Kelly 1986). However, if prenatal diagnosis is typically done with the goal of identifying an affected fetus so that the pregnancy can be terminated, then it is directive and in fact reflects discrimination against the disabled (Asch 1994; Roberts et al. 2002). While this "disability critique" (Parens and Asch 2000) concerning the eugenic agenda of prenatal diagnosis was originally directed to genetic counseling, it also applies to the issues discussed here. Fetal diagnosis in Israel is a burgeoning industry (Remennick 2006; Sher et al. 2003). Women who seek abortion are usually referred to the hospital committee by genetic counselors. The deliberations of the committee therefore continue and extend the process of genetic counseling. Do the committee's deliberations express negative or discriminatory attitudes about impairments and those who are supposed to carry them? Do they send a hurtful message to people who live with those same traits? Almost twenty years ago, Adrienne Asch (1988: 81) put the concerns this way: "Do not disparage the lives of existing and future disabled people by trying to screen for and prevent the birth of babies with their characteristics."

The traditional argument against this criticism claims that the desirability of preventing *serious* fetal disabilities has no implications for how people with those disabilities can or should be treated, and, in particular, does not justify their mistreatment in any way (Paul 1998; WHO 2002). While the validity of this argument should be empirically tested, it has theoretical problems. For example, who can or should define which diseases are *serious* or severe enough to justify abortion? Severity is a subjective term, influenced by expectations and norms. Only a few genetic disorders, such as Lesch-Nyman or Tay-Sachs disease, are so severe as to make the lives of people who have them perhaps not worth living. But what about congenital deafness or dwarfism, cleft lip or Gaucher disease, to name just a few examples? The vast majority of conditions for which fetal diagnosis is now—and will be in the future—possible are located on a confusing spectrum of probability, somewhere between mildness and severity, treatment and terminality (see also Rothenberg and Thomson 1994). The issue of selective abortion is hence replete with conflict and has generated loud and enthusiastic debates—especially in the U.S. and Europe—amongst liberals and communitarians, feminists and conservatives, human rights activists and bioethicists (Blendon et al. 1993; Gatens-Robonson 1996). Apparently, no public debate has emerged in Israel concerning this issue, despite its conflict-ridden nature (Raz 2004). This chapter sets out to examine the debates (or the lack thereof) within the deliberations surrounding applications for selective abortion following fetal diagnosis.

The Israeli Law of Abortion provides a flexible legal framework for regulating abortions. On the one hand, it sends an ideological message de-legitimizing "abortion on demand" and prohibiting abortion due to financial distress. On the other hand, it provides elbow room for the hospital committees to accept applications for abortion on the basis of medical reasons (to do with the mother, the fetus, or both) or in cases of underage or unwed mothers, or of adultery, rape, or incest. We focus here on the actual deliberations of hospital committees concerning embryopathic reasons for abortion in order to examine whether, as Hashiloni-Dolev (2006: 135) argues, "Israeli abortion policy, past and present, does not touch on the possible conflict between the interests of mothers and those of fetuses, as protection of the fetus is virtually a non-issue." The embryopathic (third) clause of the Law of Abortion, according to Shapira (1995: 24):

> appears to reveal an unmistakably lenient policy on abortion for eugenic reasons. The physical or mental defect justifying interruption of pregnancy need not necessarily be extensive or grievous. An ordinary, perhaps even a relatively minor, defect may suffice. Furthermore, the defect need only be "likely" as distinct from certain or probable.

Our question is therefore how hospital committees translate the Law of Abortion into practical decisions and negotiate its ambiguous directives.

Methodology

Since the committee deliberations are confidential, we could not access them directly. Instead, we inferred the discursive dynamics of these deliberations by juxtaposing two sources of data: interviews conducted by the first author with committee members and advisors, as well as stories on such deliberations that were reported in the newspapers. Print media reports in the three largest newspapers available to the general public—*Yediot Acharonot, Ma'arriv,* and *Ha'arretz*—were monitored by the first author who searched for stories on fetal diagnosis and requested abortion appearing from 2000 to 2006. All items indexed in these newspapers were eligible for inclusion in our analysis. The yield from these searches was 22 articles dealing specifically with requested abortion due to fetal diagnosis (see appendix for the full list). Each of the stories was analyzed to identify the stakeholders and their attitudes regarding the pros and cons of selective abortion following fetal diagnosis. Evidently, these articles represent cases that warranted media coverage because of their conflictual or otherwise extraordinary nature (Singer and Endreny 1993). We argue, however, that such borderline cases highlight the competing discourses and are likely to have implications for public perceptions and attitudes. (Rowley 1984), for example, noted that fetal screening in cases of advanced maternal age was widely adopted, in part, because extensive media coverage led to a demand for such service.

In addition to the media reports, nine representatives of the medical establishment who were members of or advisors to hospital committees were interviewed by the first author.[1] Interviews were conducted in Hebrew, usually held in the office of the respondent, and lasted between one to two hours. Respondents, who came from a variety of hospitals in Israel, were asked about their experience with and attitudes towards actual cases of requested abortion due to mild or likely embryopathy. The thematization of the media stories and the interviews, and their ensuing juxtaposition, led to the identification of key stakeholders, which we present here in a concentric order: the fetus, the parents, and committee members and advisors. In what follows we present the recurrent themes that characterized each of these stakeholders, highlighting dominant as well as minority views.

The (missing) fetus

The fetus could have been perceived as a stakeholder in the context of abortion. Even though his/her voice cannot be heard, it could have been represented by each of the other stakeholders—parents, professionals, policy-makers, jurists, or journalists. However, the main finding was an overarching lack of reference to the fetus as a stakeholder—namely a goal-directed organism with autonomy and rights. This section discusses what parents (as represented by the media), health professionals and journalists had to say (or did not say) concerning the fetus. As one of the committee advisors said (personal interview, 20/3/06): "There is a fetus in there but nobody asks what its opinion might be [. . .] the law does not recognize any fetal rights for that matter." This observation matches the academic criticism of Hashiloni-Dolev (2006: 136), who argues that the "Israeli law offers no rationale for its regulation of abortion, referring neither to the status and rights of the fetus nor to those of the pregnant woman. Thus, the Israeli fetus has no legal standing whatsoever and is not recognized as an autonomous being." In one of the cases reported in the media (report #3 in the appendix), a hospital committee refused to allow abortion following an ultrasound diagnosis implying an embryopathy of "short bones." The report describes a deliberation between committee members that centered on the question of the reliability of the ultrasound results. None of the committee members, nor the parents (who requested the abortion) or the reporter, however, raised the possibility that life with "short bones" (i.e., dwarfism) is perhaps worth living. In other reports of cases where the embryopathy was mild or likely, the dominant attitude of the parents concerning the embryopathy was similarly constituted of fear that the committee would not approve the request for abortion.

The dominant view among committee members and advisors reflected an awareness that what they were doing was eugenic, and an attempt to rationalize this. One form of rationalization hinged on perceived public pressure. As one committee advisor (a genetic counselor) explained (personal interview, 23/3/06):

> This issue of whether the fetus is deaf, okay, does it mean it has no right to live? This issue almost never comes up. We focus on the characteristics of the embryopathy and not on the person. I think people would say that even in cases of mild embryopathies, we want the child to have the best life possible. I think the common attitude is— "actually, we are doing him [the unborn] a favor."

Another form of rationalization emphasized the determination of the "client" to prefer abortion, thus removing the blame from committee members and advisors. The question whether such a decision should indeed be "client-led" was, however, ignored. As another committee member commented (personal interview, 29/1/06):

> Is the fetus present during the deliberations? No. Is it good that he is not present? The population we are dealing with here manages its reproductive decisions according to risk margins that are lower than anywhere else in the world. People here are not willing to take any risk. We are prisoners of this situation [. . .] we are hysterical and consequently there is no consideration of the opinion the fetus might have. So does he need to be present in the deliberation? I think not . . .

Another committee advisor similarly said (personal interview, 12/1/06):

> If a couple decides to go and test the fetus for deafness, which is part of the tests offered by hospitals, not by recommendation but elective, and there is a positive test result, we would refer them to the hospital committee. We cannot say at this point: "after everything we have done, now we must stop you." Why did we start with it to begin with? It's a moral decision, and moral decisions are for the family to decide, not for us.

One of the interesting cases reported in the media in this context (report #5 in the appendix) dealt with a "wrongful life" suit in which, after eight years of deliberations, the judge ruled that it was possible to prevent the birth of a baby with a congenital heart defect and a genetic disease, had the doctors acted properly and given the parents all the information. The judge commented that it would have been justified to authorize late abortion—in this case, even in the eighth month of pregnancy (see also Savulescu 2001; Shapira 1995). Once again, the report revolved around the liability of doctors and the problems created for the parents, whose right to abort had been compromised. Despite the questionable severity of the embryopathy and the viability of the fetus, none of the participants—including the reporter—thought to mention the fetus's perspective.

The issue of late abortion, which is particularly relevant to this case, represents another lacuna in the discourse on the fetus. Late abortions are performed mostly for embryopathic reasons and are far more common in Israel than in Western countries (Gross 1999). As a committee advisor said in this context (personal interview, 9/4/2006):

> Here at the hospital there are extreme cases of women undergoing abortion in a very late stage [. . .] it is like delivering the newborn and then hitting him with a big stick on the head. This is truly a viable fetus. And yet they perform abortion in such late stage. Give it one hour and it would have been a baby [. . .] on the other hand, those who know the parents realize how tough this is for them. I think one must consider this on a case by case basis.

The Israeli Law of Abortion in itself (as apposed to other abortions laws) sets no time limit for late abortion, thus overlooking the issue of viability—a pivotal source of debate in the West, but not in Israel. The Israeli Ministry of Health (memorandum #23/07, issued 19.12.07) recently decided that requests for late term abortions (beyond week 24) will be discussed only by special, high-level committees[2], and to justify termination of pregnancy the embryopathy must be medically considered severe (or moderate up to week 27) as well as probable (probability of more than 30 percent). There are still no clear-cut definitions of each classification or reference to a specific defect as mild, moderate or severe. The influence of this change in policy still waits to be studied, particularly since the new guidelines are also open for interpretation and negotiation by parents, committee members and advisors. While the recent memorandum of the Ministry of Health (2007) is an important step forward, one can ask whether the more stringent criteria regarding the severity and probability of fetal abnormality that it advances in the context of late term abortions should not also be raised and discussed in the general context of selective abortions due to embryopathies.

The only reference to the issue of the rights of the fetus was brought up in one report (#7) whose subject was intrauterine fetal surgery. The report cites a woman, whose twin fetuses were operated on in the womb in order to separate their blood systems (a life-threatening TTTS syndrome). Chances of success were 33 percent, and the woman recounted how her family and friends suggested selective abortion: "They told me: you are young, why do you need this [. . .] do an abortion and get it over with, there will be other pregnancies." In explaining why she chose to have the surgery instead, the woman commented:

> I said to myself, if you had 3-year-old twins who needed a life-saving surgery, you'd run to the end of the world to get that surgery. So, just because they are still in your womb, does it make you less responsible for them? I felt that even if they hadn't been born yet, they are still my children just the same.

Interestingly, this attitude was presented as "surprising" in the report. In contrast, the reporter cited Professor Lifshitz, head of fetal surgery at Sheba Hospital, as saying that because Israelis pursue "the perfect child," there is an overall secular tendency not to confront problems (for example through fetal surgery) but rather to terminate the pregnancy. According to the reporter, doctors do not provide all the information regarding the treatment of children diagnosed with embryopathy, and the overall inclination in Israel is to terminate every problematic pregnancy rather than to confront the problem (report #7).

The parents

When an embryopathy is found, parents face the dilemma of whether to continue the pregnancy. Report #12 describes the case of a young woman, six months pregnant, who was told that she and her husband were carrying a mutation for a disease that might harm the fetus's lungs and liver. Still expecting the results of amniocentesis, she told the reporter: "Since the beginning of this pregnancy my husband and I did twelve genetic tests. I keep asking myself, what if they find that the baby is deaf? Would that be reason enough to abort?" According to the vast majority of the reports, this dilemma is resolved through selective abortion, even in cases where the embryopathy is mild or only likely. Report #12 also mentions the story of a couple who decided to abort following a positive diagnosis for Klinefelter disease (symptoms including fertility problems and a spectrum of learning disabilities and attention deficits). The couple was cited as saying: "We didn't want to take an unnecessary risk. Especially after the geneticist told us: 'If I were you, I would go for abortion.'"

A recurrent theme in the reports and the interviews concerned the social legitimacy attributed to selective abortions due to embryopathy. In report #3, which discusses the case of the fetus that was diagnosed with "short bones," the reporter described empathetically the "heavy pressure" put on the committee by the parents. The report contained no criticism towards the parents for pressuring the committee or for taking "too many" fetal tests. Indeed, many of the reports (see for example report #10, #11) proudly comment on the "Israeli world record" in individual as well as prenatal testing: "Only 27 percent of Israeli couples did not take genetic testing before deciding to have the first child" (report #10). In another report (#12), prenatal tests are presented almost as an addiction; the reporter describes a woman who, after having exhausted the battery of standard tests, paid thousands of shekels out-of-pocket for additional tests that were not subsidized by the HMOs. "Every time a new test is out on the market, it's very tempting," the woman is cited as saying, "and as if all this wasn't enough, I added two tests for deafness and blindness."

Parents' views, as presented in the vast majority of the reports, construct prenatal diagnosis as an important and taken-for-granted part of "responsible parenthood." This new concept of responsible parenthood, representing normalization and subjugation in Foucauldian terms, also implies that parents who choose to avoid prenatal diagnosis are "irresponsible or primitive," and that parents who choose not to abort in cases of embryopathy are "crazy" or otherwise deviant (quotes cited in report #2). Such reports, presenting a dominant, positive, and pro-eugenic view of fetal diagnosis amongst Israeli parents, stand in sharp contrast to a small and laconic piece (report #13) which mentioned that parents in the U.K. tend *not* to use a screening test for colon cancer recently offered by hospitals as part of PGD (pre-implantation genetic diagnosis).

How do parents negotiate the ambivalence of the embryopathic clause? According to the vast majority of the reports, parents did not see the lenience of the clause as a problem, but rather as an advantage they could exploit. In report #16, the journalist asks: "What does a married woman who wants to abort an unwanted pregnancy have to do in order to persuade the hospital committee?" According to the report, for many women the answer is: "to find the loopholes." The reporter describes a variety of false justifications provided by women to the hospital committee, such as saying that the husband was not the father, or that the pregnancy was conceived while the woman had an intra-uterine contraceptive device, or that she has been taking medicines that could have harmed the fetus. The two latter reasons potentially increase the risk of embryopathies, thus qualifying the applicant for selective abortion under the embryopathic clause. According to the same report, committee members admitted, not for the record, that they had no desire to find out if the applicant was telling the truth. We return to this position when discussing the position of committee members below.

Committee members and advisors

We begin with the general views of committee members and advisors concerning their function in the context of the embryopathic clause, and then move to a discussion of ambivalent cases. Generally speaking, opinions of committee members and advisors towards selective abortion due to the embryopathic clause ranged from pro-eugenic acceptance of the existing situation (the majority view) via ambivalent position to outright criticism (the minority view). The following quotations from the interviews illustrate the majority view of pro-eugenic acceptance of the existing situation:

> There are so many women who sit in front of me and say: In my family there are no genetic diseases. This is bullshit; do you know how many mutations you might be carrying? We have seen so many couples who were carriers of deleterious genes, and we have prevented the birth of so many sick children. (personal interview, 10/12/06)

For this respondent, prenatal diagnosis was eugenic and was indeed supported precisely for that, since "eugenic" for them meant the improvement of the health of progeny and carried positive rather than negative connotations. As another respondent commented (personal interview, 10/12/06):

> There is no other country that competes with Israel in terms of the number of prenatal tests. I see it as a very positive thing. Women who take the tests are doing something very important. You have to do the maximum, otherwise if there's a problem you are stuck with it.

Moreover, one of the interviewed committee advisors told the first author that:

> When I fear that the committee would not approve the requested abortion, I approach members directly in order to persuade them. I tell them, once we recommended amniocentesis for this indication, and the result was positive, we must help the parents. I explain to the members of the committee the complications of the relevant embryopathy and this helps, many times. When things are ambivalent it is very useful to have such a conversation. I think that committees today are much more attentive to the needs of the parents, even in the case of late abortions. (personal interview, 10/12/06)

As this quote suggests, many committee advisors push for eugenic abortions, even in cases of mild or likely embryopathies. This could also reflect a growing fear of legal suits regarding "wrongful births" as well as a public health bias for prevention (Hashiloni-Dolev 2007). It was common to hear the respondents expressing empathy, rather than criticism, towards the parents who apply for abortion. The following quote illustrates this empathy as well as the ambivalence that comes with it (personal interview, 10/12/06):

> Sometimes I have an unpleasant feeling sitting in front of a couple who tell the committee: We are not going to be able to deal with such a child. The committee is playing God, and there is this feeling of unfairness, for me at least. The couple is right to insist that if there is a problem then it befalls on them because they would have to take care of the sick child. Who are the committee members to decide for them? I totally understand these parents. On the other hand you ask where the end is, and I don't know, I really don't know where to draw the line.

Indeed, there were respondents who expressed their difficulties in dealing with the ambivalence that comes with the ethical questions relating to the approval of abortions, especially due to mild or likely embryopathies. As one committee member said:

> It makes you very doubtful. . . That a baby will be born with a defect, and to let the parents and the child deal with a defect all their lives. . .

> On the other hand, who gave us the moral authority to decide whether or not to stop a pregnancy? Maybe the child is healthy, and even if he has, for example, short legs, he can still live full and productive life, within the limits that he would have to deal with. It brings out a very difficult ethical question. (personal interview, 5/3/07)

Some respondents also mentioned the parents and the difficulties some of them are facing in trying to deal with the decision of whether or not to abort (personal interview, 20/4/07):

> A lot of Jewish couples want the perfect child; there is no doubt about it. But I also see a lot of couples that don't. I can definitely see that making that kind of decision is actually a heart-breaking experience for them. The fear that I, with my own hands, caused the death of a healthy baby—who am I to play God? Even if he is retarded, he is still my child and I would raise him and give him everything that I can. . . I definitely see the other side, too.

In addition, a few of the respondents expressed criticism of the existing situation, pointing to the financial interest of the medical system (personal interview, 29/1/07):

> What's going on in Israel has long gone beyond medicine. It is business, pure and simple. If you think about it as business, then you shouldn't be surprised at the amount of ultrasound or genetic testing or amniocentesis per capita, with or without medical justification [. . .]. We are the only country where the medical establishment offers women to undergo amniocentesis for diseases whose frequency is one to ten thousands. Why? I have no idea. Money? Maybe also money, but not just that.

In sum, although the general opinion expressed by the respondents was a pro-eugenic acceptance of the existing situation, it seems that such acceptance is not without underlying moral and ethical dilemmas, experienced by committee members and advisors, as well as parents.

How do committee members and advisors negotiate the ambivalence of the embryopathic clause? Moving beyond the general opinions just discussed, a majority of the respondents acknowledged that some cases were indeed ambivalent:

> The truth is that I had never really given it much thought, but now that you are showing me the clause in writing, I agree it is ambivalent [. . .], what does it mean, that the child may suffer from physical or mental defect? If it's doubtful, then it is not certain that the newborn would have a defect. And how do you define a physical defect? What are the boundaries? Mental defects, these are even more complicated

> to define[. . .]. Everyone tells you that Down's syndrome is a defect, but it can be either very severe or mild. (personal interview, 23/3/06)

Committee members who have to deal with the ambiguity of the embryopathy cannot turn to the law for guidance since the legal clause regarding embryopathy is itself ambiguous. In the context of such medical and legal ambiguity, boundary negotiation often reproduces traditional normative scripts. Down Syndrome, for example, has been viewed for most of its history as a public health problem, with prenatal screening aimed at reducing its incidence (Raffle 2001). As Bryant et al. (2008) show, only relatively recently there have been efforts to promote reproductive choice rather than test uptake as the preferred measure of a screening program's success.

Other respondents added the lack of standardization among committees to the ambivalence just mentioned:

> Sometimes I tell the parents, you have better chances with a committee in the Tel Aviv area. There was this woman who applied to the committee which she thought would be the most understanding of her case. She was in her late pregnancy and there was a suspicion of small head circumference—a very ambivalent case. She applied to a committee in a central hospital and they approved it. I know of someone with a similar case whose application was rejected by another committee. (personal interview, 23/3/06)

In this case, the counselor used her inside knowledge regarding the politics of the committees in order to help her clients achieve the abortion they wanted. This quote emphasizes the flexibility of the committee system and the lack of consistency in interpreting the law.

While many of the respondents agreed that ambivalence existed, the majority was satisfied with it, claiming that the issue of selective abortion warranted flexibility:

> I am okay with this clause because it allows authorizing selective abortions even without precise or specific diagnosis. I prefer not to have ethical regulations in such issues. Let me give you an example: Let's say we have a fetus with cleft lip. That was the finding, but the extent of the risk for the fetus may be more serious. Can it be repaired? We cannot be sure. (personal interview, 29/1/07)

It seems that this ambivalence provides a welcomed flexibility that enables committee members to approve abortions even in borderline situations—an ability they view positively.

Indeed, another source of ambivalence that surfaced in the interviews concerned the issue of late abortions. As one of the respondents said:

> I think there is a difference between week 24 [of gestation] and week 35. For me, week 35 is a human being [. . .]. Somehow it is obvious that it is much easier to terminate a pregnancy in week 12, 13 than after week 30. It is almost birth. The period of pregnancy is very crucial—there was a reason for the establishment of "high level committees." (personal interview, 23/3/06)

In contrast, another respondent justified late abortions in the following manner:

> Some say it is different when the fetus is viable. I think this is true only to a certain extent. If the embryopathy was found late in the pregnancy, this is not the couple's fault. You know that if the embryopathy was found 3 to 4 weeks ago, abortion would have been approved by the committee without any discussion. Now there will be discussion only because a few weeks have passed? A 14-week fetus is no less a child than a 24-week fetus. In cases of heart defects there are always deliberations in the committee. Especially in cases of late abortion. We bring the expert opinion of cardiologists and start to deliberate whether the risk is significant enough or not. Each member has their own opinion. Somebody says 10 per cent; another one says 20 per cent [. . .]. I tend to go with the parents because it's their burden. (personal interview, 10/12/06)

As mentioned before, committee members face very hard ethical dilemmas—as a result of lack of clear standards regarding the severity of embryopathies justifying abortions. These dilemmas become accentuated in cases of late pregnancies. According to one chairperson of a "high-level committee," there are indeed many instances of loud debating amongst members (see report #4).

Moreover, some committee members told the first author that in cases of mild or likely embryopathy, especially in cases of late pregnancies, the difficulties of making the decision has led them to ask for further examination of the fetus's medical condition:

> We ask the parents to present us with the best tests in every field which is relevant to the specific defect. Only then we actually make the decision, relying on our committee advisors[. . .]. I have to say that there is a very big dilemma, and this is why we turn them to the best experts, in order to get the clearest picture possible. A lot of times you can't really get a clear picture. For example a woman that had CMV [viral infection] during her pregnancy, and expressed fear that the baby was infected and would suffer from defects. It is very very

sensitive and it is very very hard to make a decision like that (personal interview, 7/3/07)

Some parents were quoted as expressing similar dilemmas:

> Look, it is ambiguous, some parents hear that there are some dangers, and immediately, without any hesitations, ask for abortion. But there are some who would definitely check, consult with more doctors, won't take it for granted, it is very personal [. . .]. Look, they receive the genetic counseling, it's not like something is found in the ultrasound and immediately they make an abortion. It's not that simplistic. I can definitely see that there are parents who ask for more counseling, that have a very big conflict, that consult a religious scholar. I think that people do invest in it and that if they turn to the committee, they actually mean to abort (personal interview, 11/3/07).

Conclusion

The purpose of this chapter was to explore the views of hospital committee members and advisors in Israel, as well as of parents whose voices are represented in the media, regarding selective abortion due to mild or likely embryopathies. Committee members, as well as parents (as represented by the media), did not share attitudes similar to those held by some disability rights advocates in the U.S. and the U.K. Indeed, respondents in the two groups generally viewed selective abortion due to mild or likely embryopathy favorably. In other words, the majority of the respondents, and all the print media reports, subscribed to and supported the eugenic goal of prenatal diagnosis. This study thus complements a growing number of studies which characterize Israel as a pro-eugenic society.

To what extent can the particular disposition found in this study be the result of an international biomedical worldview, rather than being specifically related to Israeli culture? Comparative evidence suggests that the Israeli case is exceptional. For example, health professionals in France who were involved in abortions due to mild or likely fetal diagnoses expressed difficulties with their role, criticizing the risk of eugenic pressures (Garel et al. 2002).[3] In the U.K., obstetricians have also expressed similar worries about third-trimester termination of pregnancy (Liford and Thornton 1993; Paintin 1997; Green 1995). In contrast, such comments were not commonly heard from Israeli health professionals. Legal ambiguity, perceived as a positive state of affairs by the majority of Israeli respondents, as it provides flexibility, was negatively viewed by the majority of the respondents in France and the U.K.

This chapter described the complementary views of two groups, parents (as represented by the media) as well as committee members and advisors, concerning selective abortion in cases of mild or likely embryopathies. The vast majority of the respondents referred to a shared view of "responsible parenthood," which for them meant responsibility towards the parents' needs rather than the needs of the unborn, and was possibly also perceived in the context of "wrongful births" (cf. Skorecki 2005). Is there a linkage between the pro-eugenic discourses that dominate the attitudes of parents, as they were presented by the media, and medical professionals in Israel? Are there any connections or influences between those discourses and their main characteristics, i.e., the directivity of the medical establishment, the pro-eugenic public view of "responsible parenthood," and the parental pressure to increase the "flexibility" of committee members and advisors? Evidently, this question requires further research. The two discourses correlate, and probably also reinforce each other, at least according to our findings in the Israeli setting. Previous studies found that the way in which a reproductive issue is covered in the media can clearly influence the attitudes of the public. For example, Singer et al. (1999) found that, after the North American media became more negative regarding abortions, there was a significant increase in those saying they would not want to have an abortion in the event that a prenatal test disclosed a genetic defect in the fetus (cf. Caruso et al. 1998).

When Wertz (1998) conducted her worldwide survey of genetics professionals, she measured the acceptance of eugenics using the statement "An important goal of genetic counseling is to reduce the number of deleterious genes in the population." The majority of geneticists in 12 out of the 36 nations surveyed (including Israel, but not the U.S.) agreed with the statement.[4] This led Wertz to conclude that most genetic counseling around the world is directive (and hence eugenic), and that the ideal of "nondirective counseling" found in English-speaking countries is actually an aberration from the general practice of giving advice.

Hashiloni-Dolev (2007) further substantiated these findings in comparing Israeli and German geneticists, and the lives these two societies consider (un)worthy of living. Even representatives of Israeli disability organizations were found to support prenatal diagnosis as representing a eugenic improvement in the health of progeny, while at the same time expressing their commitment to support the needs of individuals already born with disabilities (Raz 2004). All the media reports in the last five years revealed a similar pro-eugenic approach by stating that the wide variety of prenatal diagnoses available in Israel enables the reduction of the number of births of children with embryopathies.

When the parents apply to a hospital abortion committee, it means that their decision to abort has already been made and the committee's function is to approve or disapprove it. Our findings concerning the pro-eugenic attitudes of the vast majority of committee members and advisors in cases of mild or likely embryopathies can be seen to follow from the directive approach of Israeli geneticists. Indeed, many of these geneticists serve as committee members and advisors. The categories of committee members, geneticists, and advisors often overlap; geneticists often participate in hospital abortion committees as members, and when the committee requires an expert (and/or second) opinion regarding a specific mutation, it asks for the advice of geneticists with the relevant expertise. This validates the assessment, made long ago by proponents of the disability critique, that the intention of genetic counseling is eugenicist by implication[5] and that eugenics is built into genetic counseling because of the normativity of medicine.

In seeking to understand "what mutes moral criticism of prenatal diagnosis in Israeli society" (Hashiloni-Dolev 2006: 143), several over-arching explanations have been provided by different authors. Remennick (2006) suggested that Israeli women seek prenatal genetic testing that leads to selective abortion due to a combination of factors: strong health provider support of such tests; emerging social norms that equate "good mothering" with taking "genetic responsibility"; deep intolerance towards disability; and fear of the burden of care for a disabled child. The last three issues were particularly characteristic of the views shared by the majority of our respondents, with "good mothering" becoming an instance of "responsible parenthhood." Weiss (2002) explained the Israeli zeal for the perfect child as part of the cultural script she calls the "chosen body," emanating from both Zionist ideology and Jewish religious tradition. Hashiloni-Dolev (2006) focuses on the Israeli biopolitics of the beginning of life, based on Jewish tradition and Zionism, which regard life as beginning after birth and perceive fetuses as parts of their mothers with no autonomous rights.[6] The prevalence of prenatal diagnosis leading to selective abortion among secular Israelis was explained as influenced by a nationalist Zionist ideology combining pro-natalism and veneration of the body as well as by a medical establishment that, generally speaking, legitimizes directivity (Weiss 2002; Kahn 2000; Kanaaneh 2002).

We would like to add to these general claims a practical observation emanating from our findings. On the one hand, the very existence of a penal law of abortion and the official existence of its formal gatekeepers, the hospital committees, conveys an *ideological* message of pro-natalism and the stigmatization of selective abortion. On the other hand, a closer reading of the law (for example in terms of the ambiguity of the third clause) and an examination of the leniency of hospital committees shows that *in practice*, those who want selective abortion can get it quite easily. The "muting of moral criticism" could also be located in this ambiguous gap between ideological decalartions and practical flexibility. On the one hand, the law restricts selective abortions, thus paying lip service to moral criticism. On the other hand, abortions can be easily obtained by manipulating the loopholes which are built into the system and accepted positively by medical professionals as well as the general public. This pragmatic status quo seems to have silenced public (and particularly political) debate, which nevertheless still lurks in the background.

Appendix: list of print media reports

1 "Towards pre-pregnancy diagnosis" Irit Kinor, Ha'arretz, 2 April, 2000.
2. "The desire for the perfect child," Tamara Traubman, Ha'arretz, 10 October, 2004.
3 "A mistake in the test almost caused an abortion," Hila Elroi de Ber, Ma'arriv, 9 December, 2005.
4. "The stomach turns around," Reuvan Weiss and Sarit Rosenblum, Yediot Acharonot, 9 June, 2006.
5. "Writing in memory, not in the file," Ran Reznik, Ha'arretz, 3 May, 2002
6. "New: the sex of the fetus can be determined before pregnancy," Dalya Mazori, Ma'arriv, 10 September, 2002.
7. "The person inside," Ayelet Negev and Yehuda Koren. Yediot Acharonot, 14 April, 2006.
8. "Before the semen enters the picture," Tamara Traubman and Ran Reznik, Ha'arretz, 11 August, 2005.
9. "The bond of silence," Tali Lipkin-Shachak, Ma'arriv, 17 March, 2006.
10. "Research: tens of futile abortions in Israel every year," Dan Even, Ma'arriv, 3 July, 2006.

11. "My perfect child," Yehuda Koren, Yediot Acharonot, 28 May, 2000.
12. "Passes in the genes," Ruti Kadosh, Ma'arriv, 7 October, 2004.
13. "Baby on demand," Moodi Kreitman, Yediot Acharonot, 3 November, 2004.
14. "The defect found in the 8th month, the fetus died." Anat Bershakovski, Yediot Acharonot, 6 November, 2005.
15. "Baby girl on demand," Lilit Wagner, Yediot Acharonot, 28 February, 2002.
16. "Lies I told the committee," Aviva Lori, Ha'arretz, 11 August, 2006.
17. "Preventive programs for genetic diseases in the Arab population," Dr. Stavit Shalev, Yediot Acharonot, 21 July, 2004.
18. "The police auditor tough findings," Yoav Yitzhak, Ma'arriv, 15 March, 2002.
19. "Double tragedy," Michal Goldberg, Yediot Acharonot, 29 June, 2006.
20. "Battle between religious and female Knesset members concerning abortion," Linoy Bar-Gefen, Yediot Acharonot, 5 December, 2000.
21. "The minister of health: approval of abortion without consideration," Alon Gideon and Haim Shadmi, Ha'arretz, 4 July, 2001.
22. "Survey: 17 percent think disabled people are a nuisance," Ruti Sinai, Ha'arretz, 15 November, 2005.

Notes

1. Data from print media and interviews was collected by the first author as part of her M.A thesis.
2. "High-level committees" (*va'adot al*) are special committees formed in regional hospitals, that discuss applications for late abortions.
3. The study reported by Garel et al. (2002) used interviews conducted in three tertiary care maternity units in France to explore the conflicts and ethical problems experienced by medical professionals involved in prenatal diagnosis and termination of pregnancy The French legislation governing selective abortion for fetal abnormality dates from 1975 and was amended in 1994. In quite a similar manner to the Israeli law, it allows termination without any upper gestational age limit when the pregnancy "severely endangers the mother's health" or there is a "strong probability" of a "severe" fetal anomaly. In a parallel manner to Israel, selective abortion in France has to be approved by a multidisciplinary hospital committee.

4. Note that when a slightly different phrasing was used, i.e., "prevention of diseases is a highly important goal of genetic counseling," 52 percent of the surveyed U.S. genetic counselors also agreed (Wertz & Fletcher 1989).

5. Holtzman & Shapiro (1998) argued that prenatal diagnosis followed by selective abortion has replaced sterilization as "the major eugenic technique."

6. It is not clear, however, how to reconcile Hashiloni-Dolev's claim that Jewish tradition disregards the fetus as a living person and supports the prevention of life with disability, with the *halachic* position that the fetus is considered a person after 40 days of gestation and hence selective abortion is prohibited by the majority of rabbis (thus leading to pre-marital, rather than prenatal, genetic testing and carrier matching in the form of *Dor Yeshorim*, the program implemented in the ultra-Orthodox community).

References

Amir, D. and O. Binyamin. 1992a. "Abortion Approval as Ritual of Symbolic Control." In *The Criminalization of a Woman's Body*, ed. C. Feinman. Binghampton, NY: Haworth Press. 1–25.

Amir, D. and O. Binyamin. 1992b. "The abortion committees: Educating and controlling women." *Journal of Women and Criminal Justice* 3: 5–25.

Asch, A. 1988. "Reproductive technology and disability." In *Reproductive laws for the 1990s*, eds. S. Cohen and N. Taub. Clifton, NJ: Humana Press. 59–101.

Asch, A. 1994. "The human genome and disability rights." *Disability Rag and Resource* Jan/Feb: 12–15.

Blendon, R. J., J.M. Benson and K. Donelan. 1993. "The public and the controversy over abortion." *Journal of the American Medical Association* 270 no. 23: 2871–2875.

Bosk, C. 1992. *All God's Mistakes: Genetic Counseling in a Pediatric Hospital.* Chicago: University of Chicago Press.

Bryant, L.D., S. Ahmed and J. Hewison. 2009. "Conveying information about screening." In *Fetal Medicine: Basic Science and Clinical Practice*, eds. C. Rodeck and M. Whittle. Edinburgh: Elsevier. 225–33.

Caruso, T.M., M.N. Westgate and B.H. Holmes. 1998. "Impact of Prenatal Screening on the Birth Status of Fetuses with Down Syndrome at an Urban Hospital, 1972–1994." *Genetics in Medicine* 1, no.1: 22–28.

Conrad, P. 1997. "Public eyes and private genes: historical frames, news constructions, and social problems." *Social Problems* 44, no. 2: 139–54.

Conrad, P. 1999. "A mirage of genes." *Sociology of Health and Illness* 21, no. 2: 228–39.

Foucault, M. 1976. *The Birth of the Clinic: An Archaeology of Medical Perception.* London: Tavistock Publication.

Foucault, M. 1977. *Discipline and Punish- The Birth of the Prison.* New York: Vintage Books.

Foucault, M. 1991. "Governmentality." In *The Foucault effect: Studies in governmentality*. eds. G. Burchell, C. Gordon and P. Miller. Chicago: University of Chicago Press. 87–104.

Franklin, S. 2003. "Rethinking nature-culture: anthropology and the new genetics." *Anthropological Theory* 3, no. 1: 65–85.

Garel, M., M.Gosme-Seguret, M. Kaminski and M. Cuttini. 2002. "Ethical decision-making in prenatal diagnosis and termination of pregnancy: a qualitative survey among physicians and midwives." *Prenatal Diagnosis* 22, no. 9: 811–17.

Gatens-Robonson, E. 1996. "A defense of women's choice: Abortion and the ethic of care." *The Southern Journal of philosophy* 30, no. 3: 39–65.

Ginsburg, F. and R. Rapp. 1991. "The politics of reproduction." *Annual Review of Anthropology* 20: 311–43.

Green, J. 1995. "Obstetrician's views on prenatal diagnosis and termination of pregnancy: 1980 compared with 1993." *British Journal of Obstetrics and Gynecology* 102, no. 3: 228–32.

Gross, M. 1999. "After Feticide: Coping with Late-Term Abortion in Israel, Western Europe, and the United States." *Cambridge Quarterly of Health Care Ethics* 8, no. 4: 449–62

Hashiloni-Dolev, Y. 2006. "Between Mothers, Fetuses and Society: Reproductive Genetics in the Israeli-Jewish Context." *Nashim: A Journal of Jewish Women's Studies & Gender* 12: 129–50.

Hashiloni-Dolev, Y. 2007. *A Life (un)Worthy of Living: Reproductive Genetics in Israel and Germany*. Secaucus, NJ: Springer.

Holtzman, N.A. and D. Shapiro. 1998. "Genetic Testing and Public Policy." *British Medical Journal* 316: 852–56.

Israeli ministry of health. 2007. The general office notice regarding abortion committees at the stage of viability (memorandum #23/07). Jerusalem. [Hebrew].

Israeli ministry of health. 2008. Abortions by law 1990–2007. Department of information, Information and computerization services. Jerusalem. [Hebrew].

Jennings, B. 2003. "Genetic Citizenship: Knowledge and Empowerment in Personal and Civic Health." A Concept Paper Prepared for The March of Dimes/Health Resources and Services Administration/ Genetic Services Branch Project on Genetic Literacy.

Kahn, S. 2000. *Reproducing Jews: A Cultural Account of Assisted Conception in Israel*. Durham: Duke University Press.

Kanaaneh, R.A. 2002. *Birthing the Nation: Strategies of Palestinian Women in Israel*. California: University of California Press.

Kelly, T.E 1986. *Clinical Genetics and Genetic Counseling*. Chicago: Yearbook Medical Publishers.

Lilford R.J. and J. Thornton. 1993. "Ethics and late termination of pregnancy." *Lancet* 342: 499.

Lippman, A. 1992. "Led (Astray) by Genetic Maps: The cartography of the Human Genome and health care." *Social Science and Medicine* 35, no. 12: 1469–76

Lock, M. 1998. "Perfecting Society: Reproductive Technologies, Genetic Testing, and The Planned Family in Japan." In *Pragmatic Women and Body Politics*, eds. M. Lock and P. Kaufert. Cambridge: Cambridge University Press. 206–39.

Mahowald, M.B. 2003. "Aren't We All Eugenicists? Commentary on Paul Lombardo's 'Taking Eugenics Seriously'." *Florida State University Law Review* 30: 219–34

Nelkin, D. and M. Lindee. 1995. *The DNA Mystique: The Gene as a Cultural Icon*. NewYork: WH Freeman.

Nye, A.R. 2003. "The Evolution of the Concept of Medicalization in the Late Twentieth Century." *Journal of History of the Behavioral Sciences* 39, no. 2: 115–29.

Paintin, D. 1997. "Abortion after 24 weeks." *British Journal of Obstetrics and Gynecology* 104, no. 4: 398–400.

Parens, E. and A. Asch. (eds). 2000. *Prenatal Testing and Disability Rights*. Washington, DC: Georgetown University Press.

Paul, D.B. 1994. "Eugenic Anxieties, Social Realities, and Political Choices." In *Are Genes Us? The Social Consequences of the New Genetics*, ed. C.F. Cranor. New Brunswick, NJ: Rutgers University Press. 201–9.

Paul, D.B. 1998. *The Politics of Heredity: Essays on Eugenics, Biomedicine, and the Nature-Nurture Debate*. Albany, NY: State University of New York Press.

Raffle. A.E. 2001. "Information about screening: is it to achieve high uptake or to ensure informed choice?" *Health Expectations* 4, no. 2: 92–98.

Rapp, R. 1999. *Testing Women, Testing the Fetus: The Social Impact of Amniocentesis in America*. New York: Routledge Press.

Rapp, R, and F. Ginsburg. 2001. "Enabling Disability: Rewriting Kinship, Reimagining Citizenship." *Public Culture* (special issue on "reflections on disability criticism") 13, no. 3: 533–56.

Raz, A. 2004. "'Important to test, important to support': Attitudes toward disability rights and prenatal diagnosis among leaders of support groups for genetic disorders in Israel." *Social Science and Medicine* 59, no. 9: 1857–66.

Raz, A. 2005. *The Gene and The Genie: Tradition, Medicalization and Genetic Counseling in a Bedouin Community in Israel*. Durham, NC: Carolina Academic Press.

Raz, A. 2009. *Community Genetics and Genetic Alliances: Carrier Testing, Eugenics, and Networks of Risk*. New York: Routledge.

Remennick, L. 2006. "The Quest after the Perfect Baby: Why Do Israeli Women Seek Prenatal Genetic Testing?" *Sociology of Health and Illness* 28, no. 1: 21–53

Roberts, C. D., L.M. Stough, and L.H Parrish. 2002. "The Role of Genetic Counseling in the Elective Termination of Pregnancies Involving Fetuses with Disabilities." *The Journal of Special Education* 36, no. 1:48–55.

Rothenberg, K. and E. Thomson. 1994. *Women and Prenatal Testing: Facing the Challenges of Genetic Technology*. Columbus, OH: Ohio State University Press.

Rothman, B. 1986. *Tentative Pregnancy: Prenatal Diagnosis and the Future of Motherhood*. NewYork: Viking Penguin.

Rothman, B. 1998. *Genetic Maps and Human Imagination: The Limits of Science in Understanding Who We Are.* NewYork: Norton.

Rowley, P.T. 1984. "Genetic Screening: Marvel or Menace." *Science* 225:138–44.

Savulescu, J. 2001. "Is current practice around late termination of pregnancy eugenic and discriminatory?" *Journal of Medical Ethics* 21, no. 3: 165–71.

Saxton, M. 1984. "Born and unborn." In *Test-Tube women: What future for motherhood?*, eds. R. Arditti, D. Klein and S. Minden, Boulder, CO: Pandora Press. 300–11.

Saxton, M. 1987. "Prenatal screening and discriminatory attitudes about disability." *Women Wise* 4: 8–11.

Sawicki, J. 1999. "Disciplining Mothers: Feminism and the New Reproductive Technologies." In *Feminist Theory and the Body: A Reader*, eds. J. Price and M. Shildrick. Edinburgh: Edinburgh Uni. Press. 190–202.

Shapira, A. 1995. "'Wrongful Life' Suits by Defective Newborns for Faulty Genetic Counseling," In *The Human Genome Project: Legal, Social and Ethical Implications—Proceedings of an International Workshop*. Jerusalem: Israel Academy of Sciences and Humanities.

Sher, C., O. Romano-Zelekha, M.S. Green and T. Shohat. 2003. "Factors affecting performance of prenatal genetic testing by Israeli Jewish women." *American Journal of Medical Genetics*, 120A, no. 3: 418–422.

Singer, E., A. Corning and T. Antonucci. 1999. "Attitudes toward genetic testing and fetal diagnosis, 1990–1996," *Journal of Health and Social Behavior* 40, no. 4: 429- 46.

Singer, E. and P.M. Endreny. 1993. *Reporting on Risk—How the Mass Media Portray Accidents, Diseases, Disasters and Other Hazards.* New York: Russell Sage Foundation.

Skorecki, K. 2005. "The Unborn Child: Scientific Discovery, Medical and Ethical Dilemmas," In *The Embryo: Scientific Discovery and Medical Ethics*, eds. S. Blazer and E. Zimmer. Basel: Karger. 120–42

Weiss, M. 2002. *The chosen body: The politics of the body in Israeli society.* Stanford: Stanford University press.

Wertz, D. 1998. "Eugenics is alive and well: A survey of genetics professionals around the world." *Science in Context* 3–4: 493–510.

Wertz, D. and J. Fletcher 1989. *Ethics and Human Genetics: A Cross-Cultural Perspective.* Heidelberg: Springer-Verlag.

WHO. 2002. *Genomics and World Health: Report of the Advisory Committee on Health Research.* World Health Organization: Geneva.

Chapter 9

CULTURAL VALUES IN ACTION: THE ISRAELI APPROACH TO HUMAN CLONING

Gali Ben-Or and Vardit Ravitsky

This chapter[1] presents the regulation of human cloning[2] in Israel. It describes some prevalent cultural values that are influential in policy making and legislation in this area. It then explores the Israeli legislative process leading to the "Prohibition of Genetic Intervention (Human Cloning and Genetic Manipulation of Reproductive Cells) Law 1999"[3] and its extension in 2004.[4] This process reflects unique Israeli approaches grounded in cultural values relating to the moral status of the human embryo, the importance of research leading to medical breakthroughs and the significance of scientific progress as a key to success and survival.

The Israeli context: three cultural themes

Israel defines itself as a "Jewish-democratic state," in the sense that it seeks to combine Jewish and democratic values in the shaping of its cultural identity as well as its legislative processes. In many instances Jewish values and Zionist narratives play an important role in shaping public perceptions and public policy, even with regards to novel scientific issues such as cloning or embryonic research (Prainsack 2006).

A. *The moral status of the human embryo*

A first prominent cultural theme involves the moral status of the human embryo. According to Jewish tradition, human status and personhood are not acquired at the moment of conception. In contrast to most conservative Catholic positions that treat the human embryo as a fully developed person from conception, the Jewish approach may be characterized as based on the idea of "gradual respect." Jewish tradition recognizes the embryo as progressively acquiring human status, and thus as deserving an increasing degree of respect, but it is only acknowledged as a full "person" at birth. One explicit expression of this position is that in cases of danger to the mother's life, it is permissible and even obligatory to terminate the pregnancy in order to save her life all the way until the very end of the pregnancy:

> If a woman is in hard travail, one cuts the child in her womb and brings it forth member by member, because her life comes before that of [the child]. But if the greater part has proceeded forth, one may not touch it, for one may not set aside one person's life for that of another. (Oholoth 7: 6)

According to Jewish tradition the embryo acquires the status of a "formed embryo" only forty days after conception. The Babylonian Talmud (*Yevamot* 69b) states that "the embryo is considered to be mere water until the fortieth day." Moreover, according to the Orthodox Jewish view, the status of the in-vitro pre-implantation embryo outside the womb is comparable to that of gametes, namely, it should not be wasted in vain but may be manipulated for research purposes if the goal of the research is therapeutic (Bioethics Advisory Committee of the Israel Academy of Sciences and Humanities 2001).

Consequently, the Israeli debate—unlike the heated political controversy in the U.S.—does not link the morality of embryonic research to the debate around abortion. Abortion involves the termination of pregnancy and therefore impinges on the embryo or the fetus in utero. In contrast, cloning and stem cell research involve the manipulation of the in vitro embryo, *before* implantation. In the Israeli cultural context, this distinction is of paramount importance.

B. *Curing and saving lives*

A second relevant cultural theme involves the overriding value that Jewish tradition ascribes to any attempt to cure and save lives. In general, the Jewish perspective encourages open-minded attitudes towards research efforts that have therapeutic aims. When ethical

concerns arise, the therapeutic *goal* is the key element in permitting
the research, even if the research is still preliminary. The Israeli public
debate tends to endorse the use of the term *"therapeutic* cloning,"[5] thus
emphasizing the ultimate goal of the process, even at a time when it is
still unattainable. The ethical question surrounding therapeutic cloning is thus framed as follows: "Is it ethical to use cloned human embryos in the hope of producing transplantable tissue, thus minimizing
risks of rejection of implants and saving the lives of patients?"

C. Science and technology

A third cultural theme involves prevailing Israeli attitudes that are
favorable towards scientific research and technological innovation.
Science and technology are perceived by Israelis as a unique key to
economic success and to future survival as a small state poor in natural resources. The Israeli Ministry of Education promotes science and
technology education not only as an essential part of the education
required for becoming a contributing citizen, but also as a "basis for
national and social strength" (Ministry of Education n.d.). A recent
survey found that there is nearly a total consensus (96 percent) within
the Israeli public regarding the importance of maintaining a high level
of science and technology and that Israel's achievements in science
and technology are an important source of national pride, above the
country's accomplishments in other areas (Yaar 2006). In addition,
the level of public trust in academic research institutions is very high
(71 percent) in comparison to public trust in other social institution,
such as political parties (only 25 percent).

These current public attitudes echo a long standing Zionist narrative that links scientific and technological innovation with social re-
construction and the notion of transforming the Jews into a modern
nation "like the nations of the world" (Penslar 1991). In the context of
cloning and embryonic stem cell research, these attitudes probably account for legislators' reluctance to interfere with the freedom of scientific investigation and the apologetic stance that can be depicted in the
legislative process described below, in which the underlying sentiment
is that "the legislator should not interfere with scientific research at the
level of the Petri dish in the lab" (Science Committee 1998).

Regulating human cloning:
The "Prohibition of Genetic Intervention Law"

In January 1999 Israel became one of the first countries in the
world to pass a law prohibiting human reproductive cloning with

the "Prohibition of Genetic Intervention (Human Cloning and Genetic Manipulation of Reproductive Cells) Law 1999." A legislative process that started as a dispute between politicians haunted by the prospect of dangerous scientific advances and scientists worried about restraints that would impede research, the law eventually managed to accommodate the views of both parties, as well as those of philosophers, jurists, and rabbis whose voices were heard along the way. Unlike other bills in some other countries, Israeli legislators chose not to prohibit cloning or stem cell research designed to generate human tissues for transplantation ("therapeutic cloning"), but rather outlawed only human cloning for the purpose of "creating a person" ("reproductive cloning"). The law created a five-year moratorium and enforced a repeated consideration, thus acknowledging the dynamic character of scientific investigation. Consequently, the law was extended in 2004. While its spirit was essentially retained, its prohibitions were further specified and explicated at that time.

Preliminary initiatives

Early in 1997 the world was introduced to Dolly the sheep, the first cloned mammal. Cloning immediately became the subject of intense debate worldwide. Legislators around the globe were horrified by the prospect of human cloning and numerous bills were proposed to forbid any research leading to this outcome. Like their counterparts in other countries, Israeli parliament members were troubled to such a degree that only a few days after the publication of the first newspaper article about the birth of the little sheep, three preliminary bills aiming to prohibit cloning were submitted to the *Knesset*.[6] These Bills were extremely broad and sought to forbid any experimentation related to the replication of genetic traits in human beings and animals. Of the three, only the one promoted by Member of Knesset (hereafter "MK") Haggai Meirom[7] ended up evolving into a law.[8]

The explanatory note to the preliminary bill expressed the fear that "genetic engineering could compromise the spirit, uniqueness, character and distinctiveness of the individual." It argued that cloning "represents a serious danger to the human race" and that it would "endanger fundamental moral and ethical human values." The Israeli Government, which according to the code of practice of the government has to form a position regarding private bills of Knesset members, objected to the proposal at first. In the discussion that was held by the Committee of Ministers on

Legislation, it was decided that the government would reject the proposal, even though it supported the fundamental principle that duplicating human beings should be banned, due to the fact that the prohibitions in the proposal were too broad and might impede research leading to potential treatments. Eventually, after MK Meirom agreed to narrow down the proposal, the committee decided to support this initiative, on the condition that the law would be drafted in collaboration with the relevant government ministries.

Preliminary discussions

Prior to embarking on a legislative process, the Knesset's Special Committee for Scientific and Technological Research and Development (hereafter "Science Committee") held preliminary discussions to consider whether legislation was indeed required. In one of these preliminary discussions, the Science Committee's chair sought to explore *Halachic*[9] opinions regarding human cloning and the meeting was thus held at the offices of the Chief Rabbinate of Israel. The Chief Rabbis of Israel who participated in the discussion [10] expressed their views, stating that they did not object to scientific investigation as such, but also emphasizing that some limitations should be put in place in order to prevent the misuse of certain technologies. Explicit reference was made to the Jewish experience of the Holocaust:

> Cloning might lead to a selective attitude that would be disastrous from a human, a moral and a Jewish perspective. (...) The idea of "super humans" versus "sub humans" who should be annihilated reminds us of darker days in human history. Therefore, every society, and especially the Jewish people who have experienced so much suffering, must be aware of the dangers involved.[11]

The Chief Rabbis also emphasized the important *Halachic* obligation to heal. Rabbi Yisrael Meir Lau, Israel's Chief Ashkenazi Rabbi, stressed the idea that once the permission to heal was granted to human beings, this permission is transformed into a religious imperative. By not fulfilling it, one is guilty of violating the moral principle of "Thou shalt not (...) stand idly by when your neighbor's life is at stake" (Leviticus 19: 16). He concluded by saying:

> In light of the bitter experience of the 20 [th] century, I would like us to proceed slowly. Not to say an absolute no, since that would be impractical and we should be realistic, but at the same time to be aware

of the dangers and recognize the appropriate boundaries. We should make any attempt to heal, but avoid those things that might harm the foundation of our values. (Science Committee 1997)

This quote is characteristic of the traditional Jewish mindset. It seeks a delicate balance between caution and progress, while perceiving the potential for future treatments and cures as of paramount value.

During that initial discussion, one of the participating researchers, Professor Avinoam Reches, [12] argued that:

What society needs today (. . .) is not a broad global prohibition on research, but rather a set of moral guidelines and limitations that would clarify "the rules of the game" for the coming millennium. (. . .) We do not know how things will evolve in the next fifty years. Science will keep moving forward. That is its nature. (. . .) Politicians must not, and cannot, forbid science from advancing and it would be better for all concerned—for science, politics and religion—if we work together and cooperate with one another. (Science Committee 1997)

The *Knesset* plenum also held two discussions before beginning the legislative process. There too, there seemed to be an agreement regarding the need for striking the right balance between a cautious approach towards new technologies and the protection of scientific freedom. MK Ravitz from the ultra-orthodox *Yahadut Hatora* party stated:

Judaism does not stand in opposition to technological development. Rather, within the framework of Judaism we acknowledge that God gave humans the ability to create, to do things that seem miraculous. Such scientific and technological capabilities were given to mankind to enable us to improve, help, and assist human society. (. . .) Legislation should restrain technology and science to avoid inflicting suffering on future people. (Knesset Plenum Assembly 1997: 1262–67)

These ideas were echoed in the words of MK Taleb A-Sana from the Arab-Muslim party *Mada-Raam*, who stated:

On one hand, scientific research should advance for the benefit of all and in order to find a cure for existing disease. On the other hand, we should protect creation, society, and the family. In my opinion Jewish and Arab cultures have a lot in common and we should emphasize these commonalities. (Knesset Plenum Assembly 1997: 323 [note 23])

The overall sentiment regarding the legislative process thus reflected the cultural values described above. A broad consensus was expressed regarding the need to protect scientific freedom and avoid any impediments to research aiming to cure, while the need for caution was a constant consideration as well.

The legislation

The bill of MK Meirom passed the "preliminary reading" on January 14, 1998 following a discussion in the Knesset plenum. It was then transferred to the Knesset's Science Committee for further discussion and refinement in preparation for the first reading. In this preliminary discussion, MK Meirom, who initiated the bill, made a statement that set the tone for the legislative process:

> We will not rush this complex legislation. We are striving for a law that would establish a supervising mechanism on genetic experiments, particularly in humans, and would introduce ethical boundaries. (. . .) In my conversations with scientists they have expressed their concerns that such legislation might impede research. I hereby declare that we will do our best not to impede research, and to enable it as long as it is meant to promote human welfare, health, and strength. (Knesset Plenum Assembly 1998: 4305–07)

This statement indicated the formula according to which the law was later drafted. On the one hand, a determination to implement moral boundaries and on the other, to avoid any harm to research. Although MK Meirom made this promising statement, the discussions did not follow in this spirit of collaboration.

Although there seemed to be an initial agreement regarding the need for balance, the original bill presented to the Knesset was very broad. It proposed to prohibit human cloning and to set a ban on any experimentation on humans that did not aim to cure or prevent a disease but rather aimed at duplicating genetic traits in humans. It also proposed to forbid experiments in animals that were aimed at duplicating human traits. It touched on fundamental issues involving morality, social values, and freedom of research and ended up raising profound disagreements. It was very difficult to reach understanding, and a long process was required in order to reach the goal declared by MK Meirom and to draft a law that would be acceptable both to politicians and scientists.

In preparation for the first reading of the preliminary bill, the Science Committee invited scientists, philosophers, ethicists, legal experts, rabbis, and other interested parties to contribute to the formulation of the proposal. Diverse voices were welcomed around the table. As the legislative process progressed, legislators and researchers found themselves on two opposite sides of the cloning debate. Even though MK Meirom declared that he "will do [his] best not to impede research," legislators seemed inclined to accept a broad ban on any research leading to cloning, while researchers were concerned that politicians might limit future beneficial research. The Scientific Committee thus took ten months to prepare the initial proposal for a "first reading."

During these discussions, the Ministry of Justice submitted to the Science Committee a survey regarding the regulation of cloning in others countries. The survey showed, for example, that in Germany "any person who artificially causes a human embryo to develop with the same genetic information as another embryo, fetus, living person, or deceased person," or "transfers an embryo as specified above into a woman" shall be punished by up to five years imprisonment or by a fine. [13] The United Kingdom prohibited "replacing a nucleus of a cell of an embryo with a nucleus taken from a cell of any person, embryo or subsequent development of an embryo."[14] In Denmark it was forbidden to conduct "experiments whose purpose is to enable the production of genetically identical human beings."[15] In the United States numerous bills were submitted to the Senate and to the House of Representatives with the aim of prohibiting cloning by prohibiting the technique of somatic cell nuclear transfer. [16]

Declarations of international bodies on the subject were also mentioned. *The Universal Declaration on the Human Genome and Human Rights* (UNESCO 1997) states in article 11 that "(p)ractices which are contrary to human dignity, such as reproductive cloning of human beings, shall not be permitted. States and competent international organizations are invited to co-operate in identifying such practices and in taking, at national or international levels, the measures necessary to ensure that the principles set out in this Declaration are respected." The *Additional Protocol to the Convention for the Protection of Human Rights and Dignity of the Human Being with regard to the Application of Biology and Medicine, on the Prohibition of Cloning Human Beings*, of the Council of Europe (1998), states in article 1 that "(a)ny intervention seeking to create a human being genetically identical to another human being, whether living or dead, is prohibited."

In spite of the strong scientific and academic opposition, MK Meirom held a firm position supporting the prohibition on research leading to human cloning. A sense of animosity was developing and it became clear that the discussions might not result in a solution that would be acceptable to both politicians and scientists. The legal advisors of the Knesset and of the Justice and Health Ministries tried to reach an agreement regarding the draft of the law but these efforts were not successful. MK Meirom insisted on including the regulation of animal experimentation in the law in addition to that of human beings, which was not acceptable to scientists.

Another aspect of the law that met with resistance from scientists was the establishing of a committee that would have the authority to approve genetic experiments on humans *and* animals. Scientists argued that animal experimentations were already regulated under specific legislation and that this law should address only human experimentation. Meirom's proposal distinguished cloning, which he wanted to ban, from other genetic duplication techniques, which he wanted to regulate. Scientists rejected this distinction and argued that the law should only ban the creation of a cloned human being. Government representatives felt that such intricate legislation requires collaboration with scientists and insisted that the wording of the law should be acceptable to scientists.

In an attempt to bridge the widening gap and to achieve agreement regarding the purpose of the law, a meeting was organized in one of the leading medical centers in Israel between MK Meirom and a number of prominent researchers. The meeting was attended by the general director of a leading hospital, the Dean of a faculty of medicine and prominent genetics and biology researchers. MK Meirom thanked the attendees for their willingness to help to find the right model for the law, and an atmosphere of understanding and cooperation was established. During that meeting the gap was bridged.

The first speaker explained that human cloning requires different limitations than animal cloning, since the latter might benefit humanity enormously. Another stressed that the hazards of germ line gene therapy [17] are more concrete than those of human cloning. By the end of the meeting all participants agreed to limit the law to human reproductive cloning and to accept the model of a moratorium. They also agreed that an advisory committee should be established to advise the Minister of Health on developments in the area of genetics and make recommendations regarding possible updates to the prohibitions of the law.[18]

In an interview, MK Meirom expressed his evolving understanding of the difficulties raised by his original proposal and the process by which he modified his position:

By and by we found ourselves standing in the place of prohibiting research on human beings and experiments on genetics. The more I got into the technology, and the more I saw doctors and scientists involved in the technology, I came to the conclusion that it would be very difficult to distinguish between the technologies [and outlaw some, while permitting others]. (. . .) Later on I learned that this [prohibiting all cloning techniques] may cause harm to the field of genetics, and that it might stop various technologies that were in the middle of the way [of developing further]. (Prainsack 2006: 193)

Following the meeting, a draft was sent to all the participants based on the achieved agreement. [19] This draft was approved at the first reading in the *Knesset* (Knesset Plenum Assembly 1998: 457–60) and later became the basis of the law that was finally enacted in December 1999. Since then, the Israeli law—acknowledged as one of the most liberal in the world—has gained much respect in many international conferences for its unique resolutions.

The Israeli law therefore did not prohibit specific cloning techniques as did laws in some other countries. [20] Gali Ben-Or, who took part in drafting the law as the representative of the Ministry of Justice explained that:

The legislator should not interfere with scientific research at the level of the Petri dish in the lab. A legislator should establish a general principle, a social norm. It is clear that at this time Israeli society objects to the idea of using cloning in order to bring children into the world. (. . .) We are intentionally avoiding exact definitions of specific technologies in drafting this law. Banning a specifically defined technology might entail a situation in which the legislator is in a constant race to regulate new technologies as they emerge. Our goal is to ensure that cloning does not lead to the birth of a human being, no matter the exact technology used for that purpose. (Science Committee 1998)

Moratorium or prohibition?

When the Israeli law was introduced to the Knesset plenum, it was explained that:

Since the public debate on this issue is just beginning, it is hereby suggested to establish a period of five years, during which the public debate can be expanded and the ethical, legal and social implications of these developments can be clarified. (. . .) To prevent the law

> from becoming an obstacle to scientific progress, we suggest that an
> advisory committee will submit to the Minister of Health a detailed
> annual report on these matters, thus ensuring a periodic examina-
> tion of the law and its usefulness. (Knesset Plenum Assembly 1998b:
> 457–60)

Israeli legislators thus chose the model of a moratorium rather
than that of a legal prohibition. The choice of this unique legal
mechanism originated from Knesset discussions of the proposed
law and was inspired by the report of the U.S. National Bioethics Advisory Commission, which recommended a three to five
year moratorium on federal funding for cloning (National Bioethics Advisory Commission 1997). Since the legislation potentially interfered with scientific freedom, legislators perceived it
as exceptional and unique, and they called for caution and scrutiny. The underlying view expressed during Knesset discussions
was that science advances faster than the law and therefore a
law for a prescribed period of time is the appropriate mechanism
to prevent the Israeli code of laws from becoming irrelevant and
outdated.

It was decided that this law, unlike others that are valid in-
definitely or until modified, would be enacted as a "temporary
provision" for a limited period of five years, after which it would
expire. Although the term "temporary provision" would usually
appear in the title of the law, MK Meirom insisted that in this
case it would not, due to his concern that such a title might diminish the respect for the law. The first clause of the law therefore stated:

> The purpose of this law is to determine a prescribed period of five
> years during which no kind of genetic intervention shall be per-
> formed on human beings in order to examine the moral, legal, so-
> cial and scientific aspect of such kinds of intervention and the im-
> plication of such intervention on human dignity.

Interestingly, different countries chose different mechanisms
for the regulation of issues surrounding genetics. For example,
while Israel chose the model of a moratorium on cloning, it preferred the model of unlimited legal prohibition regarding genetic
discrimination, as reflected in the Genetic Information Law of
2000,[21] which prohibits the use of genetic information for insurance purposes. Other countries chose to approach the same issue
differently. The U.K, for example, chose to establish a moratorium on the use of genetic information for insurance purposes,
and this moratorium has recently been extended until the year

2011 (Department of Health 2005). On the other hand, regarding cloning, the U.K. chose to set a prohibition that is unlimited in time.[22]

The provisions of the law

The original law of 1999 (see appendix A) prohibited human cloning, defined as "the creation of a complete human being, chromosomally and genetically absolutely identical to another person or fetus, living or dead." Unlike similar laws in other countries, Israeli legislators did not specify the technique of somatic cell nuclear transfer (by which Dolly the sheep was created)[23] as the target of the prohibition. Realizing that new techniques might emerge over time, it was agreed that the purpose of the law was to prevent the *outcome* of human cloning (i.e. the birth of a child who is chromosomally identical to another) and not some specific *process* by which such a child was created.

The law also prohibited the creation of a person using reproductive cells that have undergone a permanent intentional genetic modification (germ line gene therapy), reflecting concerns about the impact that such genetic modification can have not only on the resulting child, but also on future generations that would inherit the modified genetic trait.

With regards to this prohibition, the law created a unique legal mechanism which allows exceptions to the rule under strict conditions. According to this mechanism, the Minister of Health may permit the performance of certain types of germ line genetic interventions that are usually prohibited, if an advisory committee recommends it and if "he is of the opinion that human dignity will not be prejudiced." The rationale behind this mechanism was to allow specific uses of germ line gene therapy if it became a safe and effective way of preventing the birth of children with genetic diseases in the future. To date, this mechanism has not been used, and no regulations have been set up for its use.

The inclusion of such a unique "exception mechanism" in the law was justified based on the understanding that germ line gene therapy may become possible even before cloning does. Creating a built-in option for allowing it was recognized as simpler and more effective than having to modify the law if this indeed occurs. As in choosing the model of moratorium over that of permanent legislation, this unique mechanism reflects the view of science as dynamic and constantly progressing and the realization that it may soon carry tremendous therapeutic benefits. Here again, Israeli legislators tried to prevent legislation from interfering in harmful ways with the achievement of such potential benefits.

The UN International Convention against reproductive cloning: The Israeli position

Two years before the moratorium on cloning had ended, Israel again needed to formulate a position regarding legislation concerning cloning, this time in the international arena. In 2002, the UN began discussions regarding the proposed "International Convention against the Reproductive Cloning of Human Beings" (UN 2002–2005). While Israel wished to contribute to international efforts to prohibit a medically unsafe method of reproduction, it found it difficult to support limitations on cloning for therapeutic research and even objected to the idea that reproductive cloning fundamentally offends human dignity. Contrary to the approach of the *Universal Declaration on the Human Genome and Human Rights* of 1997 which perceives reproductive cloning of human beings as "contrary to human dignity" (article 11), the Jewish point of view does not necessarily perceive cloning *per se* as an affront to human dignity and Israel was reluctant to take such an approach (Ben-Or 2000).

The Israeli position was discussed and formulated in numerous meetings in order to ensure that it best reflected the Israeli law and the unique values of Jewish *Halachah* and Jewish culture. Participants in these meetings included representatives of the Ministry of Foreign Affairs (who represent Israel in the UN discussions), Ministry of Health, and Ministry of Justice, as well as the chief scientist of the Ministry of Science, the chairman of the Bioethics Advisory Commission of the National Academy of Science and Humanities, and a rabbi who served as a Bioethics Consultant to the Minister of Health.

Israel supported the intention to create an international convention that would prohibit human cloning. However, it interestingly emphasized the human dignity of the "newborn that may be potentially created, irrespective of the unlawful nature of the act which brought him or her into life" and urged "consideration of this unique aspect, so as to reaffirm that any child created by reproductive cloning, irrespective of the unlawfulness of the reproduction techniques which brought them into life, will be accorded the same rights as any other human being, by virtue of the human character they possess, without discrimination" in order to "prevent the possible dehumanization of any child."[24]

It should be noted that at that time, the Raelian[25] cult declared that a cloned baby had already been born (CNN 2004). The ban on human cloning was suggested because cloning was believed to be contrary to human dignity, but the Israeli delegation wanted to draw attention to the notion that treating humans with dignity means that if a baby was born using this prohibited technique, he should be considered a human being entitled to respect like any other, regardless of the method used to create him.

In these discussions, Israel was not willing to support a ban on therapeutic cloning and supported the countries that wanted to separate the proposal and concentrate on banning reproductive cloning. Eventually, none of these efforts were successful and to this day the UN has not created a convention to ban either reproductive or therapeutic cloning. Instead, the General Assembly adopted the United Nation Declaration on Human Cloning on March 8, 2005, which states: "Member States were called on to adopt all measures necessary to prohibit all forms of human cloning inasmuch as they are incompatible with human dignity and the protection of human life" (UN General Assembly 2005). Eventually, due to the circumstances at that time, Israel abstained in the vote regarding the adoption of this declaration.

Extension of the law

Prior to the expiration of the original law in January 2004, the Science Committee of the Knesset convened a discussion regarding its extension. Already in this preliminary discussion, a disagreement arose between those who supported the renewal of the law as a temporary moratorium, and those who argued it should now become a permanent law (Science Committee 2003a). The idea of enacting a permanent law stemmed mostly from a concern about the way Israeli legislation would be perceived internationally, considering other countries had passed permanent laws prohibiting cloning and only Israel adopted the model of a moratorium. One of the main supporters of a permanent law was the chairman of the Science Committee at that time, MK Polishuk. MK Paz-Pines argued the same position:

> If we leave the issue of cloning open we are proclaiming that it is not problematic. The Knesset should declare that cloning is undesirable, unless science proves that it can be channeled only toward uses that carry tremendous benefits. (Science Committee 2004)

In another discussion, Professor David Heyd of the Hebrew University, who supported the extension of the moratorium for another five years, stated:

> If it were not for the moratorium that was established five years ago, we would not be sitting here today, because no one would have bothered to revisit this issue. (. . .) It is very important that the legislator forces upon itself this gathering five years from now as well. (. . .) We know that legislators do not hurry to change laws even when public values and approaches change. Laws tend to be stagnant and persist even longer than society sees fit (. . .) It is thus difficult for me to envision a rational argument against the idea of moratorium. (Science Committee 2003b)

Eventually, after an intense debate on this issue, it was decided to extend the moratorium for five years, based on the realization that the cloning debate is far from over. The Knesset thus expressed its commitment to revisiting the issue periodically. In addition, the revised law expanded the authority of the advisory committee and stated that it should "follow developments in medicine, science, biotechnology, bioethics and law in the field of genetic experimentation on human beings in Israel and abroad," and submit an annual report on these matters, advising the Minister of Health regarding genetic experimentation on human beings and the prohibition on germ line interventions.

In the discussions regarding the extension of the law, it also became apparent that the definition of human cloning required clarification and it was thus modified in two significant ways. First, the distinction between reproductive and therapeutic cloning, which was not as clear in 1999 when the law was enacted, was now well established. The revised law thus clarified that the prohibition is solely regarding "human reproductive cloning" and not regarding experimentation that might lead to new therapies, for example cloning human embryos in order to harvest embryonic stem cells for research. In the explanation of the revised law it was emphasized that any cloning experiments for medical purposes must be conducted in accordance with the principles of research ethics and the relevant regulations, and would be approved only following a thorough examination of each specific proposal.[26]

Second, the definition of "human cloning," which in the original law was "the creation of a complete human being, chromosomally and genetically absolutely identical to another person or fetus, living or dead," was revised and now specified two elements: First, "the creation of a human embryo by means of transferring the nucleus from a somatic cell into an ovum or a fertilized ovum from which the nucleus has been extracted, in order to create a person who is genetically and chromosomally identical to another person or fetus, living or dead," and second, "the insertion of a cloned embryo into the uterus of a woman or another womb or body."

This modification was required because the original law did not specify a prohibition regarding implantation of a pre-embryo in the uterus. Critics claimed that under the letter of the law, implantation would be legal as long as there is no intention of carrying the baby to term (thus "creating a complete human being") and provided an abortion is preformed. Others claimed that if the embryo was not "absolutely identical" because of differences in mitochondrial DNA, it would also be legal even though that was not the legislator's intention. To prevent the possibility of such interpretations, the revised law explicitly prohibited "the insertion of a cloned embryo into the uterus of a woman or another womb or body," and the Israeli legislator had to abandon the previous position that the law should not prohibit a specific technology but rather prohibit the outcome.

Another modification of the original law focused on penalties. Considering the potential financial gains of human reproductive cloning, it was decided to increase the amount of the monetary fine (to an amount of over one million Shekels at the time, roughly $230,000 U.S.) and the number of years' imprisonment from two to four.

In March 2004 the final version of the revised law was accepted by the Knesset and the law was thus extended, stating as its purpose:

> to prevent reproductive cloning in humans by establishing that certain kinds of genetic intervention shall not be performed on human beings in view of the moral, legal, social and scientific aspects of the prohibited forms of intervention and their implications for human dignity, and in order to assess public policy regarding those kinds of intervention in view of those aspects, considering also freedom of scientific research for the advancement of medicine. (Knesset Plenum Assembly 2004)

Conclusion

The Israeli approach towards human cloning to date has been reflected in an intricate legislative process that involved all stakeholders and allowed a wide variety of voices to be heard. This process exhibited a struggle to protect the freedom of scientific research, in particular research that has the potential for medical breakthroughs, while still banning those specific practices that were considered unsafe or ethically dubious.

This Israeli position is grounded in unique cultural values that underlie the legislative process. The paramount value of life saving therapies is reflected in the constant effort to protect research that might lead to such therapies. The value of scientific progress as a key to national success contributes to an attitude that is reluctant to limit any type of research. In addition, the Israeli view regarding the moral status of the embryo is grounded in Jewish traditions that do not perceive the in vitro human embryo as a person deserving the same protection as a developed fetus. This makes it ethically unproblematic to allow research on cloned embryos that are created not for reproductive purposes. These cultural themes thus lead to a unique approach that is more permissive than the approaches of most Western countries.

Israel created a unique model for regulating human reproductive cloning. As shown in this chapter, this idiosyncratic approach is based on cultural, traditional, and religious values and should therefore be understood within the appropriate cultural context. Different countries legislate and regulate new technologies within their own cultural and social contexts, which makes international agreement difficult to reach, as demonstrated by the failure of the UN to reach a convention banning cloning.

Recently the UN's Institute of Advanced Studies issued a report entitled *Is Human Reproductive Cloning Inevitable: Future Options for UN Governance* (UN Institute of Advanced Studies 2007). The report's main purpose is to call upon the nations of the world to unite and ban reproductive cloning. However, the report also includes some interesting statements concerning potential cloned human beings. For example, it states that ". . . ethically as a human being any cloned individual would have equal rights under the UN Declaration of Human Rights."[27] Such statements are in line with the Israeli approach as described above. The report also suggests that programs to educate the general population and to protect the dignity of all humans, including cloned ones, should be developed. Rather than using potential discrimination and prejudice as an argument for banning reproductive cloning, the report warns that "there is danger that cloned human beings may be exposed to the risk of discrimination, which needs to be prevented . . . legal complexities would need to be carefully examined, and these are the future topics for governance of reproductive technology."[28] This report might indicate that some aspects of the Israeli approach may inspire other countries as they consider the implications of human cloning in the future.

Appendix 1: The Original Law

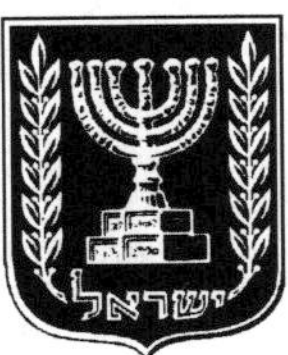

Prohibition of Genetic Intervention (Human Cloning and Genetic Manipulation of Reproductive Cells) Law, 5759–1999

Purpose of Law 1. The purpose of this Law is to determine a prescribed period of five years during which no kind of genetic intervention shall be performed on human beings in order to examine the moral, legal, social and scientific aspects of such kinds of intervention and the implications of such on human dignity.

Definitions 2. In this Law–

> "**Advisory committee**"—the Supreme Helsinki Committee appointed under the Public Health (Medical Experiments on Humans) Regulations 5741–1980;
> "**Human cloning**"—the creation of a complete human being, chromosomally and genetically absolutely identical to another person or fetus, living or dead;
> "**Reproductive cell**"—human spermatozoon or ovum;
> "**Minister**"—the Minister of Health.

Genetic intervention prohibited 3. Throughout the period during which this Law is in force, no person shall perform any act of intervention in the cells of any person with one of the following purposes:

(1) Human cloning;

(2) Causing the creation of a person by use of reproductive cells that have undergone a permanent intentional genetic modification (Germ Line Gene Therapy).

Advisory committee 4. The advisory committee shall follow up medical, scientific and biotechnological developments in the field of genetic experimentation on human beings, shall report to the Minister annually thereon, shall advise the Minister in this respect, and shall make recommendations to the Minister in respect of the force of the prohibitions set out in section 3.

Permission for certain types of genetic intervention 5. (a) Notwithstanding the provisions of section 3, the Minister may, if he is of the opinion that human dignity will not be prejudiced, upon the recommendation of the advisory committee and upon such conditions as he may prescribe in regulations, permit the performance of certain types of genetic intervention that are prohibited under section 3(2).

(b) The performance of genetic intervention permitted under sub-section (a) shall be subject to receipt of advance permission upon conditions that shall be prescribed.

(continued)

(c) The Minister shall prescribe in regulations under this section the conditions for the grant of a permit, the arrangements for granting the permit, the methods of supervising the performance of permitted genetic intervention and the obligation to make reports.

Penalties   6. A person who commits any one of the following acts shall be liable to two years' imprisonment:

(1) infringes the provisions of section 3(1);

(2) infringes the provisions of section 3(2), unless acting lawfully pursuant to a permit granted under section 5.

Preservation of   7. The provisions of this Law shall add to, and shall not derogate
Laws   from, the provisions of any law.

Validity   8. This Law shall remain in force for five years from the date of its publication.

Performance   9. The Minister shall be responsible for the implementation of this Law.

Benjamin Netanyahu   Yehoshua Matza
Prime Minister   Minister of Health

Ezer Weitzman   Dan Tichon
President of the   Speaker of
State   the Knesset

Appendix 2: The Revised Law

Prohibition of Genetic Intervention (Human Cloning and Genetic Manipulation of Reproductive Cells) Law, 5759–1999

Purpose of   1. The purpose of this Law is to prevent reproductive cloning in
Law   humans by establishing that certain kinds of genetic intervention shall not be performed on human beings in view of the moral, legal, social and scientific aspects of the prohibited forms of intervention and their implications for human dignity, and in order to assess public policy regarding those kinds of intervention in view of those aspects, considering also freedom of scientific research for the advancement of medicine.

Definitions   2. In this Law–

"**Advisory committee**"—the Supreme Helsinki Committee appointed under the Public Health (Medical Experiments on Humans) Regulations 5741–1980;

"**Human cloning**"—"human reproductive cloning"—
any of the following:

(1) the creation of a human embryo by means of transferring the nucleus from a somatic cell into an ovum or a fertilized ovum from which the nucleus has been extracted (in this law—a "cloned embryo"), in order to create a person who is genetically and chromosomally identical to another person or fetus, living or dead;

(continued)

(2) the insertion of a cloned embryo into the uterus of a woman or another womb or body.

"**Reproductive cell**"—human spermatozoon or ovum;

"**The Minister**"—the Minister of Health.

Prohibited actions

3. Throughout the period during which this Law is in force, no person shall perform any of the following acts:

(1) Human cloning—human reproductive cloning;

(2) Using reproductive cells that have undergone a permanent intentional genetic modification (Germ Line Gene Therapy) in order to cause the creation of a person.

Advisory committee— duties and powers

4. (a) The advisory committee—

(1) Shall follow developments in medicine, science, biotechnology, bioethics and law in the field of genetic experimentation on human beings in Israel and abroad;

(2) Shall submit to the Minister and to the science and technology committee of the Knesset an annual report, on the exercise of its powers and duties according to this law and a summary of the developments referred to in paragraph (1); the report and summary shall be submitted annually, no later than March 1;

(3) Shall advise the Minister on the matter of genetic experimentation on human beings and shall provide him with its recommendations concerning the prohibitions set out in section 3.

(4) The Minister shall establish regulations concerning the exercise of the powers of the Advisory committee according to this law; such regulations shall also include powers of supervision and control.

Permission for certain types of genetic intervention

5. (a) Notwithstanding the provisions of section 3, the Minister may, if he is of the opinion that human dignity will not be prejudiced, upon the recommendation of the advisory committee and upon such conditions as he may prescribe, permit through regulations the performance of specific kinds of genetic intervention that are prohibited under section 3(2).

(b) The performance of a genetic intervention permitted under sub-section (a) shall be subject to advance receipt of a permit upon conditions that shall be prescribed.

(c) The Minister shall prescribe in regulations under this section the conditions for the grant of a permit, the procedures for granting a permit, the methods of supervising and monitoring the performance of a permitted genetic intervention, and any related reporting duties.

Penalties

6. A person who commits any one of the following acts shall be liable to four years' imprisonment or a fine equal to six times the fine set in paragraph 61(a)(4) of the Penal Law 5737–1977:

(1) Performing human cloning (Human Reproductive Cloning);

(continued)

> (2) Using reproductive cells that have undergone a permanent intentional genetic modification (Germ Line Gene Therapy) in order to cause the creation of a person, unless acting lawfully pursuant to a permit granted under section 5.

Preservation of Laws   7.   The provisions of this Law shall add to, and shall not derogate from, the provisions of any law.

Validity   8.   This Law shall remain in force until March 1st 2009.[*]

Implementation   9.   The Minister shall be responsible for the implementation of this Law.

Benjamin Netanyahu   Yehoshua Matza
Prime Minister   Minister of Health

Ezer Weitzman
President of   Dan Tichon
the State   Speaker of the Knesset

---

[*] In 2009, the law has been extended once again, and is in effect until May 23, 2016. No changes to the law have been made.

Appendix 3: The Israeli Position Regarding the UN International Convention Against Reproductive Cloning: Statement by Ms. Ady Schonmann

"On a purely philosophical level, when taken to extremes complete with apocalyptic nightmares of pure evil, there seems to be unanimous support for the prohibition of human reproductive cloning. The mere thought of ever having the ability to breed mass armies of clones is genuinely reprehensible. The possible instrumentalization of humankind is equally a cause for concern. On a philosophical level, such concerns reflect a deterministic belief that humans, like objects, can be duplicated. But alongside those who believe that a person is entirely shaped by his or her genetic characteristics, there are those who believe in the existence of a soul and a spirit as part of the human identity, which can never be cloned. Most would also agree that the human being is the outcome of cultural, educational and social influences, all of which have a considerable effect on shaping a distinct identity of even those who carry an identical genetic makeup. Be that as it may, at present one thing is clear, that human reproductive cloning is absolutely unethical. . . .

The cautious approach taken by the Israeli parliament stems from the understanding that science in this field is still in its infancy, and therefore it is only natural that at this stage we have far more questions than answers. Israeli law reflects both an understanding that science should not be demonized in the eyes of the public, yet at the same time the public must be assured that the far-reaching implications of scientific development in genetic engineering, as applied in medicine, are being carefully scrutinized and evaluated for all their multi-faceted repercussions.

To some extent, Israeli law on human cloning derives its inspiration from Jewish teachings and philosophy which oppose biological determinism and emphasize both personal responsibility and the imperative to heal and save lives. The treaty of principles states that: "Everything is foreseen, yet freedom is given." Maimonides, the great Jewish authority of the 12th century and a physician himself, comments on this verse, saying that what is "foreseen" refers to men's nature, those aspects of which he has no control, such as being tall or short. But human behavior depends on man's will and responsibility and reflects God's gift of "freedom."

It is also interesting to note, that while on the one hand, the prophet Ezekiel describes the dangers of pride and hubris, referring to those who say "mine is the source of life, and I am my own creator," on the other hand Jewish tradition also provides a clear imperative to heal and save lives, as reflected in the Biblical imperative "thou shall surely heal." A modern equivalent may be found in the human right to the highest attainable standards of health, including reproductive medicine.

And finally, while my delegation supports a legally enforceable ban that criminalizes the reproductive cloning of human beings, at the same time, we also recognize that there may be those who would try to circumvent this ban and violate it, as with other criminal activity. In view of the *human dignity* of the newborn that may be potentially created, irrespective of the unlawful nature of the act which brought him or her into life, my delegation would urge consideration of this unique aspect, so as to reaffirm that any child created by reproductive cloning, irrespective of the unlawfulness of the reproduction techniques which brought them into life, will be accorded the same rights as any other human being, by virtue of the human character they possess, without discrimination. My delegation believes that a clear statement on this matter is required in order to prevent the possible dehumanization of any child."

Notes

1. *Disclosure:* Gali Ben-Or took part in drafting the Israeli prohibition on cloning law and Vardit Ravitsky participated in some of the Knesset discussions during the legislative process. Both authors participated in the formulation of the Israeli position regarding the UN International Convention Against Reproductive Cloning.

2. *Cloning* is the process of creating a genetically identical copy of cells or organisms by "somatic cell nuclear transfer" (SCNT). This process entails the transfer of a nucleus from a donor adult cell (somatic cell) to an egg from which the nucleus has been removed.
3. *Sefer HaHukim* (The Book of Laws of the State of Israel) 1697, 7 January 1999: 47.
4. *Sefer HaHukim* (The Book of Laws of the State of Israel) 1934, 31 March 2004: 340.
5. Therapeutic cloning (also known as research cloning or embryo cloning) involves taking an egg from which the nucleus has been removed, and replacing that nucleus with DNA from the cell of another organism. If successful, this results in a blastocyst (an early stage embryo of about 100 cells) that is genetically almost completely identical to the original organism. The aim is to create cells or even specific organs to be used for injection or transplant into a host for therapeutic purposes, without fear of immunological rejection.
6. Genetic Experiments (prohibition of cloning) Draft Bill, 5757–1997 (no. p/1245); Supervision of Medical Experiments on Human Beings Draft Bill, 5757–1997 (no. p/1309); Prohibition of Experiments of Cloning Human Beings Draft Bill, 5757–1997 (no. p/1379).
7. Haggai Meirom was an MK on behalf of the Labor party since 1988. Before that he was a farmer, studied law, and worked as a lawyer.
8. Bill no. p/1245 (unpublished).
9. *Halachah* is the collective corpus of Jewish religious law, including biblical law and later *Talmudi* and rabbinic law, as well as customs and traditions. When appropriate, and in particular with regard to laws that address issues with moral dimensions, the Israeli Knesset takes into consideration *Halachi* positions in the process of legislation. These positions can influence the content and the wording of the proposed law.
10. Rabbi Yisrael Meir Lau and Rabbi Eliyahu Bakshi-Doron—Israel's Chief Rabbis at that time.
11. Rabbi Yisrael Meir Lau (Science Committee 1997).
12. Prof. Avinoam Reches is a neurologist in Hadassah Ein Kerem Hospital in Jerusalem and is also the Chairperson of the Ethics Board of the Israeli Medical Association.
13. The Embryo Protection Law of December 13, 1990.
14. The Human Fertilization and Embryology Act 1990, chapter 37, paragraph 3 (3) (d).
15. Law no. 503 on the Scientific Ethics Committee System and the Examination of Biomedical Research Projects, Order No. 69 of 8 January 1999.
16. For example see U.S. Congress 1997–1998a and 1997–1998b.
17. Gene therapy is an experimental procedure aimed at replacing, manipulating, or supplementing nonfunctional or malfunctioning genes with healthy genes. Germ line gene therapy alters the DNA of sperm or egg cells. In humans each mature germ cell contains a single set of 23 chromosomes, half the usual amount. All other cells in the body—called somatic cells—contain 46 chromosomes. Germ line gene therapy

is particularly risky because it affects not only the somatic cells of an individual, but rather alters the DNA in the reproductive cells, which means the alteration will pass on to all the descendants of the treated individual.

18. Private notes of Gali Ben-Or, Minutes of Meeting of June 24, 1998, Ein Karem Hospital Jerusalem, Israel.

19. Private notes of Gali Ben-Or, Minutes of Meeting of June 24, 1998, Ein Karem Hospital Jerusalem, Israel.

20. For example, The Human Fertilization and Embryology Act 1990 (chapter 37) in the United Kingdom prohibited "replacing a nucleus of a cell of an embryo with the nucleus taken from a cell of any person, embryo or subsequent development of an embryo."

21. *Sefer HaHukim* (The Book of Laws of the State of Israel) 1766, 25 December 2000: 62.

22. Human Reproductive Cloning Act 2001 and The Human Fertilization and Embryology Act 1990.

23. Somatic cell nuclear transfer is a process of making a clone, a genetically identical copy, by replacing the nucleus of an unfertilized ovum with the nucleus of a body cell from the organism. This is the method that was used to create Dolly the sheep in 1997.

24. Comments made by Ady Schonmann September 24th 2002. Agenda 162, Working Group for the Elaboration of a Mandate to a Convention against the Reproductive Cloning of Human Beings. No publication; private notes of Gali Ben-Or.

25. The Raëlian Movement is a religious cult whose members believe that scientifically advanced extraterrestrials known as the Elohim (one of the words used to refer to God in the Torah) created life on earth through genetic engineering, and that a combination of human cloning and "mind transfer" can ultimately provide immortality.

26. *Hatzaot Hok* (Publication of Bills of the State of Israel). "The Prohibition on Genetic Intervention (Human Cloning and Genetic Manipulation of Reproductive Cells (amendment) Bill 2003," 23 December 2003: 290.

27. Supra note at page 10.

28. Supra note at page 13.

References

Ben-Or, G. 2000. "The Israeli Approach to Cloning and Embryonic Research." *Heidelberg Journal of International Law* 60, no. 3–4: 763–70.

Bioethics Advisory Committee of the Israel Academy of Sciences and Humanities. 2001. *Report on the Use of Embryonic Stem (ES) Cells for Therapeutic Research.* <http://www.academy.ac.il/bioethics/english/report1/Report1-e.html> (accessed November 27, 2007).

CNN. 2004. "Raelian Leader Says Cloning First Step to Immortality." <http://edition.cnn.com/2002/HEALTH/12/27/human.cloning/index.html> (accessed November 27, 2007).

Council of Europe. 1998. *Additional Protocol to the Convention for the Protection of Human Rights and Dignity of the Human Being with regard to the Application of Biology and Medicine, on the Prohibition of Cloning Human Beings*. <http://conventions.coe.int/treaty/en/treaties/html/168.htm> (accessed November 27, 2007).

Department of Health. 2005. "Concordat and Moratorium on Genetics and Insurance." <http://www.dh.gov.uk/assetRoot/04/10/60/50/04106050.pdf> (accessed November 27, 2007).

Knesset Plenum Assembly. 2004. "Minutes of the March 3rd 2004 Assembly." <http://www.knesset.gov.il/laws/heb/FileD.asp?Type=1&SubNum=1&LawNum=1934> (accessed December 1, 2007).

Knesset Plenum Assembly. 1997. "Minutes of the December 2nd 1997 Assembly, DK 164, Oct-Nov 1997." Jerusalem: Knesset.

Knesset Plenum Assembly. 1998a. "Minutes of the January 14th 1998 Assembly, D.K. 167, Jan-Feb 1998." Jerusalem: Knesset.

Knesset Plenum Assembly. 1998b. "Minutes of the November 2nd 1998 Assembly, D.K. 172, Oct-Nov 1998." Jerusalem: Knesset.

Ministry of Education. n.d. "Science and Technology Syllabus for Elementary Schools." <http://cms.education.gov.il/EducationCMS/Units/Tochniyot_Limudim/science_tech/AlHatochnit/> (accessed November 27, 2007).

National Bioethics Advisory Commission. 1997. "Executive Summary." <http://bioethics.georgetown.edu/nbac/pubs/cloning1/executive.htm> (accessed November 27, 2007).

Penslar, D. J. 1991. *Zionism and Technocracy: The Engineering of Jewish Settlement in Palestine, 1870–1918*. Bloomington, IN: Indiana University Press.

Prainsack, B. 2006. "'Negotiating Life': The Regulation of Human Cloning and Embryonic Stem Cell Research in Israel." *Social Studies of Science* 36, no. 2 (April): 173–205.

Science Committee. 1997. "Minutes of the March 31st 1997 Meeting." (unpublished), Knesset Library).

Science Committee. 1998. "Minutes of the December 29th 1998 Meeting." (unpublished, Knesset Library).

Science Committee. 2003a. "Minutes of the November 12th 2003 Meeting." <http://www.knesset.gov.il/protocols/data/html/mada/2003–11–12.html> (accessed November 27, 2007).

Science Committee. 2003b. "Minutes of the December 8th 2003 Meeting." <http://www.knesset.gov.il/protocols/data/rtf/mada/2003–12–08.rtf> (accessed 27 November, 2007).

Science Committee. 2004. "Minutes of the January 12th, 2004 Meeting." <http://www.knesset.gov.il/protocols/data/rtf/mada/2004–01–12.rtf> (accessed November 27, 2007).

UN. 2002–2005. "Ad Hoc Committee on an International Convention against the Reproductive Cloning of Human Beings." <http://www.un.org/law/cloning/#introduction> (accessed November 27, 2007).

UN General Assembly. 2005. "General Assembly Adopts United Nations Declaration on Human Cloning by Vote of 84–34–37." <http://www.un.org/News/Press/docs/2005/ga10333.doc.htm> (accessed November 27, 2007).

UN Institute of Advanced Studies. 2007. *Is Human Reproductive Cloning Inevitable: Future Options for UN Governance.* United Nations University: Japan.

UNESCO. 1997. *The Universal Declaration on the Human Genome and Human Rights.* (accessed November 27, 2007. <http://portal.unesco.org/en/ev.php-URL_ID=13177&URL_DO=DO_TOPIC&URL_SECTION=201.html>

U.S. Congress. 1997–1998a. "Human Cloning Prohibition Act." <http://www.govtrack.us/congress/bill.xpd?bill=s105–1601> (accessed December 1, 2007).

U.S. Congress. 1997–1998b. "Human Cloning Research Prohibition Act." <http://www.govtrack.us/congress/bill.xpd?bill=h105–3133> (accessed December 1, 2007).

Yaar, E. 2006. "Science and Technology in the Israeli Consciousness." http://www.neaman.org.il/neaman/publications/publication_item.asp?fid=757&parent_fid=488&iid=3428 (accessed November 27, 2007).

Part III

COMMUNITY:
A SELF-PORTRAIT
WITH TECHNOLOGY

ART, Community, and Beyond: Human Embryonic Stem Cell Research in Israel

*Interviews with Prof. Nissim Benvenisty
and Prof. Karl Skorecki
Interview and Introduction:
Daphna Birenbaum-Carmeli*

Introduction

The study of human embryonic stem cells (hESCs) is inherently linked to IVF. It is the extracorporeal existence of fertilized eggs in the early stages of cell division that has enabled the recent development of the study of these special cells. Comprising the primary moments in human development, embryonic stem cells offer a singular vantage point to foundational life processes.

Stem cells are distinguished by unique properties. They can divide and renew themselves for long periods. Embryonic stem cells are unspecialized but can become any type of cell (e.g., the beating cells of the heart muscle or the insulin-producing cells of the pancreas). Adult stem cells can generally differentiate only into cell types based on their tissue of origin, but can also generate replacement for cells that are lost through normal living, injury, or disease. Research on stem cells can thus look into the development of an organism out of a single cell or the replacement of damaged cells by healthy ones in adult organisms. Owing to these exceptional characteristics, some scientists consider stem cells as the basis for a new medical approach: regenerative medicine, which would treat diseases like Parkinson's disease, diabetes, and heart disease. Additionally, stem cells may become a platform for screening new drugs and understanding birth defects (National Institutes of Health n.d.).

Evidently, these issues are not related to human reproduction in any direct fashion. Rather, in the study of hESCs, IVF "products" serve as a platform for the investigation of basic questions of general scientific interest and therapeutic potential. In other words, while the two domains are inextricable—IVF being a prerequisite for hESC research—the fertilised ova are here a means rather than an end in themselves. How, then, if at all, do we relate hESC research to reproductive medicine in general and to the Israeli scene in particular?

hESC research is burgeoning in Israel. Research funds are directed to this field, cutting edge laboratories are being inaugurated, and local accomplishments are celebrated as standing out in terms of both numbers and centrality in the field. This momentous position was evident from the earliest days of hESC research, when Israeli scientists participated in the formative projects that have virtually established the field. Already in the *Science* article that reported the first ever extraction of ESC from human blastocysts, the authors, mostly American, thank an Israeli IVF clinic for providing "the initial culture and cryopreservation of the embryos used in this study" (Thomson et al. 1998). In their local laboratories too, Israeli researchers conduct key experiments and their publications are a central frame of reference for colleagues (see the Benvenisty interview below).

Israeli scientists research diverse fields of the natural sciences and participate routinely in international collaborations. Nevertheless, the domain of hESC research appears to operate by a somewhat distinct code. In comparison to other fields of inquiry, hESCs are studied within a thoroughly globalized network. Research teams are still based in particular countries, of course. However, cell lines are shared internationally, and researchers from numerous countries get together in order to set a globally accepted code of practice and to standardize an ethical approach that would be applied across settings. They also proactively encourage dissemination of knowledge and sharing of biological products (see the Skorecki interview below).

Looking at the hESC research ethos of global collaboration and sharing—as portrayed in the ensuing interviews—one may take a comparative look at the early days of IVF. When IVF was first applied in Israel, local experts were made widely known to the general public, primarily through media articles that presented them as bringing a remedy to local suffering by enabling couples to have biogenetically related offspring. The coverage had very strong national subtexts when it highlighted the Jewish Israeli identity of the doctors as well as the importance of biogenetic reproduction. The tacit reproduction of central social categories like family, ethnicity, and Jewish identity imbued public discourse on the subject.

The reality of hESC research is different. Addressing more abstract questions that are defined, at this point, as basic science, hESC researchers are less concerned with social classifications. Issues like primary cell differentiation, cell self-renewal, and hESC as a model for drug experimentation transcend not only social categories but the human species as well. Whereas IVF is imbued with issues of social equity and applied on specific individuals with particular social identities, hESC as investigated today is much more "culturally inert." If we follow this line of thought, we may suggest, very cautiously, that the globalized, sharing research culture described by the scientists interviewed here, metaphorically echoes the universal type of processes they are probing.

At the symbolic level, this mode of global collaboration may conjure greater integration of Israeli scientists within a global community. Belonging to this exclusive community of wealthy industrialized nations is a desirable consequence from an Israeli perspective, one more welcome, fresh upshot from IVF. In this sense, IVF may once again play a key role as a platform for Israeli participation in a high profile international network. However, the relative weight of national and local community in this globalized network, and its concomitant scientific and political significances, remain to be seen.

Interview with Professor Nissim Benvenisty, M.D.,Ph.D.

Professor of Genetics and Head, Department of Genetics, the Alexander Silberman Institute of Life Sciences, the Hebrew University, Jerusalem, Israel. Benvenisty is an expert in stem cell research, embryo development of humans and mammals, cancer research, and tissue engineering.

The interview was conducted in Jerusalem over two sessions in March and May, 2007.

* * * * *

Professor Nissim Benvenisty (NB): Research on human embryonic stem cells (hESCs) started in Israel in 1998, when cells which had first been isolated in Wisconsin, U.S.A., and were brought over to Israel. I had been working on mouse ESCs since 1993 and was in fact waiting for the extraction of hESCs which was, so we all assumed, imminent. When the popular Israeli press announced—one day before the publication in the professional press—that such cells had been isolated, I telephoned, very atypically of me, Professor Josef Itzkovitz, who collaborated with the group in Wisconsin. I invited him to my lab so he could decide whether he was interested in research collaboration. We presented our mouse ESC studies to him, and subsequently we started to work on the human cells together.

You have to understand that at that time, embryonic primary cell differentiation was an esoteric field. Very few researchers worked on this topic, scarcely a couple of dozen worldwide. Our funding came from cancer research. It was truly esoteric.

It was only after hESCs had been isolated that this research became a central, mainstream field of research. In fact, until today, we are still working on questions that we formulated back then, in the days of our mouse ESC project.

Daphna Birenbaum-Carmeli (DBC): What sort of ties did you have with IVF clinics at that time?

NB: At the beginning very loose. It was obvious that the source of hESCs was IVF, but we were concerned about ethical difficulties. At some point I did approach a former classmate of mine, who was a doctor in an IVF clinic, and we discussed the possibilities of isolating ESC together, but didn't move forward.

The main ethical concern with hESCs is that they are derived from human blastocysts. Since there are surplus blastocysts in IVF clinics that will otherwise be thrown away, there is no doubt that rather than discarding valuable biological material, it should be used to advance research and medicine.

Since 1998, we have managed to produce additional cell lines in our laboratory. We work primarily with sick blastocysts that have been obtained via preimplantation genetic diagnosis (PGD). So, we use the sick blastocysts that will never be implanted into the uterus, and otherwise would be discarded, to model for human genetic diseases. Fragile-X, for instance, is the most prevalent cause of inherited mental retardation in boys, and the mouse model does not apply to humans. So, studying hESCs that carry the mutation that appears in fragile-X patients is very important.

DBC: Can you tell me about the ethical regulation of hESC research in Israel?

NB: When we first started to work with hESCs, no guidelines or regulations existed. I approached the Hebrew University and requested that a committee be formed to address hESC-related ethical issues. Though the university had an ethics committee, including a section that monitored cell research, it was clear that these were no ordinary cells and needed closer consideration. The committee consisted of three professors: of medicine, human genetics, and molecular biology. Today, the American National Institute of Health (NIH) requires that any university wishing to carry out hESC research has such a committee (stem cell research oversight [SCRO] committee).

DBC: Can you locate Israel within the international landscape of hESC research?

NB: Around the year 2000, the Bioethics Advisory Committee of the Israeli Academy of Sciences and Humanities formed a subcommittee that would set guidelines for researching hESCs (Revel 2000). The guidelines, which were published in 2000,[1] are fairly liberal but not the most liberal in comparison to other countries; certainly not exceptionally liberal. Generally speaking, we divide countries into four policy categories:

1. Both extraction and study of hESCs is forbidden (Ireland, Poland).
2. Extraction of cells is not allowed but research is permitted on cells that had been extracted before a particular date (U.S.A. by public funding).
3. Extraction of cells out of "spare" IVF embryos is allowed. Creation of embryos for research purposes is not (Canada, Japan, Spain).
4. Both extraction and study of hESCs is allowed. Embryos may be taken from IVF excess or be generated for research purposes (U.S.A. by private funding, U.K., India, China). These countries also tend to be more liberal in terms of cloning policies.

Israel belongs in the third category, with countries allowing cell extraction from unused IVF embryos and research of such cells, but prohibiting the production of embryos for research purposes only. More generally, in terms of cloning, Israel allows therapeutic but not reproductive cloning. The regulations that monitor these practices are subject to reconsideration every five years, following which, approval is renewed.

DBC: How do you see the views of religious authorities on hESCs?

NB: On a closer look, the embryo is viewed as a diverse entity in the eyes of religion. *Halachah* makes fine distinctions regarding the status of the embryo throughout its development, recognizing six different stages:

1. Up to 5 days, i.e., before implantation has taken place.
2. 5 to 40 days—*golem*. According to *halachah*, during these first two stages research aiming to save lives—in the broad sense of the term—is allowed.

Then there are four more stages:

3. From 41 days to the end of the second trimester.
4. Third trimester—viable fetus.
5. Fetus moving through the birth canal.
6. Neonate, with full human rights.

The fetus's status and its rights increase as it develops. According to Judaism there is no opposition to using embryos up to 40 days old, but in fact, we do not need to go beyond the 5-day limit.

The Israeli Academy of Science and Humanities has summarized the views of representatives of the three major religions in the country (Judaism, Islam, and Christianity), plus scientists' views, and from this decided on the 14-day cut-off point. The 14-day limit originated with U.K. regulations for human development research, which we broadly adopted in Israel, and therefore carried over to the domain of hESCs. The 14-day limit designates the time when the neural tube starts to form. If the end of life is the termination of brain activity, then the commencement of brain development is the beginning of life. This principle still requires, of course, donation and informed consent. On the whole, monitoring of hESC research in Israel is very tight.

DBC: Are people generally willing to donate pre-embryos to hESC research?

NB: I don't meet the "parents" in person, but I know that not everyone donates their embryos for research, which is perfectly fine. At the moment there is no shortage of sick embryos for research.

DBC: What does limit hESC research in Israel then, if anything at all?

NB: Well, if you work with a larger population, you are exposed to more biological material and can generate more cell lines of the same disease, which can then be compared. In Israel, the biological material is relatively scarce owing to the size of the population. It's not because people refuse to donate embryos for research. Families with a genetic disease are especially aware of the importance of scientific research and understand that there is no better way to use these embryos. In fact, the first ones to approach us were a couple who had two sick daughters. A few other people with sick children came up with the same idea.

DBC: What sort of contact do you maintain with researchers in other countries?

NB: We have very tight connections with other countries. I am a member of the steering committee of the International Stem Cell Initiative, which is a world consortium, consisting of more than 15 countries. In this consortium we are trying to generate "gold standards" for hESC research. We also have an established collaboration with Harvard University, where we share information, knowledge and cell lines. At the moment we have 17 cell lines from Harvard. Additionally, I am a member of the International Society for Stem Cell Research (ISSCR) Task Force. Here, we have formulated a set of guidelines for good practice with hESCs including setting regulations for informed consent and material transfer agreement. We expect openness in sharing material with other researchers.

DBC: How many cell lines are there in existence altogether?

NB: Probably several hundred. We are now trying to create a world registry through the International Stem Cell Initiative. In fact, I am surprised myself by the scope of the collaboration. There is some competition but it is outweighed by collaboration. There was not a single laboratory we approached that refused to collaborate.

DBC: How do you explain this cooperative attitude? What do participating laboratories gain?

NB: Mainly knowing what is going on. There is the feeling of pioneering and innovation; at the beginning there was a strong sense of esotericism and ethical concern, as well as mutual help, which persists to this day. The International Stem Cell Initiative (ISCI) helps create regulations in countries that do not yet have them in place. There is still a feeling that there is work to be done in various countries. At first we were concerned that the research would weaken. In practice, the opposite has happened: there is more research, and countries have become more liberal. Maybe, I should add, with the exception of Italy, which changed its policy towards greater restrictions because of the Vatican's restrictive point of view.

DBC: What do you see as the great promise of hESCs?

NB: The public hears about cell transplantation, for instance in Parkinson's disease, diabetes, neurodegenerative diseases, and cardiovascular and liver conditions. But these will all take time, probably 5 years until the first clinical trials.

In addition, there are two other domains:

1. Understanding the primary development of humans. This is fascinating—the development of all the various tissues that later on in life decelerate in their growth, or altogether halt development. If we manage to isolate the appropriate factors, we might be able to induce the self-regeneration of these tissues.
2. The domain of genetic diseases. Today, we study these diseases on mice. However, in many cases the mouse model is unsuitable. At this point, we are starting to use human cells in research. This will allow us such procedures as screening new medications in culture by using hESCs. We are creating a human model for these diseases.

DBC: Are there any characteristics that are specific to doing hESC research in Israel?

NB: Research is fairly intensive here in this field. I'll give you an indication: Last summer, the periodical *Stem Cells*, which is the main journal in the stem cell field, published an overview of works on cell lines and their use in experimental work (Guhr et al. 2006). Among other things, the authors analysed early publications on hESCs. In the year 2000 there were just 4 papers that had reported on experimental work with hESCs. Out of these 4, 2 came from my laboratory. The article then listed the most productive countries in hESC research. U.S.A. topped the list with 125 publications, followed by Israel with 42 publications. (U.K., Korea, China, Singapore and Australia followed suit with 30, 27, 16, 15, and 13 publications respectively.) Taking a closer look at the top stem cell papers published between 1998 and 2004, the involvement of Israelis is evident. Out of the 24 most frequently cited papers on hESCs, all published between 1998 and 2004, 5 papers were from my laboratory (about 20 percent of the top papers). Four U.S.A. papers had Israeli co-authors in their teams (Guhr et al. 2006). Altogether then, there are 9 Israeli scholars or research teams among these 24 key stem cell publications. But we are gradually becoming "diluted," because more and more laboratories and scientists enter the field, and because we cannot possibly compete with the scope of funding provided in some countries, mostly the U.S.A. and U.K. In local terms, we are quite reasonably funded, but the sums are dwarfed in comparison to foreign investment.

* * * * *

Interview with Prof. Karl Skorecki, MD

Professor of Medicine/Nephrology, Department of Anatomy and Cell Biology, Rappaport Faculty of Medicine, Technion, Israel Institute of Technology, Haifa, Israel. Skorecki is an expert in population genetics and human embryonic stem cells in cancer.
The interview was conducted in Haifa in May 28th, 2006

* * * * * *

Daphna Birenbaum-Carmeli (DBC): What do you see as the main promise of hESC research?
Professor Karl Skorecki (KS): Ultimately—but I think it's going to take a very long time—hESCs will become a major source for a new field of regenerative medicine, that is, the ability to generate replacement cells for people with diseases in which their own cells can no longer support the functions of the body. For instance, heart failure is at the point where medications and drugs are no longer effective, and the person is a candidate for a heart transplant. In the future, such people will be able to enjoy the benefits of human heart cells generated from hESCs. Or, unless a preventive therapy will be found for Alzheimer's disease or Parkinson's disease, there will be recourse for those patients whose organ functions are deteriorated to re-supply the missing cells with cells derived from hESCs.
But I believe that will take a very long time, decades. There will be some early breakthroughs in less dramatic areas, for example, in bone and joint disease, in which I think it's a matter of years, not decades. I am pretty sure that'll happen. The reason it'll take so long is that there are some scientific and technical problems as well as safety issues we need to overcome. Because we are talking about biological material, we have to be sure that we are not subjecting people to potential harm; that the cells don't turn into cancer or a tumor and infect the patient.
And finally, I think it's a matter of a very short time until hESCs will be used as an experimental platform for testing new drugs, discovering the function of new genes, and understanding cancer and

cell development. I think hESCs are already useful in that regard and that's where my own lab focuses, on cancer research. . .But that's not the ultimate promise of hESC research.

DBC: What do you consider the main ethical concerns?

KS: I think scientists have to be cognizant of, and responsible towards, the society in which they are working, whatever their personal views are. There certainly is in the world a diversity of opinions about the ethical aspects of using hESCs based on their source. That's well known and a lot has been written about it. I think Israel has been in a leadership role in the world not only scientifically but also with respect to the societal and ethical concerns, and I think it has done so in a very enlightened way by taking into account the different views people have. Israel has done something that's not usually considered typical for Israel, rather atypical: civil discourse on a very high, intelligent level with respect to the societal and ethical issues regarding hESC research. Let me cite two important examples.

Way ahead of the rest of the world, around 2000 to 2001, the Israeli Academy of Sciences appointed a bioethics advisory committee chaired by Professor Michel Ravel, which produced a document based on the deliberations of a committee that consisted of a very interesting, eclectic, and wisely chosen group of individuals, including scientists, ethicists, theologians, and public individuals. The committee produced a set of guidelines which I know are used by the rest of the world, from the UN to other countries. They are still to this day one of the most important sets of guidelines ever written on the ethics of hESC research. That's one example.

The other important example: In 2002 and 2005, there were two very important international conferences, sponsored by the Technion, the Ministry of Health, the Israel Medical Association, Rambam Medical Centre and the Rappaport Institute for Research in the Medical Sciences, on ethical issues regarding the embryo. The conferences were extremely successful. And here is what was amazing: There were representatives of the Vatican, representatives of Islam, of humanistic perspectives, of scientific discourse. The Far East was not represented, but there was quite an eclectic group of individuals, and the dialogue was carried out at a very high level without screaming, yelling, with many diverse points of view. I wouldn't say there was a consensus, but there was a polite, respectful public discourse. So much so, that for the first conference we had to twist the arm of our keynote speaker, Professor Jeffrey Drazen, editor of the *New England Journal of Medicine*, to come, but then he happily came to the second conference because as he said this type of conference could not have taken place in the U.S. with its picketing, demonstrating, and political interference. And that, I think, indicates that Israel really is in a leadership position and is viewed as such in the world, attended by speakers as I mention from the U.S., England.

DBC: Was there any international reference to these conferences?

KS: The first one led to a proceedings book which was reviewed favourably in a number of medical journals, and was commended for the way it provided a picture of the diversity of opinions regarding bioethical issues related to the embryo, beginning of life and so forth, and hESC research in particular. It's interesting that shortly after the conference, many journals suddenly had editorials dealing with these issues and I believe that the conference had an effect there, although it's my own inference.

DBC: Could you identify major debates or points of disagreement related to hESC research?

KS: The main point of contention focuses on defining full person sanctity: When does it begin? There is at least a theoretical consensus worldwide—I say theoretical because we know sadly of many places where what I am about to say doesn't apply—that at least from the moment of birth, every individual should be granted full person sanctity, full protection. I think no one disagrees with that. The controversy begins prior to birth. It starts with termination of pregnancy: the late-stage fetus, mid-stage fetus, embryo in the uterus—what sanctity does that entity have? And of course there are differences in religions and laws. That confuses the public, because when you use the word "embryo" loosely, applied to the source of embryonic research, many individuals think incorrectly of termination of pregnancy, especially for hESC research. In practice, the source of the hESC is the pre-embryo, or the fertilized egg, sourced from IVF procedures—supernumerary fertilized eggs that are not going to be implanted. Under consent and appropriate guidelines, they may be used to derive hESC.

Now, the status of that entity, the blastocyst, the fertilized egg that's undergone a few cell divisions, this is the main source of controversy. Does that entity have any sanctity at all, like a fully breathing human being? Something in between? Essentially, it boils down to whether or not that entity has full personhood.

DBC: Where do you personally draw the line?

KS: I don't draw a single line anywhere. I adopt a view, which happens to be consistent with a Jewish point of view, that personhood is acquired in stages through fetal development and it's only achieved at birth. But there is an important line that relates to hESCs and that is uterus implantation. There is something dramatically different between a blastocyst or fertilized egg product that has been implanted in a woman's uterus, and one that has never been in a woman's uterus. Implantation changes that ball of cells from an entity with the potential to become a human being, but one that requires the parents' decision and a medical act, into something that can plant in the uterus and start to develop. I think that's quiet different from a frozen ball of cells in a canister in an IVF facility.

The pre-implantation embryos, up to the blastocyst stage, have very little personhood sanctity—not nothing; they should be treated with respect, but medical research with parental consent, and with ethical guidelines, has a priority over their sanctity so long as they haven't been derived for that purpose, because that violates another ethical principle by utilizing women's bodies to create a medical research product. But, in terms of the sanctity of that blastocyst there is some demarcation at uterus implantation. Now, the Catholic Church doesn't view it this way; they view the fertilized egg as the beginning of life.

DBC: And how do these diverse perspectives influence the practice of research? Is there a different reality of research in Israel in comparison to other countries?

KS: There are very clear cut differences. For example, in the U.S. at this time, it is not illegal to generate hESCs from IVF products, but one may not use federal funds to do this. One can use taxpayers' funds to do hESC research on a set of named lines which existed before, I believe, August 9, 2001, when President Bush set out the government administration policy in the U.S.

DBC: Any other research restrictions?

KS: Only the same restrictions that apply to human subject research in general, research in human tissues. By the way, a repercussion of the U.S. federal funding restriction is that a number of states in the U.S. have developed their own state funding to promote hESC research and fill in the gap. There are also some countries in Europe where the generation of hESCs is illegal. Now, let's take an extreme example, the Far East, where everything has gone way too far in being overly permissive. So, in the Far East there is almost no regulation—I am being a little general here, sorry—but there is very little regulation, to the point where in South Korea, for instance, people can take advantage of the permissiveness and pay women to have their eggs for research and so forth. That's something that

Israel has wisely prohibited. In Israel, the generation of hESCs is legal. There is a moratorium on reproductive cloning, and the generation of hESCs for research must fall under the rubric of the Helsinki guidelines as with all research involving human subjects.

DBC: Can you remember any particular research that was located in one country rather than another because of legal restrictions?

KS: I have a colleague in Texas. We have a collaborative project that involves using hESCs to study how to develop a human tumor micro-environment. We want to study human cancers in the context of human cells but not in a human being; to test anti-cancer drugs growing in a human environment but not in the human being, before the drugs are released for testing. The U.S. partner has equipment and know-how that we don't have, but we had to discuss his lab's NIH funding very carefully. The cells we have are among the cells that do have a Bush approval. However, we would have to go through quite a bit of paperwork in order to make sure that the cells could be used in his lab, or that he could use his lab equipment for hESC research. It certainly made it much more logical for us not to have his lab involved with the cells in any direct fashion, and to grow the cells here. So, we isolate DNA out of the cells and send him DNA but not the cells, whereas, under other circumstances we may have sent him the cells. But, so as not to make his life complicated, because of the federal restrictions there, we chose this particular pathway. These are the kind of practical implications involved.

DBC: What do you consider as the basis for Israel's interest and openness in this field in comparison to other countries?

KS: Religion is the most obvious basis: Islam and Judaism influence Israeli law and public opinion. There is a secular community, but still one cannot ignore the Jewish and the Islamic underpinnings of the large majority of the population. Judaism and Islam both have a clear permissive viewpoint that sort of neutralizes religious objection. Then we are left with bioethics and humanistic perspectives, which, I think, in a rational analysis also leads to a permissive point of view. There are some other reasons as well: There is a sociocultural tradition, again, partly related to Judaism and Islam, to seek health. Across all spheres, I see big differences in the attitude of Israelis from what I saw in Canada, when I practiced there, regarding the lengths to which family would go to find cures, to seek out the best surgeons, to seek out transplantations, to seek out expensive therapies, to preserve human life and health.

DBC: Are you suggesting some kind of difference in attitude between Israeli and Canadian patients and families?

KS: Yes, society in general. There is extreme emphasis here on curing, healing, prolonging life. For example, I am a nephrologist, who deals with dialysis patients with kidney failure who need transplants. I recall, ten years ago, families and also political decisions in Canada, where kidney disease patients would sometimes be allowed to die, and I didn't see society, politicians, families or communities raising money or finding solutions for their patients or family members. Not that long ago, there was a shortage of dialysis machines in Canada, and it took tremendous pressure to get more units built. And interestingly, families and general practitioners, realizing that their patients with kidney failure would not be able to enter a dialysis program, would let those patients pass away. That would never happen in Israel; the Knesset would be in uproar. The idea of the importance of saving lives and the promise that I began with of stem cell research, and the obligation to heal, are paramount in Judaism.

I think it's also true in the Arab community, and in Muslim American community. Both Judaism and Islam have a sort of fatalist point of view: Everything comes from God, etc. Despite that, there is great emphasis on saving lives, and doing research to help mankind when it comes to illness. The fact that on the roads in Israel we hurt each other and the fact there is violence—that's a great paradox. On the one hand we are spending money trying to save lives through health care research; on the other hand, unfortunately, we are not careful enough in terms of preserving life when it comes to traffic, roads and so forth. Nevertheless, I see that as another element in the so called permissive attitude to hESC research here. Other elements are that Israel wants to be recognized as being at the forefront of scientific endeavours—that's other aspect. I think those are the main reasons.

DBC: Do you personally have any concerns about hESC research?

KS: I have concerns. One is that we should not create false hopes or premature optimism. I am optimistic but we have to indicate that it will take time. I have concerns about people putting up smoke screens when it comes to adult stem cells—when people are against hESC research because of their particular philosophies or religious persuasions, and talk about adult stem cells as being a completely scientifically available alternative to hESCs, which they are not. I have concerns, not in Israel, but the rest of the world, especially the Far East, about people, scientists and even countries getting carried away with the promise or possibilities—with the temptation—to the point where they would do what was done in South Korea: falsify data, pay women to generate eggs, etc. I have some concerns about reproductive cloning: We have to be on guard to make sure no one tries to do silly and dangerous things about reproductive cloning, which isn't directly related to hESC research, but it is related. And bio-safety concerns, we have to be very careful. I think we can learn a lot from gene therapy. Gene therapy was raised in the 1990s as a great hope and it was carried away—we haven't seen a lot of successes but we've seen some tragedies. So I think we have to be very slow and careful.

I want to make one other point that goes back to what was said earlier. I talked about the Jewish perspective and the Islamic perspective. I think there is also a different view in Jewish philosophy also shared by other philosophies—that human beings are allowed to intervene in the process of the creation of life. There is no reason not to; we don't have to be afraid. The idea that the process of creating life is something only the divine God can do and humans cannot have any role in: That is something Israeli society and Judaism—and as far as I know, Islam also—rejects. Instead, they say that humans are allowed to intervene in the process of the creation of life, to intervene with nature in a constructive manner, and that is probably one of the underpinnings of the permissiveness as well.

Note

1. The report "Ongoing Research on Mammalian Cloning and Embryo Stem Cell Technologies: Bioethics of their Potential Medical Applications" was authored by Michel Ravel, M.D., Ph.D., of the Department of Molecular Genetics at the Weizmann Institute of Science, Israel. Professor Ravel is also member of the International Bioethics Committee of UNESCO. At present, the committee is chaired by Profesor Ruth Arnon of the Department of Immunology at the Weizmann Institute of Science, Israel.

References

Guhr, A., A. Kurtz, K. Friedgen, P. L. Oser. 2006. "Current State of Human Embryonic Stem Cell Research: An Overview of Cell Lines and Their Use in Experimental Work," *Stem Cells* 24: 2187–91.

National Institutes of Health. n.d. *Stem Cell Basics*. <http://stemcells.nih.gov/info/basics/basics5.asp> (accessed June 21, 2007).

Revel, Michel. 2000. "Ongoing Research on Mammalian Cloning and Embryo Stem Cell Technologies: Bioethics of Their Potential Medical Applications." <http://www.academy.ac.il/bioethics/english/articles/cloning1.htm> (accessed September 9, 2007).

Thomson, James A., Joseph Itskovitz-Eldor, Sander S. Shapiro, Michelle A. Waknitz, Jennifer J. Swiergiel, Vivienne S. Marshall, and Jeffrey M. Jones. 1998. "Embryonic Stem Cell Lines Derived from Human Blastocysts," *Science* 282, no. 6 (November): 1145–47.

Chapter 11

Medicine and the State: The Medicalization of Reproduction in Israel[*]

Yali Hashash

Introduction

Feminist and sociology researchers in Israel over the last two decades have consistently claimed that Israeli reproductive policy has always been, and remains, an expression of the State's nation-building efforts. Within this framework, two main contentions are made: (a) Israel's reproductive policy primarily aims at winning a "demographic race" against the Palestinian Arabs and is, therefore, pronatalist[1]; and (b) Israel, although pronatalist, is equally concerned with the reproduction of the "New Jew," who exhibits physical and/or cultural attributes that fit Westernized/modernistic qualitative demands.[2]

These two contentions take for granted that as a profession, medicine has assumed the role of an obedient servant of the State, lending its expert skills to the Jewish nation-building project. Further, Israeli scholarship in the field has sometimes understood gynecologists to be agents of progressive processes that allow women to gain wider control over their reproduction.[3] Thus, medicine as a profession has not only been portrayed as the loyal servant of the State in its nation-building project, but also as the servant of women in need of rescue and reproductive possibilities. Critical sociological research, on the most part, has therefore neglected gynecology as a subject of independent analysis.[4]

In this chapter, I wish to trace the medicalization of reproduction in Israel by pointing at and tracking gynecologists' interests. I will argue that beyond national, political, cultural, and ideological agendas, the medical establishment in Israel has also acted in its *own* interests in increasing its professional power and influence by continuing to deepen the medicalization of reproduction. From this perspective, ideological justification structures were instrumental, nurturing the medical establishment's ever growing power position. I will suggest that Israeli medicine cannot be understood as a mere tool used by a presumably homogenous state to promote a coherent political agenda or reflect a clear value system. As this chapter aims to expose, Israeli physicians have their own interests, which they try to promote within or *vis-à-vis* the State. Since it is my understanding that cultural explanations, such as pro-natalism, have often worked to cloud rather than clarify the understanding of such processes, this chapter will focus on more "structural" dimensions, i.e., the negotiation between Israeli medicine and the State over resource allocation and legislation regarding reproduction.

Working within the generally accepted frameworks of Foucauldian analyses of state power and doctors' professional power, my emphasis is on the continuous negotiation over state resources taking place between state agencies, and non-state actors who can potentially use bio-power and population control discourses as vehicles for obtaining professional resources (Fligstein 2001). According to this view, professionals employed as administrators within state apparatuses facilitate the production of a common language which eventually directs state agencies to embrace professional interests in their decisions and policies. This understanding applies to medical professionals as well, who in their negotiation with state agencies, and while acting from within state agencies, frequently manage to rely on scientific language to achieve almost full autonomy over the practice and funding of their professional domain (Abbott 1991).

In the domain of gynecology, professionalization and the very inclusion in the field of medicine largely pivoted on the medicalization of pregnancy during the second half of the 20th century. Barker (2003) describes how in the United States, a network of state officials and medical professionals directed state action toward establishing medical knowledge as the exclusive source of authority and jurisdiction in matters of reproduction, gradually rendering other professionals and sources of knowledge irrelevant. In other countries, medicalization has taken the aura of a national enterprise, depending on and aiming for public legitimacy, constituting itself as a vehicle in the service of national objectives. At the same time, physicians and particularly gynecologists came to occupy state administrative positions with an active role in decision-making processes (Abbott 1991).

In this chapter, my aim is to point to the professional interests that doctors and gynecologists have had in specific directions of evolution and change in Israel's reproductive policy over the years. In other words, I hope to underscore the role of doctors and medical researchers in the shaping of legislation and resource allocation. My focus is on three historical moments in the medicalization of reproduction in Israel.

Section one will examine population regulation between the 1950s and the 1970s, focusing on the issue of contraception use. Whereas traditional sociological literature has emphasized the state's ideological motivation to minimize the use of contraception as a means of population regulation, this section will suggest the medical interest in expanding the use of medical contraception, thereby creating a clientele for experimentation, while taking part in a larger debate over the appropriate size of families in Israel.

Section two will examine the medicalization of pregnancy termination, as it developed during the 1970s. This section reveals the abortion debate as an arena for legitimizing an existing medical practice, as well as furthering the medicalization of pregnancy and reproduction in general.

Section three examines the converging debates over human cloning, stem cell research and oocyte donation that are currently underway in Israel. It reveals the major influence that the medical community has had on legislative processes in this area, particularly the effort to ensure scientific access to human oocytes and to remove legal hindrances to scientific cloning research.

These processes, and medical pressure aimed to influence legislations in general, are not necessarily covert. Indeed, the Israeli Medical Association (IMA) openly lists this sphere of activity as part of its role and mission.[5]

I: Reproductive medicine and population regulation in Israel

In the 1960s and 1970s, population regulation was discussed by various state-appointed professional bodies in Israel. Although it is traditionally thought that the Arab-Jewish "demographic race" was the major focal point of these discussions. The diversity within the Jewish population and the state population policy with regards to the various Jewish groups was at least equally important in most professional deliberations, in which doctors played an active integral part (Hashash 2004).

The national family planning program was among the major issues that were discussed. Research has usually commented on the scarcity of family planning in Israel, interpreted by researchers as an expression of the State's pronatalist policy (Portugese 1998). In contrast to that approach, I shall analyze not the absence, but rather the presence of family planning in Israel, in order to explore its medicalized characteristics, and the medical influences on its shaping.

During the 1950s, the first decade of the Israeli State, population regulation was a major concern for many countries in the West, as well as for other population policy-makers globally. Different population policies that were endorsed were motivated by either strong eugenic objectives, or aspirations for social reform. Medical establishments responded to population regulation policies by offering medical means to implement state policies, as well as medical opinions as to the healthy size of a family and the medically-recommended time interval between pregnancies.

The interest in population regulation programs was crucial for the development of the medicalization of reproduction, primarily because it constructed a legitimate working field for practitioners. But its importance was also conceptual. Population regulation encapsulated the very idea of planning, which is the basic tool of any professional intervention. As such, the idea of planning future fertility trends or family size constitutes a favorable *a priori* for anyone who wishes to legitimize a professional intervention in that field.

Israeli doctors were quick to join the developing field of medical contraception. The Hebrew-language professional magazine *Harefu'ah* [Medicine] reported that an Israeli gynecological study had become one of two pioneering publications in the area of contraception as early as 1959 (Vego & Shapira 1968). However, Israeli doctors' interest in the subject was not necessarily national; indeed, it was at least partly related to the activity of international bodies, such as the Population Council established by Rockefeller in the United States in 1952. In order to address global population growth, the Council worked to encourage research on contraception in various places around the world. In 1963, it included Israel in its statistical assessment of IUD clinical data worldwide (Schindler 2007; Vego and Shapira 1968). The U.S. Department of Health was also interested in funding family planning programs and research in Israel. With the help of American funding, Israeli gynecologists were able to take part in the newest research on medical contraception that was being conducted in several clinics and hospitals throughout the country during the 1960s.[6]

Although there was already medical interest, a legitimate clientele under medically supervised contraception was still lacking. Hence, doctors negotiated with the State, which, in the mid-1960s, was still ignorant of these developments.[7] This was soon to change, but not before global interests would be translated into the rhetoric of national concerns.

Israel is an immigrant society. Between 1948—the year of its establishment—and 1960, about one million Jews immigrated to Israel from different countries in Eastern Europe, Southwest Asia and North Africa. The non-European immigrants were referred to as belonging to Mizrahi [Oriental] communities. These communities were culturally and economically marginalized by the hegemonic Ashkenazi (mostly East European) society and government. In the early 1960s, it became clear that Mizrahi Jews were beginning to form a demographic majority within the Jewish population of Israel.[8]

In 1962, demographer Professor Roberto Bachi was appointed as director of the Natality Committee (NC), which was to advise the government on aiding large families, most of whom were Mizrahi, as well as on addressing the issue of the allegedly low Jewish fertility rate.[9] The fertility discussions, as I have argued elsewhere, were not necessarily designed to solve any demographic issue. The NC defined its goal as a one of regulation intended to equate fertility rates between the different Jewish ethnic groups and to create a homogenous fertility pattern. Yet, as was well known to the experts in the committee, a homogenous fertility pattern was already rapidly forming with no governmental intervention, with Mizrahi fertility declining from nearly 6 to roughly 3 children per woman over the decade after immigration, and Ashkenazi fertility registering a slight, yet consistent increase. Therefore fertility discussions were used to address issues of the State's economic and cultural makeup, and formed a site where professionals and representatives of the middle class Ashkenazi public fought over the allocation of State's resources (Hashash 2004).

The NC, whose seven members included the director-general of the Health Ministry and a senior doctor from Israel's largest HMO (*Kupat Holim*), suggested that public funds allocated to enhance Jewish fertility rates should be directed only to smaller, better-off families that were economically and "culturally" able to afford a third or a fourth child, but whose own financial calculations made them reluctant to have this birth. This reluctance, it was claimed, might change with proper public support.[10] The committee explained that larger families do not plan the size of their families and, therefore, should not be eligible for birth incentives (NC Report 1966: 39). The NC also advised the government to distribute information on family planning as a social justice agenda (ibid.: 50).

Thus, it was the NC that was in charge of officially introducing family planning as a recommended means of fighting poverty, eventually recommending how to supplement small families' income.[11] In that way, it contributed to the creation of a legitimate clientele for new medical contraceptives. The cautious yet clear dictum of applying family planning as a major weapon to fight poverty and to prevent deterioration in the quality of the population resonated with the American Population Council agenda, enabling doctors to openly engage in medical contraceptive research and practice with a legitimate target population: women of Middle Eastern descent with several children.

The head of the Gynecology and Obstetrics ward of Rehovot Hospital, for example, published an article in which he explained that the IUD was primarily suited to "women who have given birth, and in particular women who finished giving birth and were of low educational level." The pill, he tried to point out, was suitable to all "but primitive women who are not able to take it responsibly every day" (Lancet 1970: 69).

The establishment of the Demographic Center in 1968 worked to expand this process. The Demographic Center's propaganda campaign was designed to mobilize "families with two children to increase their families to 3–4 children, and advise large families on family planning." The Center's active committee members frequently referred to the national threat of burdening the public with population growth in the lower strata.[12]

The NC and the Demographic Center helped in creating a legitimate clientele for medical contraception. But, concrete state apparatus was still amiss if family planning would be established as a nation-wide practice that was medically managed. From their power position as participants in state apparatuses that addressed population regulation issues, fertility doctors worked to influence decision-making towards a national, medically managed family planning program.

Thus we find that Dr. Polishuk, head of the Women and Labor Ward at Hadassah Hospital in Jerusalem and member of the Demographic Center, recommends, in a letter from 1968 to Dr. Gajevin,

the director-general of the Health Ministry and himself a member of
both the NC and the Demographic Center, a plan to add family planning and pregnancy-supervision programs to maternity care centers
so that women who should not get pregnant due to medical and
social difficulties could be given an IUD or hormonal contraception,
and so that these women "and their reproductive organs" could be
monitored. The plan, Polishuk suggested, would attract U.S. Department of Health funding.[13]

Perhaps the most enthusiastic medical advocate of family planning
was Professor Yitzhak Halbrecht, a leading gynecologist and fertility
researcher,[14] who was a member of the Demographic Center's Council. In the late 1960s, Halbrecht gathered a group of gynecologists and
started the Family Planning Association. In 1974, he obtained funding from the International Planned Parenthood Society and turned
the small association into the Israeli Family Planning Association
(Zafrir 1981). Through this association he advocated the American
idea of "each child a wanted child" and stressed the health hazards to
those who were not careful to space their pregnancies by a period of
2 to 2.5 years. At the Demographic Center, which supported his project (Zafrir 1981), Halbrecht had strongly advocated family planning,
stating that "it is doubtful that unplanned and therefore unwanted
children would be wanted by the state" (CEPA Report 1974: 491).

In 1974 the NC and Demographic Center family planning advocates received support from the opposite side of the political spectrum: the Katz Committee. The Katz Committee (officially named
the Prime Minister's Committee for Youth in Distress) was appointed by the government following ethnic and social riots that spread
from Jerusalem to the entire country. The Black Panthers, as they
called themselves after the American movement, protested against
the discrimination of Mizrahi population and accused the government of encouraging social gaps based on ethnic criteria. Unlike the
NC, the Katz Report that was submitted in 1974 advised the government on allocating budgets for welfare, education, and cultural
activities in underprivileged neighborhoods and townships in the
country. Like the NC, it linked poverty and a large number of children, and advised the establishment of a national family planning
program as a remedy. That same year, the Health Ministry decided
to cooperate with Halbrecht's association, and to incorporate family
planning services into already-existing medical services—maternity
care centers and gynecology wards (Zafrir 1981)—giving a governmental push to the medicalization of family planning.

So, while several political agendas were at work—the NC's quasi-
eugenic one, and the Katz Committee's social one—it was medical

professional interest that could be mobilized through and for the convergence of global and local interests. Thus, local social concerns were defined in terms of quality and quantity, as coined by foreign institutions (e.g., the Population Council; the Planned Parenthood Association), so as to contribute to the growing local medical expertise in the field of contraception, and to facilitate local participation in the research and development of medical contraceptives. Non-medical considerations were put under the umbrella of medical jurisdiction, and social reasons were cited in order to mobilize research funds.[15]

The medicalized character of family planning has been further strengthened through the following decades, so much so that in her 1996 survey on the availability of contraceptives in Israel, Larissa Remmenick (1996: 26) reported that:

> This topic [birth regulation] in Israel is based on medicine, probably to a larger extent than in other countries. . . Modern contraceptives are represented in reproductive clinics by 3–5 types of pills and a similar number of IUDs, while popular non-medical contraceptives are not perceived by doctors as relevant to their profession. . . . The potential of some of these non-medical measures, like the diaphragm and the condom combined with spermicides, is not properly used, as doctors have no incentive to recommend them.

II: Induced abortion

The previous section explored doctors' role in introducing and shaping family planning in Israel. It has been suggested that the inner logic of gynecology as a profession required dissemination of the idea of planning in order to justify medical intervention in reproductive processes. Medical attempts to influence the public demand for such intervention were also explored. Approaching the medical establishment as a site of power with a significant degree of autonomy allows us to re-examine pregnancy terminations as well, and explore their role in the medical process.

The conceptual acceptance of the possibility to terminate a pregnancy is a vital component in the medicalization of reproduction. This section will follow the medical establishment's efforts to legalize abortion under medicalized conditions, and the construction of the abortion debate as a site for advocating further medicalization in the future.

Amir has systematically examined the politics of induced abortion in Israel (Amir 1989; Amir and Benjamin 1992). In her accounts of the various political forces struggling over a local resolution that would enable a relatively consensual practice, gynecologists are rarely seen as political agents. Instead, they are depicted as either progressive in relation to women's interests or neutral in relation to the political debate. Despite her reference to physicians as her informants for the various organizations that have contributed to the shaping the practicalities of abortion, Amir (1989) virtually never dwells on the possibility that the gynecologists could have been using their power positions in state administration or in the local health care system to promote some vested interests of their own.

In 1972, the Health Ministry established the Committee for Examining Prohibitions on Abortion (CEPA). Similar to other state regulations concerning reproduction that have benefited doctors' interests, the CEPA may also be viewed as having advanced the distinct interests of the medical establishment.

Up until the early 1970s, the Abortion Law was legally based on a British Mandate law from 1936, which was enforced along lines drawn by the Israeli attorney general in 1952. The law stated that a prosecution could take place only if the abortion was performed against the woman's will, caused her death, was performed negligibly, or was performed by anyone other than a licensed physician. The issue was discussed by a gynecologists' sub-committee of the NC, which advised the NC that abortion was a risky medical procedure and therefore should not be allowed unless conducted under medically accepted criteria. Similarly, the 1974 CEPA report argued forcibly for the need to make abortion a legal medical procedure, and for the need to prohibit it under any other circumstances. The bill it proposed recommended the following (CEPA Report 1974: 432):

> *No charges* of criminal responsibility will be brought against the person performing the abortion if the procedure was carried out in a *recognized institution* receiving the written *approval of a medical committee* [emphases added] on the grounds of one of the following reasons:
>
> a) Continuing the pregnancy could cause risk to the pregnant woman's life.
> b) Continuing the pregnancy could cause the woman mental or physical damage.
> c) There is a risk that if born, the offspring would have physical or cognitive impairments.
> d) Conception occurred as a result of rape or incest.
> e) The woman is under the legal age for marriage or over 45 years old.
> f) Severe damage might be caused to the woman or her children because of extreme social conditions, including a large number of children in the household.

Similar to the circumstances surrounding family planning, abortions were in this way to be accepted under limited, medically supervised instances, allowing non-medical issues to be captured within a medical veneer.

The proposed bill argued for the enforcement of a controlled space to carry out abortions, as this would ensure "that abortions will be performed only by those who have the special expert skills required for this medical procedure." Whereas the requirement for "expert skills" can be accepted at face value, the bill did not explain why the procedure had to be conducted in hospitals only and why the decision regarding each specific case depended on institutional medical approval. One of the main features of the bill was the immunity from state interference or potential legal liability that it endowed those possessing the "expert skills." It also legalized a procedure already practiced by physicians.

Beyond the abortion procedure, the CEPA also strove to institutionalize the decision-making process leading to an abortion as primarily a medical procedure. The nature of the guidelines proposed by the CEPA, of which only the first three involve medical considerations, raises a question. If alternative procedures can easily be used to certify that the relevant medical considerations are taken into account, why should the committee be a medical one? Amir and Benjamin (1992) suggest that the importance of this directive lies primarily in ushering gynecologists into non-medical issues. The committee exerted symbolic control over women asking for an abortion. Noticeably, the committee, which was designed to interrogate the woman on her misuse of contraception, approved almost every request for abortion, and thus had no real influence on the actual decision to abort.

But the CEPA could have achieved more than the medicalization of abortion and the exertion of symbolic power over women who sought its approval. It could form the abortion debate as an infrastructure for future medicalization processes. In an addendum to the NC's 1974 report, Halbrecht, then head of the women's ward at Hasharon Hospital, proposed to set up a comprehensive center for controlling all reproductive-related processes: pre-pregnancy, during the course of pregnancy, during birth, and after the birth. The opening statement of Halbrecht's document (CEPA Report 1974: 490) reads:

> The future of the State of Israel depends on its number of citizens and their quality—both aspects depend on the magnitude of immigration from various countries of origin on the one hand and the natural increase of the local population. . . . To these two foundations we need

to add the need to care for our people's physical and mental well being and health. The health of our people who come to this country from all over the world, will be critical for our fate in our war for survival, facing multiple dangers from without and within.

Halbrecht thus positioned the medical establishment as one of the main national forces in the war for the survival of the Jewish people and the State of Israel. The set of practical suggestions he lists is much less national and much more medical in nature: constructing a comprehensive family health center that would handle problems like family-planning counseling; eugenic and genetic counseling; diagnosis of inherited diseases before and during pregnancy; monitoring pregnancy and the effects of environmental factors on its quality; conducting amniotic fluid tests for the detection of fetal defects and inherited diseases during pregnancy; treating infertility; and finally, treating sexual deviance. Connecting this range of medical reproductive activities to national goals, Halbrecht (ibid.: 494) summarized his suggestions as follows:

> The duty to heighten our efforts and exploit our resources and the immense potential to improve mothers' and children's health—is ours to shoulder. We need to act to continue the trend of a decrease in maternal death and infant mortality as well as improving our ability to prevent thousands of children from the suffering caused by damage occurring during abnormal pregnancies and births—turning them to invalids crippled for life as well as into a heavy burden on the family and society.

By hinting at the mutual interests of the individual, the family, and the State, Halbrecht positioned himself and other doctors as possessing the professional knowledge and skill to serve these mutual interests.

Halbrecht's vision had a concrete aspect. In 1974, the same year the CEPA was established, he established the Institute for Reproductive Research and Embryo Development at Hasharon Hospital. It was his plan to further develop this institute into the comprehensive center that he portrayed in the NC report. Although he himself retired in 1975, the model whose foundations he had laid mirrored the medical establishment's professional ambitions in reproductive health, and reproductive centers that would spring up later on would include all of the elements he had portrayed and more.

Upon concluding this section, it needs to be reiterated that doctors' control over both family planning and abortion could not have been accomplished without acceptance of the notion of pregnancy planning or termination, which imply approval of human intervention in the reproductive process.

III: Stem cell research, cloning and oocyte donation

The last site I wish to visit enables us to follow closely both overt and tacit medical and scientific influence on policy-making processes through a study of the debates that took place in the Science and Technology Committee of the Knesset regarding cloning and oocyte donation. The following section will depict the convergence of two legislative processes that took place in Israel since the late 1990s. The first is the law that regulates human cloning; the second is the oocyte donation bill.

In November 1998, Thomson et al. published an article on their success in producing the first embryonic stem cell line.[16] Using fertilized oocytes derived from an IVF procedure, the scientists were able to create a line of unspecialized cells and induce them to regenerate. The potential was immense: In principle, these unspecialized cells were able to differentiate into any of the specialized embryonic tissues and be useful in "drug discovery, and transplantation medicine" (Thomson et al. 1998: 1146–47).

At the time the debates depicted in the following took place (summer 1999–spring 2007) there were two sources of embryonic stem cells available: the first was from embryos cultivated *in-vitro* through the insemination of an oocyte. The second was through a method known as therapeutic cloning or research cloning.[17] Both methods require female oocytes, and each attempt to create such a line consumes large numbers of oocytes. However, since the end of 2007 scientists were able to achieve constant progress in inducing human somatic adult cells into pluripotent stem cells (iPSC) that imitate embryonic stem cells without using embryos, and therefore oocytes (Yamanaka 2009).

Because of the many ethical issues connected with using human ova and with creating and destroying human embryos, hESC research received legislative attention worldwide. Israeli legislation concerning stem cell research in Israel is included in the law that prohibits genetic intervention.

Barbara Prainsack (2006), who analyzed the legislative processes dealing with cloning and embryonic stem cell research in Israel, depicts the Israeli law as so permissive—it allows practically everything, except for the actual cloning of a fully developed human being—it sometimes draws comments from bioethics counterparts in Europe and the U.S. as being immoral. Prainsack suggests that this liberal legislation reflects a specific value system, rather than a lack of values. It is a system that draws on two cultural-political factors that jointly explain the State's permissive attitude toward genetic research. The first factor, according to Prainsack, is Jewish law, in which, unlike Christian teachings, an embryo outside the uterus has little status, and human attempts to intervene with nature are not condemned but encouraged. The second factor is the demographic-pro-natalist explanation. The pronatalist discourse in Israel is discreet and yet internalized by civilians, who exhibit Foucauldian self-governing and interpret the "creation of new individual bodies" as "saving the collective body" (Prainsack 2006: 188). These two factors, Prainsack claims, define the discursive range of the permissible and the prohibited regarding reproduction technologies.

While rejecting Prainsack's conclusions, I find her data supportive of my argument. In March 1997, an expert body—the National Council for Research and Development—was convened to discuss ethical issues concerning cloning. Prainsack describes the way scientific experts repeatedly approached a politician who had initiated a bill for State control in the field—Member of Parliament Hagai Merom—informing him in a friendly, respectful manner of his lack of understanding in science and his confusion regarding science and morals. Merom wished to ban human cloning altogether, and to restrict cloning research, while the scientists insisted that his restrictive proposals hampered scientific attempts to help humanity. As a result of this pressure, MP Merom changed his mind, and the law that was finally approved granted vast research autonomy to medical experts, thus making the Israeli law in this field one of the least restrictive in the world. The cloning of a full human being was only prohibited for a five-year moratorium, and not altogether. Prainsack quotes Merom in the aftermath as saying that these frequent meetings with scientists and physicians persuaded him that any restriction would impede genetic research.

At the end of 2003, the five-year moratorium was about to expire, and the Knesset's Science and Technology (S&T) Committee had convened several times to discuss the re-approval of the genetic intervention prohibition bill. The need of oocytes for cloning research was also debated. I now turn to follow closely the debates and eventual legislation concerning these two distinct yet related issues: the extension of the five-year moratorium on cloning, and the oocyte donation bill.

A. *Contesting politicians: the battle for the moratorium*

The central question in the discussions of the genetic intervention prohibition bill was whether to prohibit the cloning of a human entirely or to prolong the moratorium that the 1999 law enacted. The Knesset members (MKs) varied in their stance on the question, whereas the scientific community's representatives all objected to a total prohibition and advocated prolonging the moratorium. The issue of cloning research, and the need for women's oocytes for that research, arose from time to time during these discussions.

Nearly all of the committee's meetings were characterized by a high attendance from the scientific community: stem cell scientists, managers of genetic institutions or wards, fertility doctors, etc. In fact, at most of these meetings, the scientists outnumbered the MKs. Following the pattern that Praisnack describes, the scientists dismissed some of the MKs and other participant's concerns as stemming from a non-scientific, moral, and emotional attitude that might jeopardize scientific progress.[18]

The meeting of November 12, 2003 drew the presence of Professor Bolslav Goldman, who was head of the large Sheba Medical Center, chairman of the Supreme Helsinki Committee for Genetic Experiments on Humans, and manager of a genetic institution. A reading of the protocols of this and other meetings that Goldman attended shows that his main concern over the legislation was to ensure that Israeli scientific development would not be hampered, although his other professional positions might have called for a more complex set of concerns. "We have gone a long way to enable this law," he said, and continued:

> My fear is that once you start making changes, they can go in all kinds of directions, and may put on hold and delay a development that to me and most of my friends in the scientific-medical world is a most important one.[19]

When relating to ethical questions that other participants of the meeting raised, Goldman said:

> I was very disturbed by the apocalyptic picture that was presented here: man's dignity, woman's dignity, oocyte and all these issues. . . . [A]ccording to this position we must stay still and do nothing.[20]

Carmel Shalev, a member of the Supreme Helsinki Committee and a researcher of gender and reproductive health, as well as Meira Weiss, a professor of cultural anthropology and sociology at the Hebrew University, tried to raise such ethical questions in the next meeting. Weiss claimed that cloning and scientific progress could not be addressed without looking into Israel's position on human organ trafficking and the trade in oocytes. Organs are being taken from the poorer populations all over the world in order to meet the needs of the affluent, Weiss said. "Israel's involvement in purchasing oocytes from young, poor women. . .makes me very worried," she continued, claiming that the State has not dealt at all with the issue of oocyte donors.[21] Such practices, Weiss advised, contribute to Israel's isolation in the world. Professor Joseph Itskovitz, a leading stem cell scientist, commented that if the researchers were left alone to research, instead of being intimidated by the "slippery slope," they hoped to be able to clone oocytes, so that they would no longer need to extract them from women.

Shalev proposed that cloning research be prohibited for a year, since Israel had not yet regulated the field and lacked monitoring bodies and regulations. Michel Revel, head of the National Bioethics Council, warned that this position might hurt science and, specifically, the international scientific connections that Israel enjoyed. Like Goldman, Revel took the position of a science guardian, putting all other bioethical dilemmas aside. Furthermore, his role as a bioethicist was used to reassure concerned MKs. During the meeting of December 31, 2003, for example, the issue of prohibiting the in vitro development of an embryo after the fourteenth day arose. Revel asked that the law not specify a certain day, because "science keeps finding out new things" that should not be limited by legislation. MK Peaness felt uneasy, saying he had heard only supporters of the bill. Revel tried to reassure him that "there are representatives of bioethics committees, the Helsinki Committee, and the Health Ministry that do nothing but supervise research, and we have considered the matter, not as users of the methods but as supervisors of the ethics of science."

The last two sessions of the S&T Committee on the cloning law were stormy. Chairwoman Moli Polishuk, who considered herself "pro-scientist," felt herself attacked because of her categorical objection to cloning a human being:

> As to what the three committee experts have decided, I want to say that . . . these are the same people on the three committees, so you can relate to them as one group of scientists. . . . I have also heard from some of the [non-scientific] people that sit on the committees . . . that those who had a different opinion were hushed up. I myself repeatedly felt how those who think differently are being silenced. I have never seen in the Science Committee's meetings so much passion generated and pressure exerted by one particular group on another as in this matter. . . .To say that it's not interest driven, maybe; ideological concern for research purposes, maybe. . . . I felt very bad and think it is improper. . . when you speak of different views that people hold and say. . . that they are moral and not based on knowledge, when I have reiterated so many times that not the slightest harm is being done to research.[22]

Although some of the MKs said they would favor a permanent prohibition, others declared their faith in the scientists. Ultimately, the committee voted on March 1, 2004 to recommend the extension of the five-year moratorium on the cloning of a full scale human being.

B. Contesting politicians: In search of oocytes

With the extension of the moratorium, which ensured the legality of cloning research, doctors and researchers could finally make their case for oocyte donation, which meant adding research as a legitimate ground for oocyte donation.[23]

Several oocyte donation bills have been forwarded by different MKs since 1999. A special experts committee was assigned to discuss oocyte donations, issuing the Halperin report. However, those suggested bills, as well as the Halperin Committee's report, never involved donations for research. Furthermore, some measures were taken to protect the health of the donors and to supervise the operating medical staff.[24]

The debate among the scientific community's delegates, parliamentarians, and others present at meetings of the S&T Committee reveals the use of rhetoric embedded in different value systems to overcome objections to oocyte donations for research. It also reveals the ways in which rhetoric created an inaccurate impression.

On March 24, 2004, Professor Joseph Itskovitz appeared before the S&T Committee to lobby for legislation that would allow women not going through IVF treatment to donate oocytes for research. Itskovitz, the director of the Obstetrics and Gynecology Department at the Rambam Medical Center in Haifa, established its IVF section in the 1980s. He is also director of the Stem Cell Research Center, which he initiated in 1998, and was a member of the first team in the world to extract an embryonic stem cell line.[25]

During the meeting, Itskovitz stressed that current Israeli legislation was "killing" all prospects of research, whereas science elsewhere in the world was developing rapidly. What research really needs, he said, is not surplus oocytes, but new, unfertilized, and high-quality oocytes. He suggested that any woman who wished to contribute to science should have freedom of choice to do so. He stressed ("I guarantee") that the oocyte extraction procedure today is simple, safe, and gentle, and downplayed any medical risks that may be involved in subjugating women to intensive hormonal treatments. Superfluous donations did not even begin to satisfy research needs, Itskovitz stated. He then went on to stress the nationalist motivation: "We should not conceal that bio-technological developments are a national-state goal, and not only a personal goal for the researcher who will take the 'stash' and go home."

In a meeting held at the end of the following year, Professor Benjamin Reubinof, a leading stem cell researcher and head of the Stem Cell Research Center at Hadassah Hospital, presented the S&T Committee with a review of global developments on cloning.[26] "The first problem I wish to emphasize," Reubinof said,

> . . . is the availability of human oocytes for the process. . . . It is clear that the availability of human oocytes for the procedure of somatic cell transplant . . . is a crucial phase. . . . These developments can only occur in countries that allow the donation of oocytes for research. . . . In our opinion, the donation of oocytes for research into advanced and effective treatment of severe diseases has an ethical justification no less than . . . for fertility. . . .There will be many women who will be interested in contributing to science and not to fertility.

The committee chairman asked for ethical remarks. Professor Michel Revel responded: "Oocyte donation belongs to the domain of organs donation . . . and can be seen as an altruistic deed for the health of another person."[27]

"Is an oocyte defined as an organ?" the chairman asked. Stressing the fertility rather than the research need for oocytes, Revel answered: "It is also a contribution to the improvement of health and life. If you look at infertility as a disease, you can certainly look at an oocyte donation, which allows another woman to give birth, as an organ donation for her health." The bill that the committee then suggested was, however, very far from the organ donation legislation that forbade anonymous donation and required strict supervision in order to avoid trafficking.

Nira Lamai of the Future Generations Commission insisted: "But an organ donation bill has just been passed. It never mentioned oocytes." In reply, Revel encouraged her to look at stem cell research as a life saver, thus justifying the donation ethically. Lamai was not pleased. She insisted that the issues arising from cloning should not be handled exclusively by the scientific community. "The question should be referred to the Health and Justice Ministries," she advised. "Have you estimated at all what would happen if you allowed oocyte donations? How many women will come forward? What are the possibilities of the development of illegal trafficking, of a black market?"

Again, Revel played a soothing role: "We have in Israel bioethics institutions . . . a very strong ethical basis . . . several committees. . . . I think we all want a good society."

Eventually, the Knesset passed an oocyte donation bill on its first reading on May 8, 2007. The bill lacked supervision over doctors and reduced the protection for donors that was available in previously proposed bills.

The study of the protocols of the S&T Committee reveals that physicians exerted constant pressure on politicians to pass the bill in order to establish legitimate procedures of oocyte donation and a legal infrastructure for future scientific development. To this end, they used their status as professionals, and as members of national committees, to further their own interests. Though cloaked in nationalist ("bio-technological developments are a national state goal"), humanitarian ("It is also a contribution to the improvement of health and life"), or even gender-equality terms (women's right to choose to donate), these demands have unfailingly been compatible with medicalization, and the needs of bio-medical research of reproduction. What has been consistently downplayed, and mostly ignored, is the physical toll on women, as well as the ethical and social consequences of their objectification.

Subsequent to theses debates, the S&T Committee approved a new version of the oocyte donation bill. That version lacked any safeguards for the donors. At the same time, it allowed doctors to extract oocytes without any state regulation. The Knesset has approved this bill and it now awaits its second and third calls. Between 2007–2010 feminist intervention in the legislative process and the decline in the need for oocytes in hSC research enabled the introduction of major corrections to the bill, and the corrected version now awaits its 2nd and 3rd calls.

By way of conclusion

The preceding accounts have illustrated the role of the medical establishment and the scientific community in Israel as the initiators of developments, rather than executers of pre-deliberated State policy: Family-planning concerns began in hospital wards; a comprehensive State program of prenatal and natal care was suggested by physicians; and legislation for oocyte donations for research was written to meet scientific demands.

The medical establishment has been shown to negotiate state facilitation of its professional interests through their integration into Israeli local value systems. In addition, the interest in medical advances has been shown in its connection to an agenda much wider than the national agenda, whether it was the American interest in population control or the global race for new therapies and drugs based on human embryonic stem cell research. Aside from the appropriation of non-medical areas into the medical realm, the medical establishment has constantly used negotiation with the State to build an infrastructure for future growth. We have seen this "expansive" attitude in Halbrecht's vision, as well as in the pressure exerted by scientists to prolong the cloning moratorium, and in Revel's insistence on avoiding specific clauses in legislation that might limit future developments.

We have also seen that gynecologists and scientists have been in a position to influence legislation through the central role they play in different public committees. The success of the scientific community's negotiations with the State depends to a large extent on the existence of a close network of professionals and administrators who are either scientists or doctors themselves, or who otherwise share common interests. Cooperation with other state professional officials, such as the head of the NC in the case of family planning, or the legal advisor to the Health Ministry in the case of cloning legislation, has also been a factor.

The state, as Fligstein (2001) has proposed, is a complex entity, comprised of different agencies that continuously negotiate among themselves as well as with other non-state actors. The extent to which the state hands over the reproduction of its citizens to the medical profession depends upon the ability of medicine to negotiate the scope of its domain and to promote its interests through being incorporated into various administrative capacities. It also depends, as Abbot (1991) has remarked, on its competitive ability to assume authority in the field. In order to better compete, medicine had to win public legitimacy and so had to take on social and national agendas. It also had to be part of the state's decision making apparatus. Gynecologists' ability to achieve a great measure of autonomy is ubiquitous, and is a subject of growing literature. It also has its particular history and context-dependent power configurations, as this chapter has tried to depict.

Notes

*   I wish to thank Professor Daphna Birenbaum-Carmeli and Professor Yoram Carmeli for their generous encouragement, patience, and

remarks; Mr. Nick Denes, Professor Chris Corinn and Miss Mali Furman-Assa for reading the first drafts and offering their very useful and wise remarks. I am particularly in debt to Dr. Orly Benjamin, who has so kindly and willingly been a mentor and a friend throughout the long process of writing this article.

1. See for example Portugese (1998) and Berkovitch (1997).
2. See for example Melamed (2002) and Remennick (2006).
3. Amir (1989), for example, implied the existence of such a progressive role by referring to gynecologists as "liberal" when practicing abortions.
4. Smadar Sharon (2006) has suggested that architects and city planners were equally motivated to serve the hegemony as well as to work in accordance with their field's inner logic, the outlines of which are more often drawn outside of Israel. A scrutiny of the medical establishment concerning reproduction can be found to an extent in Carmeli and Birenbaum-Carmeli (2000), Shalev and Gooldin (2006), and Remenick (2006). However, these analyses are deeply entrenched in cultural interpretations.
5. "The Israeli Medical Association represents doctors in the legislative house [. . .] The IMA's activity in the Knesset focuses on proposing bills on its behalf, overseeing the process and promoting it. IMA representatives participate regularly in sessions taking place in Knesset committees, present its view on the matters at hand and work to promote doctors' welfare, health and medicine in Israel. . . . The committee of scientific and technological R&D promotes research issues, science and technology, against the backdrop of the rapid development of these issues in the world. . .and the IMA is a partner to all the bills discussed in this committee" (Israel Medical Association n.d.).
6. In 1963, Dr. Einhorn concentrated on experiments in IUD at the Tel-Aviv City Council clinic. In 1965, the gynecology departments of Ashkelon Hospital and Beer-Sheva's Soroka Hospital received vast supplies of IUDs from an American agency—the Pathfinder Foundation. According to Avraham Doron, studies in this area were conducted that year at other hospitals in Israel as well (1976: 19–22). Since the devices were quite new, their implementation caused various degrees of inconvenience to the women taking part in the research; 5.4 percent of them experienced severe disturbances requiring extraction of the device, and others suffered "minor" disturbances, such as irregularity in their periods, bleeding, or stomach aversion (Vego and Shapira 1968: 252–54).
7. Correspondence with the Israeli Health Ministry reveals that there was little awareness of medical contraception in that ministry in the mid-1960s (see Israel State Archive, Gal 2091/1: To Dr. Rivlin from Dr. H.S. Halevi, on family planning, 9.6.1964; To Optex from Dr. Tuastein, on IUD, 5 July 1964).
8. Professor Roberto Bachi, the country's chief demographer at the time, issued a demographic report stating that "the percentage of children in families from Europe has decreased greatly while the percentage of children of Asian and African descent has risen, so that today, they are the majority of the children being born in Israel." As a result, Bachi

continued, most children are being born to "un-educated and culturally inferior mothers" (ISA, Gimel 2976/14, "A review of current demographic trends in the world, the Jewish People and Israel").

9. "Allegedly," since the actual data shows quite clearly that after immigrating to Israel, European Jews were slightly, but consistently raising their fertility rates, while Sephardic women were largely and consistently lowering it, thus creating a consistent Israeli fertility trend that was much higher than in the West (Halevi 1959; for more on Bachi's manipulation of demographic data, see Hashash 2004).

10. The smaller families that have a "reasonable income [and] proper lifestyle" and "live cultural lives" were felt to be the ones that would benefit society "immensely" by reconsidering their family planning (Knesset Archive, Sixth Knesset, a meeting of the Public Services Committee, November 26,1968).

11. Programs for direct payments to large families were considered by the NC to be an undesirable method that would "reduce the will to work" (NC Report 1966: 39–40); at the same time, tax breaks designed to benefit the upper strata were enthusiastically recommended and eventually accepted by the government (NC Report 1966: 48, 51–52; ISA g/6/2091, Prime Minister Eshkol's speech to the Knesset on pronatal measures).

12. For example, Ziona Peled, a member of the Demographic Center's Council, warned, "If we push the public to create larger families to solve the demographic problem we will entrust our existence to a public that may be bigger but lower in quality, much like that of the countries that surround us" (Minutes of the Demographic Center's Council, vol. 4: 40).

13. ISA, Gal/2077/3, "A plan to change the content of work in maternal care centers," to Dr. Gajevin from Dr. Polishuk, March 4, 1968.

14. As chairman of Kupat Holim's Medicine Council from 1947 to 1967 and head of its research committee, Professor Yitzhak Halbrecht founded the Getaniu Reproduction Research Center and the Israeli Society for Fertility Research. In 1968, he presided over the Sixth World Conference for Fertility Research, which hosted 1,500 researchers from all over the world. He was an advisor to the International Health Organization (IHO) on reproduction from 1968 to 1974, and a member of its Special Committee on Congenital Defects in 1972.

15. An extreme example involves the studies conducted by Adler and colleagues in Beer Sheva, a southern town in Israel. The writers stated that their major concern was the welfare of humanity and the need to reduce its population-growth hazards. They also stated that it was necessary to implement family planning in specific populations. Their specific population consisted of North African Jewish women. In their three-year study, the doctors received over 1,000 women in two clinics: a psychiatric clinic and a gynecology center. Their patients were mostly mothers of four to eight children, mothers who suffered from various gynecological problems that were regarded by the researchers as psychosomatic in nature and resulting from too many pregnancies. They saw themselves responsible, as doctors, for family-planning education and recommended contraception to

all their patients. In particular, they stressed the value of implant-
ing IUDs to alleviate mental dysfunctions, such as depression and
psychosomatic pain, as well as a variety of gynecological problems
(Adler et al. 1975).

16. "Stem cells are immature unspecialized cells that renew themselves for
    long periods through cell division. Under certain conditions, they can
    be induced to become mature cells with special functions, such as the
    beating cells of the heart muscle or the insulin-producing cells of the
    pancreas" (Hadassah Medical Organization n.d.).

17. Research cloning refers to a process in which a nucleus from an adult
    donor cell is inserted into a recipient oocyte from which the nucleus
    has been removed. The nucleus provides all of the necessary genetic
    information, in the form of DNA, for a cell to function and divide. The
    cell is then stimulated to divide, resulting in embryonic stem cells that
    are genetically identical to the adult donor cell. These can potentially
    evolve into a cloned human being.

18. The delegates of the scientific community were comprised of scientists
    from the private sector, as well as state appointed specialists or public
    sector scientists, some affiliating to both.

19. Meeting of the Science and Technology Committee of the Knesset, No-
    vember 12, 2003 (all references to the Science and Technology Com-
    mittee of the Knesset can be found at the Knesset's website: http://
    www.knesset.gov.il/protocols/search.asp).

20. Meeting of the Science and Technology Committee of the Knesset, No-
    vember 12, 2003, on examining the need to extend the law on genetic
    intervention.

21. December 8, 2003 meeting.

22. January 12, 2004 meeting.

23. In theory, the transplanting of somatic cells into a human oocyte was
    not outlawed. However, the law clearly prohibited the extraction of
    oocytes for any purpose other than fertility, and in that respect was
    unfriendly to researchers who wished to engage in cloning research.
    The Israeli law also prohibits women who are not going through fer-
    tility treatment from donating oocytes because of the risk of hyper-
    stimulation and the procedure's purported connection with cancer.
    Two reports were prepared by the Knesset's research center on the
    risks in extracting oocytes. The most common risk is hyperstimu-
    lation of the ovaries syndrome, suffered statistically by 25 percent
    of women. The syndrome can result in severe disturbance requiring
    hospitalization, but it rarely causes death (in 0.1 to 0.2 percent of
    cases). The more aggressive the treatment, the likelier women are to
    be subject to hyperstimulation, hence the need to avoid a conflict of
    interests.

24. For a comparison of the government's 2007 bill and the Halperin rec-
    ommendations, see Kanyon, Mishori, and Hashash (2007). For an
    analysis of the protocols of the Halperin Committee and the construc-
    tion of donors and recipients of donation as different types of women
    see Bassan (2006).

25. Itzkovitz also holds several lines and has submitted three patent requests to the U.S. patent registry.
26. November 22, 2005.
27. Revel's remark is puzzling, since he had always been one of the advocates of oocyte donations for research, which means that oocytes are regarded as human tissues, and not like organs. Organ donation requires much stricter rules and is not allowed to be made anonymously.

References

Adler, T.S., M. Katz and A.Yehezkiel. 1975. "An Interdisciplinary Programme for Family Planning among North African Families in the Developmental Towns of the Negev," *Israel Annals of Psychiatry and Related Disciplines* 13, no. 2: 105–16.

Amir, D. 1989. *The Politics of Abortion in Israel* [Hebrew]. Discussion Paper Series, Discussion Paper No. 13–89. The Pinhas Sapir Center for Development, Tel-Aviv University.

Abbott, A. 1991. *The System of Professions: An Essay on the Division of Expert Labor*. Chicago: University of Chicago Press.

Amir, D. and O. Benjamin. 1992. "Abortion Approval as a Ritual of Symbolic Control," in *The Criminalization of a Woman's Body*, ed. Clarice Feinman. New York: The Haworth Press.

Barker, K. 2003. "Birthing and Bureaucratic Women: Needs Talk and the Definitional Legacy of the Sheppard-Towner Act." *Feminist Studies* 29, no. 2: 333–52.

Bassan, S. 2006. *Shortage and Commodification—Reimbursed Egg Donation from a Donor who is not going through IVF Treatment*. M.A Dissertation, Haifa University, Haifa.

Berg, M. 1997. *Rationalizing Medical Work: Decision-Support Techniques and Medical Practices*. Cambridge, MA: MIT Press.

Berkovitch, N. 1997. "Motherhood as a National Mission: The Construction of Womanhood in the Legal Discourse in Israel," *Women's Studies International Forum* 20, no. 5: 605–19.

Carmeli, Y. S. and Birenbaum-Carmeli D. 2000. "Ritualizing the 'Natural Family': Secrecy in Israeli Donor Insemination," *Science as Culture* 9, no. 3: 301–24.

Clarke, A. E., J. K. Shim, L. Mamo, J. R. Foster and J. R. Fishman. 2003. "Biomedicalization: Technoscientific Tranformations of Health, Illness and U.S. Biomedicine," *American Sociological Review* 68, no. 2: 161–94.

CEPA Report. 1974. "Committee for Examining Prohibitions on Abortion Report" [Hebrew]. *Briut Hatzibur* 4: 427–504.

Corea, G. 1985. *The Mother Machine: Reproductive Technologies from Artificial Insemination to Artificial Wombs*. New York: Harper and Row.

Doron, A. 1976. *Family Planning, Israel—Report VI*. Jerusalem: State of Israel.

Elston, M. A. 1991. "The Politics of Professional Power: Medicine in a Changing Health Service," In *The Sociology of the Health Service*, eds. J. Gabe, M. Calnan, and M. Bury. London: Routledge.

Estes, C. L., Charlene Harrington and David N. Pellow. 2000. "The Medical Industrial Complex." In *The Encyclopedia of Sociology*, eds. Borgatta E.F. and R.V. Montegomery. Farmington Hills: MI Gale Group.

Fligstein, N. 2001. *The Architecture of Markets: An Economic Sociology of Twenty-First-Century Capitalist Societies*. Princeton: Princeton University Press.

Foucault, M. 1990. *The History of Sexuality, Volume I: An Introduction*. London: Penguin.

Foucault, M. 1991. "The Politics of Health in the Eighteenth Century." In *The Foucault Reader*, ed. P. Rabinow. London: Penguin.

Freidson, E. 1970. *Profession of Medicine: A Study of the Sociology of Applied Knowledge*. New York: Harper & Row.

Gooldin, S. and C. Shalev. 2006. "The Uses and Misuses of In-Vitro Fertilization in Israel: Some Sociological and Ethical Considerations" [Hebrew], *Nashim: a Journal of Jewish Women's Studies and Gender Issues* 12: 151–76.

Hadassah Medical Organization. n.d. "Human Embryonic Stem Cell Research Center." <http://www.hadassah.org.il/English/Eng_SubNavBar/ Departments/Clinics+and+Institutes/Gene+Therapy/Human+Embryoni c+Stem+Cell+Research+Center/> (accessed February 25, 2008).

Halevi, H.S. 1963. "The Influence of World War II on the Demographic Trends of the People of Israel" [Hebrew] (PhD. dissertation, Hebrew University, Jerusalem).

Halperin, Sydney. 1990. "Medicalization as a Professional Process: Post War Trends in Pediatrics," *Journals of Health and Social Behavior* 31: 28–42.

Hashash,Yali. 2004. "Ethnicity, Class and Gender in Israel's Fertility Policy, 1962–1974" [Hebrew] (MA thesis, Haifa University).

Israel Medical Association. n.d. *Website*. <http://www.ima.org.il/> (accessed February 25, 2008).

Kanyon S., D. Mishori and Y. Hashash. 2007 "The Geese who lay Golden Eggs: A Critical Review of the Government's Bill 'Donation of Eggs— 2007'" [Hebrew], *Refua UMishpat* 36: 161–179.

Lancet M. 1970. "Choosing the Right Birth Control Method" [Hebrew], *Rofe Hamishpaha* A, no. 1: 69–72.

Melamed, Shoham. 2002. "The Double Demographic Threat: Gender, Ethnicity, Nationality and the Politics of Fertility in the 1950s in Israel" [Hebrew] (M.A thesis, Tel Aviv University).

Portugese, Jacqueline. 1998. *Fertility Policy in Israel: The Politics of Religion, Gender and Nation*. Westport: Praeger.

Prainsack, Barbara. 2006. "'Negotiating Life': The Regulation of Human Cloning and Embryonic Stem Cell Research in Israel," *Social Studies of Science* 36, no. 2: 173–205.

Quick, Sharon. 2006. "Stem Cell Research and Cloning: Science and Ethics" Paper presented at the American Academy of Medical Ethics Annual Meeting, Washington, D.C.

Remennick, Larissa. 2006. "The Quest for the Perfect Baby: Why Do Israeli Women Seek Prenatal Genetic Testing?" *Sociology of Health & Illness* 28, no. 1: 21–53.

Remennick, Larissa. 2000. "Childless in the Land of Imperative Mother-hood: Stigma and Coping among Infertile Israeli Women," *Sex Roles* 43, nos. 11/12: 821–41.

Riessman, Catherine K. 1983. "Women and Medicalization: A New Perspective," *Social Policy* 14: 3–18.

Schindler, S. 2007. "Case 24: Curbing Global Population Growth: Rocke-feller's Population Council." In *The Foundation—A Great American Secret: How Private Wealth is Changing the World*, eds. Joel. L. Fleishman, J. Scott Kohler, and Steven Schindler. New York: PublicAffairs.

Sharon, Smadar. 2006. "The Planners, the State and the Shaping of the Na-tional Space" [Hebrew], *Teoria Vebikoret* 29: 31–57.

State of Israel. 1966. *The Natality Committee Report*, Vol. I. Jerusalem.

State of Israel. 1970. *Demographic Center's Council*, Vol. 4 [Hebrew]. Jerusalem.

Thomson, J. A., Joseph Itskovitz-Eldor, Sander S. Shapiro, Michelle A. Waknitz, Jennifer J. Swiergiel, Vivienne S. Marshall, and Jeffrey M. Jones. 1998. "Embryonic Stem Cell Lines Derived from Human Blasto-cysts," *Science* 282: 1145–47.

Vego, T. and H. Shapira. 1968. "An Experiment in Using IUD for Birth Con-trol" [Hebrew], *Harefua* 74, no. 7: 252–54.

Yamanaka, S. 2009. "A fresh look at iPS cells," *Cell* 137(1): 13–17.

Zafrir, J. 1981. "Family Planning in Israel: Policy and Reality" [Hebrew], *The Israeli Family Planning Association Bulletin* December: 1–2.

Chapter 12

THE MIRTH OF THE CLINIC: FIELDNOTES FROM AN ISRAELI FERTILITY CENTER

Susan Martha Kahn

Assisted conception is so unprecedented and the consequences for beliefs about reproduction so uncertain that we anthropologists have had our plates full as we try to construct theoretical frameworks with adequate explanatory power. Much of the recent anthropological work in the Israeli context follows these trends, often using Foucauldian frameworks to illuminate the complex social processes inherent in the social uses of new reproductive technologies. I draw particular attention to the works in this volume. To date, however, little has been written about the routinization of conception enabled by these technologies and the everyday experience of the people who work in Israeli fertility clinics—the nurses, the clinic staff, the laboratory technicians. In this chapter, I depart from the usual attempts to explore the profundity of these technologies and instead focus on how they are enacted in the workplace. By imbedding the activities of conception in the context of work, I hope to draw attention to the dynamics between and amongst the people whose daily work lives are devoted to achieving conception. I argue that by focusing on the daily lives of fertility clinic workers, we can see assisted conception more clearly for what it has become—less fantastic, more routine, and in fact banal.

Fertility clinics in Israel, like all fertility clinics, employ men and women who wake up every morning, have their coffee, commute to work, and set about the often repetitive tasks that constitute their piece of the complex puzzle that is conception. Some are receptionists who greet patients and process paperwork. Others are nurses who collect blood and sperm samples from nervous, and sometimes recalcitrant, patients. Some are lab technicians who spin sperm in centrifuges and prepare eggs for fertilization. Others are biochemists or endocrinologists who peer into microscopes while injecting sperm into human ova. Some are nurses charged with the task of choosing anonymous donor sperm for individual women or matching egg donors with egg recipients. And at the top of the clinical hierarchy are the doctors, who evaluate embryos, surgically extract ova from ovaries and undertake countless other conception-enabling tasks during their regular workdays.

Numerous other social actors populate these clinical spaces: the people who clean up after these procedures (assisted conception generates a great deal of detritus in the form of disposable syringes, Petri dishes, sterile gloves, etc.), the people who wheel the patients in and out of the operating rooms on gurneys, and of course, the patients themselves, who move from operating room to recovery room to laboratory with various degrees of freedom depending on the clinic. In Israel, there are additional personnel present in many clinics: trained observers called *mashgichot* (plural; *mashgicha*, singular) who oversee conceptions to ensure they conform to Jewish law.

Clearly, a fertility clinic is both like and unlike any other workplace. Personalities conflict, political opinions clash, unexpected alliances are formed, hierarchies are reinforced and railed against, mundane discussions are commonplace, jokes are shared and enjoyed. And yet the post office it's not; it's the context for human conception. Profound moments are ubiquitous, and awe is a daily occurrence. The staff at the clinic in which I did fieldwork routinely expressed irony, irreverence, and impatience; they also appeared to experience profound compassion, heartfelt identification, and intense joy. These affectations did not make the fertility treatments more or less successful than at other clinics, but it did distinguish their workplace routines from other more ordinary jobs. In other words, assisted conception may have become banal, but it has not become mundane.

I hope this chapter reinforces the power of ethnography for making sense of these technologies, particularly in the Israeli case, where the sense of place infuses these processes so vividly. A few caveats: the fieldnotes on which this chapter is based are dated—and the relative disorganization and atmosphere of informality that characterized the clinic I describe may well have changed. These fieldnotes are based on participant-observation in mid-1990's; through a series of lucky coincidences and stubborn persistence, I made the necessary arrangements to sit in a fertility clinic and lab and watch people work. I was given almost entirely free run of the labs and clinics.

The mirth of the clinic

Day 1

I arrived at the sperm-processing lab in the morning. It was an unassuming concrete building with a discreet sign. The lab was adjacent to the hospital, where many of the primary lab procedures took place, such as the in vitro fertilizations and micromanipulations—it was also where the operating rooms were, for egg harvesting and cesarean sections.

There was one woman in a white lab coat working in the lab when I got there—I introduced myself, as did she. Her name was Avital and she was the biochemist in charge of sperm preparation. I described my work rather tentatively and she seemed very interested. I explained that I had made an arrangement with the doctor in charge to sit and observe what went on there. She showed me around enthusiastically—there was a table in the center of the room with a few metal chairs around it—there were counters surrounding the table, each filled with various kinds of laboratory equipment. There was a refrigerator for sperm and a refrigerator for food and drinks.

Rachel came in shortly afterwards—she introduced herself as the *mashgicha* on duty. She was a large, affable religious lady, wearing a wig and a dress with long sleeves. We sat at the table and drank coffee and talked. I asked her about her job and she said she was there to make sure that Mr. X and Mr. Y don't get mixed up. I asked her if she was trying to prevent adultery and she said she was just trying to prevent the mixing of the pipettes. Avital was working quietly at one of the lab benches behind us as we talked.

Avital prepared some test tubes and showed me how they prepare the sperm for "swim-up," a process in which they put the test tube in an empty cottage cheese container at a 45 degree angle and then place it in the refrigerator.

There were lots of liquids on the counters and surrounding shelves, both inorganic and organic: a whole range of reddish liquids that were measured and prepared and combined with the genetic material, either to make it more inert or to make it more active. Avital explained all the various items to me and their uses.

When the sperm is delivered she checks it for volume and motility. She uses a slide with a grid on it and examines the shape of the sperm's head and the tail. Then she stains it with different stains and counts it. When she prepares sperm for intrauterine insemination, she uses three different preparations:

1) "Swim-up," for good sperm. She puts the sperm in a test tube, places it in a cup at a 45 degree angle and lets it "swim up" for an hour and a half.
2) "Percoll wash," for low-quality sperm: She puts percoll solution in a test tube with the sperm, puts the test tube in a centrifuge and then the best sperm becomes concentrated at the bottom.
3) "Wash," for very bad sperm. For sperm for which there was not much hope. It also involved a wash and a centrifuge.

If these methods failed repeatedly, then Avital referred the sperm for micromanipulation, in which they only need to isolate a few good sperm in order to attempt conception.

All of the equipment, save the microscopes, was disposable. From the microinjection pipettes and the syringes to the catheters, the test tubes, the Petri dishes and the vials: everything was only used once. The lab generated an enormous amount of garbage.

After an hour or so, Avital took me into the hospital to see the main laboratory where they do the actual fertilizations. We walked down a long corridor, past the lines of patients, the shelves filled with prayer books, through the double doors that led to the laboratory and the adjacent operating rooms. There was another *mashgicha* there, Yael, and two additional lab technicians, Ronit and Tali. They were sitting at adjacent microscopes while Yael sat on a stool behind them, watching them work.

Apparently only women worked in the clinic—the technicians were all secular, the *mashgichot* all religious. Everyone was very friendly and welcoming. The atmosphere in the lab was very relaxed, and they were all very chatty and curious about my work—and about me. Was I married? Was I moving to Israel permanently? Did I have any family there? All questions I had come to expect after living and working in Israel for a number of years. I answered in the negative.

Ronit, one of the lab technicians, let me look through the microscope at some eggs. She was preparing some Petri dishes for IVF and
micromanipulation by removing the cumulus surrounding the ova
so that it would be easier to fertilize.

I asked about the difference between IVF and micromanipulation and she explained: "In IVF the sperm does the work, in micromanipulation we do the work for him." The micromanipulation
itself was fascinating. The micromanipulator was a large, mechani-
cal microscope with a video attached so that you could watch a video screen to see what was happening under the microscope. There
were multiple controls and it clearly required a great deal of expertise to operate.

In the micromanipulator, they slowed down the sperm in a chem-
ical solution so that they could "catch" one with microscopic tongs.
They then manipulated the controls so that the sperm was inserted
into the egg. The covering surrounding the egg was very elastic and
it was hard to puncture it with the micropipette and withdraw it
without having the egg's cytoplasm leak out.

The process looked something like this: Tali sat at the controls
of the micromanipulator and watched the magnified image of the
sperm under the microscope. She deftly tried to coax a sperm into
the micropipette by twisting dials. We all watched attentively. As
Tali successfully isolated a sperm, the *mashgicha* said: "Oh, he's the
lucky one!" Tali then used different controls to orient the egg so
that its "polar body" was stable; this was apparently the optimal
position for inserting the sperm. We watched the video image of
the egg as Tali operated the sperm controls in an effort to jab the
sperm-bearing pipette into it. Once the egg had been penetrated
with the pipette, Tali pressed a control that released the sperm
and withdrew the pipette—a successful fertilization. We all commended her.

After the micromanipulation, Ronit performed IVF on three
eggs, a decidedly low-tech procedure by comparison. She just drew
some sperm in to a syringe and squeezed it out on to each egg in
a Petri dish; then they placed the Petri dishes in the lab's incubator. They invited me to come back the next day to see if they had
made embryos.

We were, five women, sitting in blue coats, gauze hats, and
paper shoe coverings, surrounded by machines, calmly chatting
while placing drops of sperm in Petri dishes and making sure egg
cytoplasm didn't seep out of micropunctures. Between procedures, Yael was saying psalms from her prayer book, and when
I asked her if she was saying psalms for the procedure or for

herself, she laughed and said "for myself!" Apparently I had a lot
to learn.

Day 3

I arrived in the lab to find Avital using the centrifuge to concentrate
sperm. No one else had gotten to work yet.

The phone rang and she picked it up—it was someone who needed to bring in a sperm sample. She said: "It's nicer for you to do it
at home, just bring it in within forty minutes." But he lives an hour
away, so she tells him: "you can come and give it here, just know
that it's a bathroom not a hotel room." There's a pause, then she
said, "No, of course no one will enter when you are in there."

A few minutes later there was a knock at the door. It was a religious man in a long black coat with a black hat. She pointed to the
adjacent window where they accepted sperm samples, then closed
the front door, walked a few steps, and opened the window. I heard
her saying to him: "Do you want to do it now or do you have it with
you?" He hesitated and I think I heard him saying he'll bring it later.

Sperm is delivered to the lab every day, either by husbands or
wives, and the lab technicians love to recount the various imagi-
native ways that sperm has been delivered: In ketchup bottles, in
vases, in pickle jars, in condoms carefully laid out on trays, in jars
swaddled in silk scarves. Generally it is brought in small plastic cups
that are given out by the lab. They admitted that sometimes it is
disgusting to check the sperm, when it arrives in a soiled condom,
or in a cup with hairs floating in it. One very religious man would
bring in a condom with the whole top end cut off; his sperm was
first diagnosed as having absolutely no motility and instead of undergoing the repeated embarrassment of the diagnosis, he would
just continually say he misunderstood the instructions and cut the
condom practically in half so there would be no sperm to check,
motile or immotile. Miri, another lab technician, told a story about
this one big macho guy who came in, shirt open, hairy chest, chains
around his neck, pistol on one hip, mobile phone on the other. He
brought in his sperm like a trophy and when they checked it there
was absolutely no sperm in it, just seminal fluid.

These sperm delivery stories highlight the various ways that men
behaved during this sensitive transaction. They were alternately recalcitrant, inventive, macho or shy. Women patients, by contrast,
did not display a similar range of affective states. They moved in and
out of the clinic more silently and invisibly, more passively and com-
pliantly, because of the very different functions their bodies must

perform in assisted conception. Women were routinely anesthetized during various procedures, such that unconscious women lying naked on gurneys covered only by thin sheets were a daily sight at the clinic. The raw biological differences in procuring sperm and eggs were always on vivid display and yet they were never discussed or commented on during the span of my fieldwork. The men's behavior during sperm delivery was the source of much amusement; the trials endured by the women patients never so. The vagaries of sperm donation as opposed to egg donation clearly had something to do with this difference, but the fact that the clinic staff was entirely female played a role as well—the clinic staff unsurprisingly replayed gender stereotypes common outside of the clinic.

This dynamic was reinforced in the daily background chatter at the clinic, which covered the stereotypical range of women's domestic concerns—diets, children, hair-coloring, shopping, and so on.

For example, one day Ronit brought in pictures from her son's birthday party and everyone in the lab looked at each picture intently, commenting on what cute children she had, and asked who was who. "This is Grandpa Albert, this is my mother's sister, this is my brother's baby, my other brother's wife," and so on. "This is the party at the kindergarten, this is the party at home, Eran is naughty, Nadav is fat, Guy is a real Mamma's boy." One of the *mashgichot* also brought pictures of her daughter's wedding: She has eight children. We all looked and again wanted to know "who was who." "Which is your husband, which is your son, which is your daughter's cousin's sister," etc.

We talked about families as we tried to make families. We talked about Chana's bar mitzvah in Beer Sheva and the wedding she was going to in England. We talked about where Ronit's son was stationed in the army. Suri was on the phone with her husband or her mother every hour. We were swimming in family relationships there.

That afternoon, there was a Cesarean section. The *mashgicha* Yael explained to me how rare this pregnancy was: Not only did they have to harvest her eggs, but they had to do electroejaculation on the man to get sperm. Only one doctor in Israel does this procedure; apparently, it was very rare, "a real miracle," she explained. (Electroejaculation involves the application of electric current to stimulate ejaculation in cases of erectile dysfunction, traumatic injury, or other afflictions that make normal ejaculation impossible).

When the lab workers heard that "X" was coming in for her Cesarean section, everyone in the lab was overjoyed. "She's one of ours, she's one of ours," meaning that they did the IVF which fertilized the ova that became the embryo that got implanted. We all rushed over to the operating room. It didn't take long before the doctor emerged with the baby, a girl. Yael burst into tears: "Finally after seven years, thank God." Even Ronit and Tali were crying. It was very exciting; even I teared up with the emotion of it. For seven years they had been trying to have a child, and everyone in the lab felt so proud. They called up Avital in the other lab and told her. As the doctor was scrubbing down before the operation, she yelled back to me: "Now you will see the results of our work!" When the baby came out, the other doctor leaned over her and yelled: "Welcome!" Everyone was gathered around, and then the father came out to look, and everyone said *mazal tov* to him. Then the doctor placed the baby in his arms and said: "Go show Mommy. Hold her strong, like a Torah scroll!" The father was awed. He just looked sort of stunned and speechless, and brought the baby in to see her mother.

These rare moments, when babies were born who had been conceived in the lab, were compelling interruptions to the lab's daily routines. The whole clinic staff felt unified in their collective success—and delighted for the new parents. At these moments, these working relationships were transformed into a fictive kin network, as unrelated people experienced a remarkable and unprecedented social bond created by their success in achieving conception.

The clinic staff's joy after the birth of a baby was not unvariegated from what I observed. While they were always pleased when a baby was born, they seemed more pleased when the couple was long-suffering—and Jewish. This is not to suggest that Palestinian patients received unequal treatment; they certainly didn't. But the clinic staff seemed to react to these births differently—with a sense of accomplishment, but not with a sense of joy.

Day 6

A few days later I spent a long time chatting with the *mashgicha* Yael in the lab while the lab technicians were busy with a micromanipulation—they had 17 eggs that were taken out of a Palestinian woman in the morning, and they were trying to fertilize them.

Yael the *mashgicha* kissed the *mezuzah* on the doorpost every time she walked in and out of the lab. She described to me how they have discovered some kind of material that helped the sperm enter the egg and some kind of material that closed up the egg after a sperm had entered so that more don't enter. "It's amazing what the Holy One does," she said. We talked about Jewish law; she told me it's forbidden to ask a second rabbi a question if the first gives you an answer you don't like. For example, if you ask one rabbi if you can use IVF and he says no, you can't go ask a second rabbi so that he will say yes.

Later, the lab technician told me things were not going so well for the Abraham family, the ones whose eggs were micromanipulated on Friday. There was indeed a fertilization and now the woman was in the operating room for the embryo transfer. But there was some problem with her womb being shrunken and they couldn't get the embryo catheter in. As we were talking, the nurse brought the used embryo catheter back and just tossed it in the garbage can.

For the embryo transfer, Ronit unwrapped a disposable catheter and placed it on the end of a syringe. Then she pulled a Petri dish containing the embryo out of the incubator and placed it under the microscope, sucked a little bit of pink liquid into the syringe, then drew the embryos into the syringe. She then placed the syringe with the embryo-bearing catheter into the catheter's paper wrapping, being careful to hold it upright. The nurse came in to the lab and took the syringe into the operating room, where the doctor inserted it into the woman's vagina and pressed the plunger to release the embryos into her womb.

Then it was time for a coffee break back in the sperm-processing lab. I sat with the technicians and the *mashgichot* and enjoyed some cold Nescafe and rice cakes with avocado. We talked about diets and they asked me more questions about my research; we talked about *halachah* and what the rabbis say about egg donations. Ronit explained that they only ask for egg donations from secular women or Sephardim. The Palestinians aren't allowed to give, nor are the Ashkenazim. Intrigued, I followed-up on this point later with one of the doctors known for his knowledge of *halachic* issues, and he confirmed that there are different norms for giving and receiving egg donations amongst religious Ashkenazi and Mizrachi Jews (see Kahn 2000).

Yael said that she knew of a case where a Jewish woman gave birth to two children using the eggs of a Palestinian woman. They all said that they would not give eggs themselves, that they would feel like it was their child. We chatted and drank more coffee. In these moments, I felt as if I could have been working in almost any kind of Israeli office, where in my experience coffee breaks are common, and expressing one's personal opinions is *de rigueur*. Often these chats became quite spirited and funny. For example, Ronit said that all fertility doctors are short—to compensate for their lack of manliness they become fertility doctors. We all agreed that you had to laugh or otherwise the work was impossible. Not just that you should laugh, but that you had to laugh. Avital was very animated and told funny stories about her mother driving, and the horn she has for yelling curses out the window of her car. Sometimes these chats would take sudden serious turns, particularly around elections, recent suicide bombings, or other political events—which were frequent in Israel. We all spoke in Hebrew, often with lots of slang, though the *mashgichot* often spoke Yiddish to each other if they didn't want to be understood by everyone in the room.

Day 10

I just hung out in the sperm-processing lab today, eating pomelos, drinking Diet Sprite, talking about politics, who got married and who's going where on vacation—the usual. Tali showed me how they check the sperm for antibodies; Ronit described how they do a postcoital test just to check sperm quality, not in order to collect sperm for artificial insemination or IVF. Thursday is going to be a busy day and I will return then. There is a certain pleasure in the boredom of sitting around with the biochemists and the *mashgichot*, chatting.

Avital took me aside to explain to me that she was worried about how I might represent the clinic, particularly because of the way that one *mashgicha* felt that she was invested with holiness—that her job was holy—and that she thought the biochemists were just technicians. She said that this *mashgicha* had problems—that she was a bit of a fanatic and I should take everything she said with a grain of salt. She wants the clinic to stay open and doesn't want the impression to be given that they are catching all kinds of mistakes at the last minute. I assured her that I would try not to create a false impression.

Day 11

Five of us were in the lab today: the two lab technicians, Suri the *mashgicha*, and myself. Suri's prayer book sat on the micro-manipulator. We were waiting for sperm so that Ronit could get started with the intracytoplasmic sperm injection. The woman patient was having her ova harvested in the adjacent operating room and we needed sperm pronto in order to fertilize the eggs while they were still fresh. Ronit called the husband at work, and said "we need more sperm!" Apparently he'd left a small sample at the lab that morning and explained he couldn't give anymore until tomorrow. So she said: "If you want to succeed, we need more sperm now." Apparently he refused. So there was a bit of a fight and she hung up the phone and said "Men! A woman would never do that if her husband just went through an oocyte pick-up and got only six eggs."

"You have to understand, sometimes they can't do it more than once; you have to understand," the other technician explained. So they kept calling him on the phone at work and telling him that he has to come in, he had to at least try, that they didn't have enough sperm.

The nurse came back and forth from the lab to the operating room with little vials containing the woman's eggs and ovarian liquid that was all reddish, and as the nurse kept bringing them in, they kept asking: "So? Where's the husband? Why won't he give again? What kind of husband is this?" "It's a physical problem; it's not his responsibility. What can he do?" said Suri.

So it became a big discussion what to do—whose responsibility is it. The doctor then came in to the lab and said: "Just do micromanipulation on the eggs we have with the sperm we have." Discussing different strategies for coping with the man's recalcitrance about bringing in more of his sperm seemed to have a team-building effect amongst the clinic staff. Soon another nurse came in and asked Ronit: "How many times did you ask him? I'll call him!" The other nurse called and succeeded, she announced: "He's coming in an hour to give more sperm!" Regardless of which individual staff member ultimately succeeded, the victory was one for the team—all were relieved that the man had finally relented and the arduously-acquired eggs would not go unfertilized.

The radio was on, playing *mizrachi* music in the background. The incubator whirred, everyone was busy.

Day 12

I put on my surgical scrubs and entered the operating room. An inert, anesthetized patient, her wig covered with a gauze surgical hat, lay there as her eggs were harvested.

During an egg retrieval, the woman is wheeled in to the operating room awake and they anesthetize her with general anesthetic. They prepare an ultrasound probe with jelly and a plastic covering, and attach an oocyte retrieval needle around it. Then they probe around while watching a video screen, looking for follicles, which they aspirate. The anesthesiologist explained it to me: "Come closer, you can't see anything! You don't always get an egg inside a follicle." After the egg-retrieval, the woman is rolled out on the gurney—an oocyte-free, unconscious lump.

The anesthesiologist sat behind her, holding a mask over her nose and mouth, and gave a lecture on Jewish history. He asked the nurse whether she thought it was possible to build a state according to the Torah. Without waiting for her answer, he said: "The rabbis just want power; it's just a question of power." Then he started to talk about the *Baal Shem Tov*, and about how most Jews have always been regular people and the rabbis have always tried to control them. He said he follows the laws of Moses, not the rabbis, who are just interested in power. Soon, he said, we will all be robots, androids, like in the movie *Blade Runner*. "Whatever the mind can imagine will happen. There will always be Jews without religion. Israel's survival depends on those who think about defense and economics." He gave this and related oratory as he sat holding the mask over the woman's face while she had her eggs surgically removed. The woman's legs were up in stirrups, her vagina totally exposed, the doctors took turns probing around with the ultrasound with the aspirating needle attached. We watched the ultrasound monitor to see where to suck the eggs out of her ovaries.

The contrast between the hectoring, indifferent anesthesiologist and the exquisitely vulnerable, passive patient was overwhelming. The fact that this was a "training" egg retrieval only heightened this effect, as the doctors took turns jabbing the aspirating needle through the woman's vaginal walls in order to retrieve egg follicles from her ovaries.

This did not feel like a fictive kin network, harmoniously coming together to achieve conception—this felt like a clinical gang rape in which I participated as a prurient observer. I felt sickly relieved that the patient had been oblivious throughout this ordeal—she would only be interested in how many eggs they managed to harvest and her subsequent chances for successful conception. Indeed, that measure of success was the only one anyone would pay attention to— the metaphorical resonances of the encounter, the ethical problems of the medical practices that day, the emotional reality of the patient had she been cognizant of how her body was being treated, were all seemingly irrelevant to everyone except the visiting anthropologist. Yet, I did nothing to alleviate, explore, or counteract any of it. What could I have done right then and there? Change the way doctors learn to perform egg retrievals?

Day 14

Slow day. Everyone's sitting around reading the Friday papers. I was in the operating room for another embryo transfer. A woman came padding into the lab in her patient gown and the doctor said: "Selya wants to see her children." Ronit showed her the Petri dishes with the embryos floating in them. Then Selya went into the operating room, Ronit sucked the embryos up into a catheter, and the nurse came in and took the syringe into the operating room, where the doctor used it to shoot the embryos up inside Selya. The nurse then brought the catheter back and Ronit pushed whatever was left in the syringe out into a Petri dish under a microscope, to make sure that the embryos were released. A second later the woman was wheeled out, wide awake.

Back in the sperm-processing lab, the *mashgicha* helped with patient reception in a way that would be familiar to anyone who has sought assistance in an Israeli state agency: lackadaisical, confrontational, begrudging.

The technicians and *mashgichot* chatted about Jerusalem Day. Yael and Tali complained that they were at the clinic until midnight the night before doing micromanipulations. Yael said she opened the lab window last night and watched the fireworks. We did some sperm prep, ate some yogurt, and drank instant coffee.

Day 20

The big thing today was the ZIFT (Zygote Intrafallopian Transfer) embryo transfer on a religious woman with cerebral palsy—apparently her second child. Her husband, also with cerebral palsy, sat outside the operating room saying psalms. Tali told me later that she was a real *nudnik*, but that he was very smart.

I put on my scrubs and went into the operating room. I thought they would do the ZIFT with a catheter through the vagina, but they did it with a laparoscopy. The aforementioned anesthesiologist read the newspaper through the whole thing and "oohed" and "aahed" over a picture of Brigitte Bardot. It was again a teaching procedure; the doctor was teaching two residents how to do a laparoscopy.

One resident kept trying to insert the surgical instrument into the woman's stomach, but to no avail—he jabbed repeatedly into and around the patient's belly button. Finally the doctor had to do it. I learned that the key to enduring these procedures was to identify with the doctors and not with the patients—to have intellectual curiosity about what was happening, and to think of yourself as the one in control. Clearly this was how the doctor thought of it. The door to the operating room was left ajar and swung open and closed. One of the residents left the light probe on the sheets that covered the patient until the light started to burn a hole in the sheets and to smoke. Not an auspicious day in the operating room.

Back in the lab a nurse came down and told us that so and so was pregnant. "*Mazal tov*" said the *mashgichot* and the technicians in unison in genuine pleasure.

We sat for hours in the sperm-processing lab today, just chatting about the upcoming elections, about my research, about this and that. Then we all got concerned because Ronit's son hadn't phoned from his army base, which he was supposed to do, so we all got a bit anxious. Finally he phoned, and then we discussed, not coincidentally, how to punish children when they misbehave.

Day 30

Today I saw the doctor put her hands into a woman's abdomen and pull out two live baby boys. I put on my surgical scrubs and just walked into the operating room without asking anyone; I stood against the wall, at the foot of the operating table and watched the cesarean—I almost fainted when the blood surged out everywhere.

The doctor and I walked out of the operating room together. She said that the woman had been infertile for 22 years. Everyone was overjoyed with the successful outcome—another heartfelt victory for the team.

When I got back to the sperm-processing lab I must have looked white, because Rahel, the *mashgicha*, sat me down and made me a cup of tea. She said she's a grandmother so that she knows what do to for someone. She was very interested in the Cesarean and what it was like. Then Miri came in, who delivered all three of her children by Cesarean, and she said it hurts more than you can possibly imagine. Rahel was very worried that I was so traumatized by the Cesarean section that I wouldn't have any children of my own. She said that would be terrible; that I shouldn't get myself traumatized and not have children. Then she told me about her niece who had some kind of traumatic childbirth and was traumatized until this day about it. I assured her that I would recover.

The *mashgichot* make tea, take the sperm out of the centrifuge, answer the phone, and give out sperm collecting cups with brown paper bags. Some guy named Levy rang the doorbell, got buzzed in, and then Rahel gave him a cup and a bag, wrote his name on it, and sent him on his way. Fifteen minutes later he came back with the goods.

Day 31

The lab chats today were about pregnancies. Rahel was very nice to me after yesterdays' Cesarean section trauma. We talked about traffic accidents and how terrible they are, and then we talked about politics. There are real political differences among the ladies, and they are not shy about stating their political beliefs. The secular technicians are of course more left-wing; the religious *mashgichot*, more right-wing. Then Suri came in and told us this horrible and vivid story about an abscess she had in her ear on *Shavuot* and how it popped.

As we were talking someone brought in a condom for a sperm check and I watched as Yehudit put a syringe in and withdrew sperm—not an enviable task.

Day 41

They were all exhausted from having stayed up all night watching the elections—it is all anyone can talk about today. The big surprise is how many mandates the religious parties got. All the technicians are sad, even two of the *mashgichot*. So, as they prepare sperm and do egg retrievals and embryo transfers, everyone is talking about politics.

There was another Cesarean section today—the anesthesiologist was talking through the whole thing, as usual. The woman having the Cesarean was a Palestinian, and she was moaning and crying. He kept saying to her: "Ssh, it's okay, Mengele is dead, what are you crying about?" Then she cried: "*Ima, Ima*," and he said: "Yeah, that's normal, now she's crying for her mother." It was a complex irony that the Jewish Israeli doctor pretended to comfort the anesthetized Palestinian patient by reassuring her that Hitler's doctor, known for heinous medical experiments on Jews, was dead.

It wasn't until the baby was pulled out, a boy, and Tali and I were in the hallway looking at the baby, that the anesthesiologist came by and said: "See, our 'syringe' still works well, not just yours." He was, of course, referring to the penis, for this baby was conceived via sexual intercourse, not through IVF. The anesthesiologist was quite taken with his own wit.

It turned out that this Palestinian couple lived in the Occupied Territories, and I wondered how they managed to get across the border because I knew there was a closure. I decided to go ask the ladies who work at the reception desk if they were the ones who wrote the letter that allowed them to pass through the checkpoints. They said: "Why, do they bother you? Do they bother you?" And I said: "No, I just wanted to know how they got letters to pass through the checkpoints." I asked if they bothered her, and she said: "It doesn't matter what I think. I have no choice. There's no choice."

This brief encounter hinted again at the much broader set of issues implicit in Israel's fertility policies, policies which necessarily but uneasily serve to enfranchise infertile Palestinians in the Israeli fertility enterprise (Kahn 2000). While I was at the clinic, I observed many Palestinian patients receiving fertility treatment, but they did so in an environment where some clinic staff members, particularly the receptionists, were routinely indifferent or cold to them. The larger political situation directly shaped individual attitudes and behaviors in many professional encounters between Palestinians and Israelis—not surprisingly the same held true in the fertility clinic.

There was a lot of activity today in the lab. I missed the fine needle aspiration, in which they withdrew sperm from the testicle of a paraplegic ultra-Orthodox man. I did see the egg retrieval they did on his wife, but they only managed to retrieve one egg from her.

During the procedure, they were talking about politics good-naturedly. The nurse told us about her mother who doesn't speak Hebrew and who was given a ride to the elections by the Likud. The driver came in with her and chose votes for her. Then they talked about how many old people must have voted that way.

It has actually become quite boring. Miri prepared the droplets of medium for the micromanipulation; Ronit aspirated the cumuluses off of the eggs; Tali stared into space in between procedures; Suri said psalms next to the microscopes; the radio droned on in the background with election results and continual commentaries. I feel the boredom and routine of it even during the procedures, which have become quite predictable.

Day 47

I was getting increasingly bored. I watched the *mashgichot* watch the procedures in the lab, and tried to maintain interest in yet another egg retrieval, but I've seen many egg retrievals.

During this one, the doctor discussed her vacation plans with the anesthesiologist while sucking follicles dry of the patient's eggs. "You're going diving?" the anesthesiologist asks through his surgical mask. "Yeah, and I can't wait," the doctor responds, her voice similarly muffled by the surgical mask. "The diving is supposed to be great off the coast of Egypt."

Suction, suction. The red ovarian fluid passes through the tube attached to the ultrasound probe and fills up the small vial at the other end.

"I got a great deal," the doctor continues. "Three nights, four days, four dives, including the hotel and flight, for only $400 a person."

"You missed one," the anesthesiologist says, leaning over and pointing at the ultrasound monitor.

"That's not a follicle, it's a cyst," the doctor says. They joke about who is doing the procedure, the anesthesiologist or the doctor. The anesthesiologist seems a bit bored; he checks the patient's pulse under her chin, he plays with the knobs on his anesthesia machine, he calls me over and tells me to stand closer, that I can't see from where I am standing, and then he points to the ultrasound screen and starts to explain to me what is what. The doctor tells me not to listen to him, that he doesn't know a follicle from a cyst. They laugh.

The nurse detaches the vial from the suction machine and brings it into the lab next door to have it checked for eggs. "How many?" the doctor asks the nurse when she comes back. "Six, so far," says the nurse. They are referring to the number of eggs that the biochemists have found in the woman's ovarian fluid. "That's it?" the doctor asks, and continues to mine for more.

Back in the lab, Miri and Ronit are waiting for the eggs. Suri is saying psalms and I am writing in my notebook. Suri is also talking on the phone, of course. They pour the vial of egg-containing bloody fluid into Petri dishes, and swish them around in search of eggs under the microscope.

The doctor said they are getting a new freezer, and that the key to storing embryos is to have a good freezer.

Day 50

The doctor called a meeting with the *mashgichot* (Suri, Yael, and Rahel) to boost morale and try and do something for good work relations. The lab technicians were also there. The doctor began by telling them how much she appreciated their work, and that she was doing her best to be a good and friendly boss. She said they needed to boost their success rates, that she didn't want to go full speed ahead in neutral, and that's what they were doing by treating all of these "hard cases"—she meant older women or women who had already been through treatment elsewhere. She wants the *mashgichot* to talk up the clinic in their religious communities, because many of the people who successfully conceive children through IVF, particularly micromanipulation, don't talk about it—they don't want to be known as infertile, and they think that a child so conceived will be stigmatized in some way.

One of the *mashgichot* said that she wouldn't want her child to marry someone who was conceived in vitro. One problem is the fear that they will pass on infertility to their children, so, it is hard to get business from word of mouth because it is not something that people in the ultra-religious community talk about. The doctor said that obviously if a religious couple doesn't have a child it is not because they don't want one, and if finally they do have one, people will want to know how. So the doctor urged them to say good things about the clinic because they need the business. Then she praised them some more for their good work.

Then Suri asked why the clinic has to operate on *Shabbat*. Yael, who is the one who comes in on *Shabbat*, said something about turning on lights, and Suri said that the time she worked on *Shabbat* it was difficult for her as a religious woman to be seen entering a hospital to work. Suri asked, why, in any case, the unit had to operate on *Shabbat*. The doctor replied: "What do you want me to do, to tell a woman for whom it is her last period that we won't treat her because it's *Shabbat*? With some of these difficult cases you can't wait three extra days, you have to time it perfectly." So there was some discussion of this, and of the *halachic* principle of life and death. Basically, the doctor said it was important for them to stay open on *Shabbat* in order to provide the best service.

The atmosphere of the meeting was cordial. The doctor paid for cakes and soda to be brought in, and said that if there were any problems or questions that they should be addressed to her and that the *mashgichot* should not to be put off if she seemed busy or was rushing around.

When we went downstairs, after the meeting, Suri didn't seem to take this answer so well. She said that when the doctor wants to go on vacation or something for *Shabbat*, then there are no treatments. It's all a question of money, she said, running her thumb and forefinger together, and that the doctor also wants to give good service to her private patients. It is certainly not the *mashgichot* who profit from *Shabbat* work; in fact they are not allowed to take money for work they do on *Shabbat*.

Downstairs there was an argument after the meeting: Apparently Ronit and Yehudit had done a sperm preparation without a *mashgicha* present. Ronit explained that they waited for twenty minutes, and that they didn't know how long the meeting would take, so they just went ahead and did it. Suri was furious, saying: "Why didn't you wait? Why didn't you call one of us down? You knew where we were; it's not like we had gone home or anything! We were here in the building!" Ronit responded that it was an exception, that it doesn't usually happen, and that it didn't seem like the end of the world for them to do a sperm prep without the *mashgicha*. To which Suri responded: "So what am I here for? Why don't I come in every morning at nine instead of eight if it's not so important that I'm here—why don't I just skip a few days? The point is that a *mashgicha* has to be here *every* time, not just most of the time, that's the whole point of there being *mashgichot*!"

Ronit tried to stay her course and repeated: "We waited but we didn't know how long the meeting would last, and it was only once." Then the doctor came in and asked Ronit, "Really, why didn't you call them?" So Ronit got up and said she was going home; she had a headache.

Day 52

I came in today and they were all sitting around the table, just schmoozing. There was not any work. We talked about research on embryos for a while. There was an article in the *New England Journal of Medicine* about it that Avital brought in for me. Ronit had to go to a funeral, and Avital had to go deal with the plumber at her house, so the rest of us sat there and talked about face cream and toilet paper and recipes—very boring chit chat. Then a new *mashgicha* who Suri is training came in—a big Lubavitch lady who teaches *Tanach*. Suri explained to her what happens in the lab, about how people come in and bring their sperm, about the checks, about the incubator, about how and when it is important to watch and make sure they don't mix up pipettes.

The new *mashgicha* asked if she could ask questions about the procedures, and Suri said no, that she just had to know what to watch. Then Ronit said she could and should ask questions. I was trying to pay attention to what she said, although I have gotten so used to the ins and outs of the lab. It all sounded very normal and unexceptional to me, except that Suri talked about the lab as "ours" and everything that happens is what "we" do. Apparently she has been working there almost four years. "We" check the sperm, "we" wash the sperm—everything that the technicians do includes her.

Then we walked over to the operating room for the embryo transfers, of which there were three. Suri explained to the new *mashgicha* everything that happens—where the embryos are kept, how everything is sterile, what the Petri dishes are, how the Petri dishes and everything are written on with the names of the woman undergoing treatment. She asked if their identity numbers were written down also, and Suri said no, just their name and family name.

Just after we arrived, the nurse started buzzing around for the first embryo transfer. Then the doctor came sailing in, in a good mood since her scuba diving trip. The first embryo transfer went very smoothly—Tali put the embryos into the catheter and brought them into the nurse. I watched through the door as the doctor expertly inserted them.

I heard the doctor wish the patient good luck, and I helped wheel the bed back into the patient's room. The woman who was waiting for her own embryo retrieval in the adjacent bed also wished her good luck. We wheeled the second woman in, and after her, a third.

Before every embryo transfer, the nurse yells back the name of the patient and then Ronit says, "Cohen, right!"—that's how they make sure it is the right embryo. Suri said, thank God, they have never put the wrong embryo into the wrong woman, and that they should never do it—God forbid!

I helped wheel the third patient back to the room. She had gorgeous bronze hair spread out around her head like a halo, and she was all smiles. She had a woman friend waiting for her. She had to lie there for four hours before she could go home.

Day 53

Today was one of those days in the lab where everyone was in a good mood and laughing about things. Tali, Ronit, Suri, the new *mashgicha*, and I were sitting in the lab by the operating room, waiting for the egg retrieval, but apparently they couldn't find any eggs on the ultrasound so it was taking a long time. So we sat and chatted.

I asked Suri if she thought that religious couples were praying less these days when confronted with infertility problems. She said she thought it was easier for religious couples who have fertility problems because they believe that everything comes from God, so they don't get involved in blaming each other.

She said that no one stops praying because of the treatment—it all goes together, it all helps. She told us a story about a woman who was having trouble getting pregnant, so she consulted someone who told her to light candles before the *mikveh*, after the *mikveh*, at home, all kinds of candle lighting. Nothing happened, so she went back to the person and said, "Look nothing is happening," and the other person said, "Don't forget you have to have sex too!" That's the thing that people forget she said, with all the praying and remedies, that the main thing is to make sure that you have sex with your husband! Then the new *mashgicha* said that the problem is that people come too young. Like if a couple gets married at 17, and by 19 they don't have children, they are already coming in for fertility treatment.

Finally the nurse came in and asked where the sperm was. Tali said he was still out looking for a "parking place" to do it in. Once the sperm came there was a problem with it—there was no motility. Tali said that sometimes if someone hasn't had sex for a long time that's what happens on the first shot. So, Ronit went out into the waiting room and told the guy that he had to give another sperm sample. While we were waiting for the next portion, we took bets on how much motility there would be. I put 5 shekels on 50 percent motility, Ronit said 20 percent, and Tali said 30 percent. When the sperm came in and "we" checked it under the microscope, I won! 50 percent motility!

Then there was a problem with the egg retrieval, the one follicle they thought they saw turned out to be a cyst, so they prepared the sperm for intrauterine insemination.

My notes from this extended period of fieldwork continue in this vein—with occasional anecdotes interspersed throughout what became a very banal routine of conception.

Conclusion

Assisted conception has elicited an outpouring of scholarly analysis and has inspired intense bioethical conundrums; and it has been the subject of passionate religious debate and the source of profound personal joy (when successful). What I hope this chapter has illustrated is how assisted conception has also become routinized in the workplace and how the people who work to achieve conception have come to see their tasks as entirely ordinary, occasionally frustrating, and often intensely satisfying. Banality is the mark of normalization, so while we may continue to argue about how natural these technologies are, we must recognize how normal they have also become.

References

Kahn, Susan Martha. 2000. *Reproducing Jews: A Cultural Account of Assisted Conception in Israel*. Durham, NC: Duke University Press.

Chapter 13

Between Reproductive Citizenship and Consumerism: Attitudes towards Assisted Reproductive Technologies among Jewish and Arab Israeli Women

Larissa Remennick

Fertility doctor counseling young Israeli couple: "Well, you've completed six IVF cycles to no avail. Now, why don't you try to conceive in the old-fashioned way?

—A joke told by a focus group participant

Introduction

Some recent sociological analyses of reproduction approached the relations between women as mothers and various social institutions (legal and medical systems, labor market, social welfare, mass media, etc.) within the continuum between reproductive citizenship, on one hand, and individualism/consumerism, on the other. Thus, Bryan Turner (2001) has defined the concept of reproductive citizenship as a route to active social participation through reproduction, all the more important in the times of general erosion of other traditional forms of citizenship (such as worker-citizen and warrior-citizen). Reproductive citizenship is a reflection of nationalism and demographic interests of the state, which has a stake in individual reproductive decisions (especially in the context of ethnic diversity) and tries to regulate who can reproduce and under which conditions (Richardson and Turner 2002: 37–40).

The Israeli social landscape, marked by sharp ethnic divisions and ongoing political and military confrontation, has been especially conducive to ethno-nationalist discourses of reproduction on both sides of the conflict (Amir and Benjamin 1992; Berkowitz 1997; Yuval-Davis 1997; Rouhana 1997; Kanaaneh 2002; Remennick 2008). Yet, more recent analysis of women's perceptions of their fertility and motherhood (Birenbaum-Carmeli 2003; Remennick 2000, 2006) points to the ongoing merger of childbearing matters with the general agenda of individual rights and all-embracing consumption, with the ensuing expectation of the welfare state to provide quality social and medical services such as ART, subsidized daycare, and support for parents of disabled children. I called this gradual withdrawal of parenting from public jurisdiction into a private domain, with a receding importance of ethno-national motives in childbearing decisions, "privatization of parenting" (Remennick, 2000). The moral tension between reproductive citizenship and private parenting driven by individual psychological needs and consumer choices forms the main axis of analysis in this chapter.

The prevalence of infertility treatments in Israel is the highest in the world and spans all population sectors due to the country's generous financing from the public medical budget. Social forces that propel Israeli women to utilize ART *ad maximum* include overmedicalization of pregnancy, valorization of modern technologies, and the social imperative of motherhood for all able-bodied women, including singles and lesbians (Birenbaum-Carmeli 2003, 2004; Shalev and Gooldin 2006). Although alternative family forms are emerging on the Israeli social landscape, the nuclear heterosexual family with an average of three children is still hegemonic among secular Jews, and the number of children grows on par with religiosity (Fogiel-Bijiaoui 1999). Given ART's limited efficiency, especially for older women, many clients leave reproductive clinics after many months, even years, of trial without a baby, having paid a high price for the hope of motherhood: losing career and educational opportunities, challenging significant relationships, and facing emotional and health risks (Remennick 2000; Haelyon 2006).

Most previous social studies of ART in Israel addressed the experiences of the hegemonic population group—Israeli-born Jewish women, with little attention to other ethno-cultural groups of this mosaic society. Drawing on the tension between civic and consumerist dimensions of reproduction, this study tried to explore beliefs and attitudes of Israeli women of different ethno-cultural backgrounds towards fertility treatments in the general context of nationalism, familism, and majority-minority relations. Given the different social locations of the women as natives or immigrants, Jews or Arabs, with respective distance from the core Zionist ethos of reproduction as a vehicle of nation building, we expected them to exhibit differential maternal identities and understandings of the promise and peril of ART.

Study participants and methods

This research, informed by the qualitative research paradigm, sought to elicit women's own interpretation of social reality and their private experiences. This paradigm does not claim statistical representation or universal applicability of findings, but promises to glean deeper insights into women's subjective realities that are hard to capture by using standard quantified tools (Reinharz 1992). My empirical field work comprised nine focus group discussions including the total of 73 women who volunteered for the study. Participants were drawn from the pool of women of older reproductive age (30–45) who sought (in)fertility counseling and treatment in public gynecological or IVF clinics in three cities with ethnically mixed populations—Haifa, Nazareth, and Jaffa. The women belonged to three distinct sectors of Israeli society: Israeli-born Jews; post-1989 immigrants from the former Soviet Union (FSU) who comprise 20 percent of the Jewish population; and Arab women with Israeli citizenship, who also comprise about 20 percent among the country's female population (CBS 2003). These three ethnic groups represented disparate locations on the Israeli political and cultural hegemony scale: Native Jewish women belong to its core, representing the cultural master narrative, while Russian-Jewish immigrants are more marginal due to their newcomer status, limited command of Hebrew, and socio-economic downgrading upon migration. Arab women are even more distant from the Zionist master narrative due to their precarious status as a religious and ethnic minority in the Jewish State. At their first point of contact with the medical services, all eligible women were handed a letter explaining the nature of this study and calling for participation. Those who agreed left their details with medical offices and were later contacted by the research assistant.

The discussions were conducted in ethnically homogeneous groups (i.e. Hebrew, Russian, and Arabic in each city) in the participants' native language; Hebrew and Russian groups were mediated by the author, while Arabic ones were mediated by her research assistant, who is of Arabic origin. The groups typically included between six to nine discussants and their average duration was two hours. After group discussions all participants filled out a brief socio-demographic questionnaire and were ascribed alias names (which are cited in the quotes). Most participants in all groups were married, and were secular or moderately religious ("traditional"); all but few had at least high school education and most were employed outside the home. Almost one-third of native Jewish women and some Arab women had at least one child (usually from a previous marriage), while all but one of the Russian immigrants were childless. Native Jewish women were also more advanced in the number of IVF cycles already taken in the current round of treatment (see table 13).

The discussions were held during the 10 months after the participating women's initial contact with the clinic; some of them had just started their first IVF cycle, while others had completed their third or fourth cycle (the mean number of cycles among all participants was 1.9). Focus groups took place in clinical conference rooms during off hours; they were tape-recorded with participants' permission and subsequently transcribed verbatim. While it was not easy to recruit participants and ensure their arrival to the discussions (most had to be rescheduled a few times), once seated together in a private room and given the opportunity to speak their minds and hearts, women were prolific in their expression and often hard to stop. Apparently, for many of them this was a unique opportunity to share their experiences and opinions with "pals in need" on the issues that are otherwise silenced and locked inside. Facilitators used vignettes (describing typical women's accounts of IVF) to break the ice and start a discussion, and subsequently relied on the thematic guide prepared in advance. Some topics came to the fore spontaneously, while others, potentially more sensitive or politically charged, had to be prompted by the researchers in the form of open questions. Yet, researchers kept their intervention at bay, trying to remain as sympathetic and non-judgmental as possible and to involve all the participants into discussions (which is a known challenge in focus groups).

Table 13 Socio-demographic characteristics of focus group participants (absolute numbers; N=73)

	Native Jewish (N=28)	Immigrant Jewish (N=23)	Native Arab (N=22)
Age			
30–37	18	16	18
38–45	10	7	4
Marital status			
Married or partnered	23	19	21
Single/divorced/widowed	5	4	1
Religiosity			
Secular	14	21	9
Traditional/ moderately religious	11	2	10
Very religious	3	-	3
Education			
Less than high school	2	0	7
High school/vocational training	20	9	14
Academic (BA+)	6	14	1
Employment (before IVF)			
Full-time	17	19	5
Part-time	6	2	11
Unemployed/homemakers	5	2	6
Living children			
None	19	22	17
One child or more	9	1	5
Mean No. of IVF cycles taken (in the current round)	2.8	1.2	1.3

The thematic analysis ascended from topical to conceptual categories drawing on the code-book method of transcript reading described by Crabtree and Miller (1999). This approach draws on a pre-constructed menu of analytical categories (code-book) reflecting research questions and interview or focus group topics; the code-book is constantly revised and updated to incorporate new thematic units emerging from the field. Final coding and integration of the discussion data was performed by two readers to ensure greater objectivity of interpretation; inter-coder agreement was about 80 percent. Below I present the key findings organized by selected thematic categories that reflect both our pre-constructed discussion topics and those that emerged from the field. I have tried to keep the same order within every thematic item, starting from the common motifs in women's accounts and then detailing inter-group differences moving from Israeli-born Jewish women (identified in the quotes by the code *H* for Hebrew), to the native Arab women (marked by *A* for Arabic) and, finally, to former Soviet immigrants (*R* for Russian).

ART and the supreme value of motherhood

An unquestioned supreme value of motherhood and a rejection of childlessness as demeaning emerged as an overarching theme in all group discussions. Some women had a prior or current experience with ART, others heard about the treatments from other women, and most realized that the process was not going to be easy or brief. Women from all three groups underscored their readiness to endure all the difficulty of ART and pay a high personal price in time, discomfort, pain, health risks, etc., for the baby they desired. Most participants construed motherhood in essentialist and primordial terms, as an intrinsic feminine propensity or "basic instinct," although when prompted by a facilitator, many of them admitted to the societal norms and external pressures (from family, friends) for motherhood. Thus, Liat from Nazareth (H, 37) said:

> I don't know how to decouple my own intrinsic wishes from what is expected from me as a woman. After all, you want to be like everyone else in your social circle: All my friends have at least three children, and I stopped at one because of my divorce. Now that I am with a new partner I must have another baby to confirm that I am still worth something as a woman.

Although most native Jewish women underscored the personal meaning of motherhood in their lives, the motifs belonging to the public agenda and macro-level political discourse on ethnic relations were easy to discern in their accounts. For example, Miri from Haifa (H, 42), who was childless despite three years of IVF treatment in the past, said:

> Jewish women in Israel cannot afford to be selfish, like their counterparts in Europe or U.S. It may be easier to live without children or

to suffice with a single child—this leaves you more time and money for your own pursuits. But for Jews in this part of the world such individualism is especially immoral, as it puts in jeopardy the future of our people. [This comment met approval of three other group participants]

Anita from Jaffa (H, 39), who had one child from her first marriage, thought aloud about motherhood as a mission one cannot really choose but is conscripted to by the virtue of being a woman:

As the song goes, *yeladim ze simcha* [children are bliss] but they are also a lot of work and sleepless nights; the bigger they are the more you worry about their army service, personal problems, driving habits, etc. They never leave you alone, and you are there for them as long as you are alive, at least that's how it is in Jewish families. It gets burdensome at times, but I see no other way for a woman; motherhood is our chief mission in life.

Israeli-born Jews often referred to children as having collective value at the level of an extended family or peer group they belonged to. Tali from Haifa (H, 42), who had two children from her first marriage, said:

For me, family only makes sense when there are many children around, coming together at holidays, or going to nature trips and outings with friends. Israeli society is built for families with children, and if you don't have any, or have only one, you feel excluded.

A few other native women implicated demographic or nationalist ethos, exemplified by Noa from Nazareth (H, 40), who had one child:

If we stopped bearing children by whatever means—natural or medical—what would become of this country? Israel is doomed if Jewish women do not wish to be mothers.

In the Hebrew groups, such comments often caused mixed reactions, with some participants showing skepticism, often by non-verbal means (i.e. by giggling, shrugging, raising eyebrows, etc.). And, a few participants openly countered the speakers representing the traditional Zionist ethos, exemplified by Shirly (H, 33), a childless woman who responded to Noa:

What you say just shows how brainwashed we all are by the state ideology. Some women have more children than they can handle and they grow up neglected or even become deviant. What good will it make for the Jewish people? When we decide on having children, we should weigh our own abilities and resources, not the state interests.

Many women criticized Israel's shrinking welfare support of families and advocated a rational cost-benefit approach to childbearing, free of any ideological loading:

> The state propels us to have several children and then deserts mothers to struggle on their own. Where are all the promised benefits for mothers—daycare subsidies, tax breaks, etc.? I don't think I'd like to have more than one or two kids in the current situation. (Debby from Jaffa, H, 34)

Let me stress that most critical voices did not stem from the anti-nationalist, egalitarian stance (few were ready to challenge the tenet of the Jewish demographic majority) but rather from the critical view of the lack of public support for motherhood. None of the native women questioned the motherhood imperative as such, the disagreement being mainly about the numbers of children one can afford in the current public climate.

Arab women (of whom all but a few were Muslims) saw motherhood as a collective value and children as a guarantee of the continuity and economic power of an extended family or a kin network (*hamula*) and the national Arab community in general. Nadira from Nazareth (A, 33), who had one child, asserted:

> Giving children to one's people is the most important contribution a woman can make. Arab women are ready to sacrifice their own wishes and selfish interests for the sake of being good mothers.

Other Arab women stressed the role of children, especially sons, in keeping their husband satisfied and not divorcing them or taking an additional wife in a society where polygamy is common. For example, a woman with one daughter said:

> Bearing at least one son is essential to keep your dignity as a woman and also to keep your husband. A woman who does not have sons can be easily discarded and replaced. I'd do anything to give a son to my husband. (A, Haniya, 31)

Thus, the maternal identity of the Arab women was rooted in both their personal status in the family and community and their contribution to the collective good of the nation, mainly by reproducing the ranks of men—breadwinners and potential fighters for the Palestinian cause.

Russian immigrants, coming from a low-fertility culture that stresses the quality of parenting (Remennick et al. 1995), seldom sought ARTs if they already had at least one child. In fact, all Russian participants were childless and responded to the promise of ART reluctantly after all natural means of procreation had failed them. Explaining their decision to use medical intervention, they largely cited private reasons rather than the need to assert themselves as normative Israeli women belonging to the Jewish nation state or meet social expectations. Immigrant women often referred to financial troubles and other privations they experienced upon resettlement as a cause for childbearing delays, which resulted in difficulty getting pregnant by natural means. None of the Russian participants advocated "blind rushing into motherhood no matter what" (as put by Natalie, R, 38), but always adjusted their wish for a child to their actual circumstances and resources. Natalie continued:

> Being a mother is a big responsibility. We were just not ready for it during out initial years of adjustment in Israel. I couldn't bring a baby to a damp basement apartment we had rented, having no stable job, with a husband on the verge of nervous breakdown. . .

Most Russian women underscored that the child they desired was purely their own personal asset. Dina (R, 35) said:

> I want a baby for myself and my husband, not for the State or its army. On the contrary, if I have a son, I'll do all possible to keep him from the military.

As opposed to Jewish and Arab native women living on the two sides of the conflict, none of the 22 immigrant women voiced a motive implicating ethnic, national or any other "macro-level" reasons for their personal childbearing wishes and plans.

Although women of different ethno-cultural backgrounds emphasized different aspects of motherhood as a social role, family function or private experience, the theme of sacrificing other goals and interests for the sake of a baby was overarching in most women's accounts. Russian immigrants often mentioned that they risked losing their jobs as a result of the tight schedule of IVF clinic visits for tests and procedures that mostly occurred in the morning, i.e., during work hours. Some Arab women lived in the nearby villages and traveled long hours to reach the clinics; both groups of minority women had lower access to cars and often had to rely on public transport (not always dependable in Israel) and be late for work, studies, and other errands. Many women who were in the midst of IVF cycles noted that their whole life was overhauled or even "hijacked," in one woman's wry definition, by the treatment regiment, taking a toll on their physical shape, mental well-being, time schedules, etc. For many, being an IVF client became an indispensable part of their identity as "women on the way to motherhood." As long as they remained under treatment, the stigma of childlessness was lifted or attenuated, making the prospect of ending it at some point without a baby especially intimidating.

The right to parenthood and entitlement to ART services

Reflecting the pro-natalist social climate, the right to parenthood is considered a basic human right in the Israeli legal discourse, and is accompanied by generous public funding of infertility treatments (Shalev and Gooldin 2006). The sense of entitlement for ART services was conveyed by most women, who did not question their claim for a fat chunk of the national health care budget and did not compare their own privilege with the limited access to costly ART services in other countries. The assertion that subsidized or free access to ART is, and should always remain, an inalienable right for all Jewish couples as an alternative way of procreation was expressed in stronger terms by native Jewish women. To cite Ariella (H, 36), who had no children, "The state owes us this service for free if it expects us to bear the children that it needs—as workers, as soldiers, as citizens. . . . " Later she added:

> Women who are in IVF treatment pay a high enough price with their pain and submission to all these highly unpleasant procedures, you can't expect them also to fund reproductive services out of their own pockets.

Dana (H, 38), who had no children, argued along similar lines:

> Most Israeli women are giving two or three years of their youth to the military or national service; I think it is only fair that they get this aid for free in return when they are unable to mother children by natural means.

Comments by Ariella and Dana point to their understanding of give-and-take relations with the Israeli state, a kind of implied social contract between the state and the women who are providing the invaluable service to the state by giving life to new Jewish citizens despite high personal costs—in exchange they expect the state to give them a hand in achieving fertility. A breach of contract by the state (i.e., withdrawing free access to IVF) would mean a reduction in Jewish birth rates, with multiple negative ramifications for the economic and political future. Dana pointed to another aspect of the social contract between the Israeli state and its women, military or national service, by which most of them contribute to the national cause. It seems only fair that the state would assist these women to further contribute to the common good (and meet social and family expectations) by becoming mothers.

The Arab women did not speak of the right to motherhood for themselves, and were reticent when this issue was raised by the facilitator. It was apparent that the very language of rights was rather foreign to them. They typically construed ART as part of women's health services they were entitled to as Israeli citizens, and some of them even defined ART as critical or life-saving care, given the severe ostracism of childless women in Muslim society. Several women said that maternity is a privilege rather than a right and expressed gratitude for being given access to ART. Aziza from Jaffa (A, 33) who had no children, said:

> This is my last chance to save my marriage. As long as I receive IVF treatments, there will be hope for a baby and my husband will not leave me. I could never afford a private clinic, so I am very grateful that this hospital is taking me on.

A few participants (all of them educated urban Arab women) asserted that they saw no difference between themselves and Jewish women as far as free access to ARTs was concerned. In the words of Tarika (A, 33), a teacher from Jaffa:

> I am glad that at least in this respect there is no sheer discrimination of Arab citizens. The Jewish doctors may not like facilitating higher Arab birth rates, but they are polite enough not to show it.

When asked by the researcher why she believed that Jewish doctors did not like serving Arab women in IVF clinics, Tarika replied, "I just know it by their attitude, some comments between doctors and nurses you can overhear, all very subtle, but quite tangible for me." The last comment shows that many Arab women expect almost by default some form of substandard treatment from Israeli institutions, and even when explicit discrimination is unapparent, they look for the implicit signs of prejudice or contention on the part of providers.

Russian immigrant women, especially those who left the Former Soviet Union more recently, did not take for granted their access to ART, being aware of the high costs of infertility care in their former countries. Thus, Vera (R, 35) who had been in Israel for three years, said:

> I do appreciate being able to get this counseling and testing, let alone the treatments, almost for free because I had tried IVF in my city in

Ukraine and could only afford one cycle. There, this option exists only for rich women but in Israel we are all covered by public insurance, and this is very generous.

When asked by facilitator if they believed in the "right for parenthood" for all, some immigrant women were puzzled by this question and said they had never thought about parenting in legal terms. Sasha from Haifa (R, 39) reflected on this question:

> This sounds weird and somewhat demagogical to me: A right is something you can claim from the state or government as a citizen, but having children is rather a matter of biology and personal destiny. Some women cannot get pregnant or carry to term no matter what—who can they sue for that—God? Medical science can give you a second chance, but still there is no guarantee. . . .

Angela (R, 40) from the same group added:

> I understand mutual legal obligations between parents and children when they are born. I can also grasp the right for motherhood in the sense that no one can pressure a woman to terminate the pregnancy she wants. But a universal right to get pregnant—this sounds like a long shot to me.

Further probing by the facilitator made it clear that most Russian-speaking participants understood reproductive rights mainly as the right to keep or abort an existing pregnancy, as well as access to birth control and sex education. The Israeli legal notion of the essential entitlement of every human to become a parent *by means of medical intervention backed up by the state* (when natural means fail) seemed puzzling and far-fetched to most of them. Most Russians perceived fecundity and birth (like other vital events) with a trace of fatalism: Some couples are meant to be childless no matter what. Their take on ART was more pragmatic and subdued, and it lacked the heroic and sacrificial overtones voiced by many native Jewish women.

The issue of who should be entitled to free ART services is apparently very sensitive in Israeli society, tainted as it is by a deep ethno-religious rift between the Jewish majority and the Arab minority. In the Hebrew-speaking Jewish groups, several participants cautiously stated their reservations about equal access to costly IVF treatments for Arab women (this is where the issue of cost to the taxpayer came to the fore), given high natural increase rates in the Arab sector. Tami from Jaffa (H, 42), who had no children, put it like this:

> I think that democratic states with accessible medical care should define their priorities. There is no shame in calling Israel the Jewish

State, and therefore I see no flaw in supporting Jewish fertility and larger family size. It is no secret that Palestinians on both sides of the Green Line [i.e. in Israel and occupied territories] have many more kids than the Jews, and their share in the total population is growing much faster. To my mind, it is insane on the part of the State to offer Arab women free infertility treatments at the expense of Jewish tax-payers. As always, we are acting here against our own interests.

Miri from Nazareth (H, 40), also with no children, offered along similar lines:

I know this a very politically incorrect thing to say, but I think there should be limits in our generosity towards Arab citizens. They do not serve in the army, they pay less taxes, only a minority of their women work—why should they get the same costly services for free? Do we want to pay thousands of dollars for yet another Arab baby who will grow to hate us and maybe will turn his weapon against my son? There are enough private clinics for the Arabs to use.

These and similar assertions caused dissent among other discus-sants, who insisted on the principle of equal entitlement for all med-ical services for all citizens, regardless of their ethnicity. Sherri from Haifa (H, 36), who had no children, said:

If you start excluding Arabs from reproductive services, then what comes next—expensive heart and brain surgeries? Transplants? This would be a step towards a true apartheid society, in which I don't want to live.

Apparently, any dispute on the issues of fertility and family size in the Middle East eventually turns to ethnic relations and politics. Being aware of the potentially divisive nature of this topic, most women in all groups tried to avoid discussing the "Other" in the context of reproductive rights, but as the above-cited quotes show, the issue still came up every now and then. Typically enough, it was mainly women who belonged to the hegemonic majority who could allow the discussion to move toward these potentially dangerous places; with few exceptions, Russian and Arabic participants tried to avoid political overtones altogether. This reflects their insecure location on the margins of Israeli society (although admittedly on different margins and for different reasons) with the resulting reti-cence in the public expression of their true opinions. While Russian women mainly tried to avoid the clash between different political outlooks of participants (many of them openly stated their distaste for political disputes), Arab women possibly felt limited by the set-ting of the study and therefore self-censored their speech. However, a few angry comments were made by some Arab women (see, for example, Fatimah's quote in the following section on the public and private aspects of fertility).

Doctors and nurses as heroes and "procreators of the nation"

Israeli-born women also tended to glorify medical workers, particularly IVF specialists and especially men among them, for their heroic endeavors to give babies to women striving for motherhood. Some of them attributed supernatural powers to medical science and its practitioners (almost priests), and often had unrealistic expectations as to the success rates of IVF treatment. Several participants of Hebrew groups also voiced the motives of the "noble mission" these medical practitioners carried out to ensure continuity of Jewish families, and hence Jewish demographic majority in the land of Israel. Ayelet from Haifa (H, 39), who had no children, said:

> Reproductive medicine is not just another medical specialty; it has a salient role in the life of Israeli Jews. I see it as special and even sacred (*kadosh*). As more women get married later and have difficulty with natural conception, ART specialists are their main hope for motherhood and a good family life.

Ilanit (H, 33), who had one child from previous marriage, mused:

> For me, my IVF doctor is going to be my idol, the second most important man in my life after my husband. He [the husband] has low sperm count and we'll need help with sperm selection and fertilization. So the doctor who will do this for us will become sort of a third parent, an essential figure for the future of our family.

This kind of romantic or spiritually-loaded attitude toward IVF specialists was missing in the accounts by the Arab and Russian women. Their take on the role of ART practitioners was more down-to-earth and pragmatic, drawing on the information they had obtained on success rates of different procedures (more typical for educated Russian women having good access to the Internet and other data sources) or simply the expectation of quality service upon request (expressed more often by Arab women). Nahaya (A, 35), a childless teacher from Nazareth, said:

> I view IVF doctors like any other gynecologists who have treated me before. I am not even sure that they do all the complex manipulations with ova and sperm themselves, there are probably skilled lab technicians for that, whom we never meet. But their role behind the scenes may be even more important for the final result.

Victoria (R, 38), a computing specialist from Haifa, reflected along similar lines:

> I am not trying to develop a special relationship with the doctor, although I hope he or she is decent and competent. This is a public clinic, and you cannot expect too much attention or the special treatment that women with means can get in private ART centers. My best hope is that my doctor will have enough experience and good conscience so that I am spared the abuse of hyper-stimulation or harvesting too many ova. [The latter remark refers to the widely publicized medical scandal over egg donations and trade in some Israeli clinics a few years ago].

Like these participants, most other Russian and Arab women construed IVF doctors as regular medical professionals who are human and sometimes prone to error and misconduct. They did not have high expectations from the public IVF clinics they had to use, realized that infertility treatments are mass-scale and impersonal, and hoped mainly for decency and competence on the part of providers, as well as good luck (or God's will—*insha'alla*—the way many Arab women put it). Stressing a clear distinction between the "natural" and "artificial" in reproductive matters, Muslim and Russian immigrant women showed more similarity than difference in their perception of the ART services. As opposed to the women molded by mainstream Hebrew culture, women from both minorities were clearly ambivalent about the perils of medical technology and did not blindly trust their medical providers. By virtue of their greater realism (often with a tint of fatalism) and mixed feelings toward ART, they also seemed to be better prepared for a possible failure of IVF—not a minor psychological advantage, given its moderate success rates.

Between the private and public aspects of (in)fertility

Fertility and motherhood in Israel carry both private and public value, and are often discussed in the broad context of the national future and ethno-religious conflict in the Middle East (Portugese 1998; Kahn 2000; Remennick 2008). The rift between public and private aspects of ART emerged as a recurring theme in our discussions; the cultural and political gap between the groups was especially clear in the ways women reflected on these boundaries and their meaning. Israeli-born Jewish women were more attuned to the public expectations of successful motherhood as a condition of their full membership in the mainstream collective (i.e., active reproductive citizenship). Eti (H, 43), who had one child from a previous marriage, said:

> If childless women become more common, this is not just a private matter; this is a social problem for Israel. We as a society need more children to ensure our future. No wonder that the state is ready to pay a lot of money to help women become mothers.

Conversely, Arab women seemingly downplayed nationalist motives in childbearing and underscored family pressures and women's own interests in motherhood as the principal way to increase their social status and economic security. Suha (A, 36), a social worker with one daughter, said:

> In our society, a woman cannot be respected if she has not borne at least one son, a family heir. This is a deep-running tradition, also among educated and non-religious people, and I must do everything possible to achieve this goal. My husband needs a son to be respected by his siblings and co-workers, and I cannot fail him in this natural wish.

Only two participants in three Arabic focus groups raised nationalist motives, as exemplified by Fatimah from Nazareth (A, 39), a teacher with one daughter:

> Just like Jewish Israelis are concerned with their national future, so are Palestinian citizens. We live in our own country and want our offspring to live here. As long as ethnicity and religion do matter in Israel, Arab women will try to have as many children as they can. We are not going to ask anyone's permission for this.

Yet, most Muslim women avoided the politically contentious ground of the demographic race, probably due to the context of these discussions, which took place in medical facilities, run by the Jewish majority, that provided these women with vitally important services. Presumably, in a more neutral setting more Arab women would have felt free to speak out and assert their civil reproductive rights.

Russian women never mentioned the public contribution of mothers to the common good or demographic future of the Jewish people and, when prompted in this direction by the facilitator, many said that for them motherhood is a purely private matter located within the boundaries of the nuclear family. Lydia (R, 40), an economist from Jaffa, reflected:

> Bearing children for the state, or the nation, sounds like a Bolshevik idea to me. Yes, I think it is a totalitarian idea. You hear this slogan from the party bosses in places like Cuba and North Korea. In

democratic countries having or not having children is a private decision and no one should pressure women, one way or the other.

Genia (R, 43), an engineer from the same group, agreed:

> When you have a child, especially as an older mother and after dif-
> ficult treatment, the last thing you want for him or her is to become a
> toy in the hands of corrupt politicians. Your child is precious for you
> and you don't want to see him wounded in the army or being used by
> the state in any other way.

These quotes reflect a strong sense of personal autonomy and
resistance to any kind of state involvement in private life, a clear
separation between the public and private domains typical of former
Soviet citizens after many decades of forced collectivism.

Another common theme across group boundaries was the increasing public visibility of infertile women with the advent of ART that
can often reinforce rather than mitigate the existing stigma. Many
women pointed to the thriving discourse on infertility in the Israeli
media, which often presents ART as an efficient and painless solution, compelling women to seek treatment and implicitly reproach-
ing those who don't. Raisa (R, 33), who had no children, said:

> A woman's body is now drawn from the privacy of her bedroom to
> the public space of the infertility clinic and subjected to assessment
> and manipulation. Private pain and deficiency is becoming visible to
> everybody who is curious. . . .

Rotem (H, 39) endorsed her statement, adding, "Since IVF became
widely available and common in Israel, a childless woman can no
longer remain in the shadow, she is expected to step into public
spotlight and seek solutions to her private problem." The media coverage, often unbalanced and driven by the interests of the IVF industry, both exposes this formerly private and hidden suffering and
creates unrealistic expectations in older women. The latter point
was repeatedly stressed by many participants in their 40s, who were
themselves misled by the ostensible promise of ART and were starting to come to their senses after several futile IVF cycles.

At the same time, some women noted that not just their hidden
flaws and related suffering, but also the heroic effort to overcome
them and achieve pregnancy at any personal cost, are becoming
public knowledge. Quite a few Jewish women of either origin, but
not Muslim ones, construed their uptake of IVF cycles as a brave endeavor that should be made known to their milieu: "I will not conceal my intention to start IVF from colleagues at work and friends;

on the contrary, I am gong to tell everyone: Being in treatment makes me a better person, a woman on the path to motherhood," said Ayala (H, 41), who had no children. Most Arab women intended to keep their relations with Israeli IVF clinics discrete and present the pregnancy (if achieved) as a natural one to their extended family and neighbors. For instance, Nadira (A, 36) said:

> No way, I will keep this as private as possible. If I could possibly keep my husband out of this affair I would, but unfortunately he must be involved. Making a test-tube baby is not a great honor for a Muslim woman; our babies should come around naturally [laughs].

Nadira's remark in fact typified many women's wish to take sole responsibility for infertility and keep their male partners "untainted" by it. This tendency was found across ethnic groups; it signifies a popular view of childlessness as a woman's problem, despite growing knowledge that men are almost as often the faulty party (Remennick 2000). Both Jewish and Arab women spoke of their wish to save their husbands the stigma and suffering they experienced themselves, mainly for the sake of their masculine self-esteem and social status in the community. Most participants were reticent in the face of the researchers' questions about the causes of their infertility, and only a few women openly stated that it was the low sperm count of the husband that was the problem. This defensive stance also applied to the husband's necessary physical participation in the ART-related procedures, such as giving sperm in the clinical premises. Some women said that they brought their husbands to the clinic in the evening or early in the morning, when their privacy could be ensured. As for the male partners' routine participation in IVF care and support of their wives (e.g., giving them daily hormonal shots, driving them to and from the clinic, etc.), it varied across ethnic sectors. Judging by the participants' reactions to this query, native Israeli men were most supportive and involved and Arab men tended to stay out of this business, while Russian immigrant men exhibited most variability in this regard.

Concluding thoughts:
IVF as a token of reproductive citizenship

Our findings underscore significant inter-group differences among Israeli women's attitudes towards the contemporary social project of ART. Both the sense of entitlement to access these costly treatments and the perception of ART as a legitimate and respectful way to achieve motherhood were most pronounced among native Jewish women, members of the hegemonic majority. Our limited empirical evidence shows that women socialized under the Zionist master narrative of Jewish motherhood as national mission (Berkowitz 1997) expressed fewer reservations toward ART and were gladly submitting their bodies to medical control in order to achieve pregnancy at any personal cost. Women who were more distant from this master narrative (members of the Muslim minority and Russian immigrants) were more reserved and critical, did not necessarily valorize and trust reproductive clinics, and resorted to ART only after prolonged attempts to conceive naturally. These women manifested a weaker sense of belonging to the Jewish state and construed their bodies and reproduction (also when gone awry) as their own private matter, which they were ready to share only with their partners and immediate families (for Russian women) or with the extended family (for Muslim women).

In my earlier research on the stigma of infertility (Remennick 2000) and prenatal genetic testing (Remennick 2006), I pointed to the on-going "privatization of reproduction" among Jewish Israeli women, whose narratives usually lacked clear reference to the ethnic or national motifs as part of their personal wish for children generally, and healthy, "quality" children specifically. In this study, which included comparison among native Israelis and two groups located on the margins of the master narrative, the theme of motherhood as both an entitlement and an expression of reproductive citizenship could be discerned rather clearly, but mainly among the Jewish natives. Although Israeli-born women of today embrace fertility and motherhood mainly as sources of personal fulfillment and accomplished family life, the themes of ethnic solidarity and contribution to the public good (themes which dominated motherhood narratives of the earlier decades [see Berkowitz 1997; Yuval-Davis 1997; Amir and Benjamin 1997]) are still present, at least for some of the women we met during this research. Another ongoing attitudinal shift represented by our findings is from serving the nation by childbearing, to claiming state support of parents as a civil right and as an indispensable part of consumer culture. Apparently, the perception of the Jewish State by its citizens has evolved from the collective ideological project of the past to a more instrumental service provider, and its less than perfect performance is this role causes a lot of resentment.

A vivid expression of this consumer-rights driven sense of entitlement was native Jewish women's lack of qualms about the financial burden of ART to the taxpayer (at the expense of other unmet needs) regarding their own treatment. Yet, some of them objected to equal entitlement for the Arab women, referring to high public costs and proliferation of children and youth among Palestinians. This selective view of civil rights was perhaps the most tangible expression of the hegemonic sense of entitlement and ethnic rifts in the discussions we examined. Palestinian women were more reserved in expression of the national motives in childbearing, probably because of the Jewish and medical setting of the study, on which they were dependent for access to ART and their desired pregnancy. Yet even so, some of them (usually more educated and articulate ones) voiced their sense of civil rights and entitlement to make free reproductive choices as citizens of a democratic state and residents of their own historic land. Most Palestinian women were well aware of the demographic apprehensions of the Jews and assumed that Israeli medical providers were less than happy to offer them costly infertility treatments. It would be interesting to examine this assumption by interviewing Jewish ART professionals in future research. Regardless of these negative attributions, Arab participants expressed no qualms about using IVF services provided by the "Zionists." In this respect, my findings partly resonate with the more explicit and radical voices of the Arab women interviewed by non-Israeli researchers in Kanaaneh's (2002) book *Birthing the Nation.*

Russian immigrant women have emerged in this research as largely detached from the mainstream discourse on reproductive citizenship. They neither construed childbearing as public or national matter, nor claimed state support of ART as part of their "natural right" for parenthood. The very language of rights and entitlements was generally alien to former Soviet participants, and they always took the discussion to the more private space of relationships and domesticity. They saw children as a personal accomplishment of the parents (when they grow up educated and successful) and rather wanted to protect them from the encroaching hand of the Zionist state and its military. They avoided politically charged discussions as best they could, and when driven to these topics by other discussants, expressed subdued and moderate opinions that accommodated rather than criticized "the Other." Interestingly, Russian women's opinions on many accounts (e.g., the dislike of the artificial interventions in their reproductive lives; a cautious and realistic attitude towards the clinics and their staff) were closer to those of the Arab Israelis than to fellow Jewish women. It can be argued that Russian immigrants had completed the process of the "privatization of reproduction" before their migration to Israel, and their individualism was not attenuated but rather enhanced by the Israeli context of ethno-national conflict and contested motherhood.

References

Amir, Delila and Orly Benjamin. 1997. "Defining Encounters: Who Are the Women Entitled to Join the Israeli Collective?" *Women's Studies International Forum* 20, nos. 5–6: 639–50.

Benjamin, Orly and Haelyon, Hila. 2002. "Rewriting Fertilization: Trust, Pain and Exit Points." *Women's Studies International Forum* 25: 667–78.

Berkowitch, Nitza. 1997. "Motherhood as a National Mission: The Construction of Womanhood in the Legal Discourse in Israel." *Women's Studies International Forum* 20, nos. 5–6: 605–19.

Birenbaum-Carmeli, Daphna. 2003. "Reproductive Policy in Context: Implications on Women's Rights in Israel, 1945–2000." *Policy Studies* 24, nos. 2–3: 101–113.

———. 2004. "'Cheaper Than a Newcomer:' On the Social Production of IVF Policy in Israel." *Sociology of Health and Illness* 26, no. 7: 897–924.

CBS. 2003. *Statistical Yearbook*. Central Bureau of Statistics of Israel: Jerusalem.

Crabtree, Benjamin and William Miller. 1999. *Doing Qualitative Research*, 2nd ed. London: Sage.

Fogiel-Bijiaoui, Sylvie. 1999. "Israeli Families: Between Familism and Post-Modernism." In *Sex, Gender, and Politics: Women in Israel* [Hebrew], eds. D.N. Izraeli, Sylvie Fogiel-Bijiaoui, Ariella Friedman, and Orly Benjamin. Tel Aviv: Ha Kibbutz Hameuchad.

Haelyon, Hila. 2006. "Longing for a Child: Perceptions of Motherhood among Israeli-Jewish Women Undergoing *In Vitro* Fertilization Treatments." *Nashim* 12: 177–202.

Kahn, Susan. 2000. *Reproducing Jews: A Cultural Account of Assisted Conception in Israel*. Durham: Duke University Press.

Kanaaneh, Rhoda Ann. 2002. *Birthing the Nation: Strategies of Palestinian Women in Israel*. Berkeley: University of California Press.

Portugese, J. 1998. *Fertility Policy in Israel: The Politics of Religion, Gender and Nation*. Westport, CT: Praeger.

Reinharz, Shulamit. 1992. *Feminist Methods in Social Research*. Oxford: Oxford University Press.

Remennick, Larissa, Delila Amir, Yuval Elimelech, and Ilya Novikov. 1995. "Family Planning Practices and Attitudes among Former Soviet New Immigrant Women in Israel." *Social Science and Medicine* 41, (4): 569–577.

Remennick, Larissa. 2000. "Childless in the Land of Imperative Motherhood: Stigma and Coping among Infertile Israeli Women." *Sex Roles* 43, (11/12): 821–841.

———. 2006. "The Quest after the Perfect Baby: Why do Israeli Women Seek Prenatal Genetic Testing?" *Sociology of Health and Illness* 28, (1): 21–53.

———. 2008. "Contested Motherhood in the Ethnic State: Voices from an Israeli Postpartum Ward. *Ethnicities* 8 (2):199–226.

Richardson, Eileen and Bryan S. Turner. 2002. "Bodies as Property: From Slavery to DNA Maps," in *Body Lore and Laws*, eds. A. Bainham, M. Richards and S. Day Scalter. Oxford, UK: Hart Publishing.

Rouhana, Nadim. 1997. *Palestinian Citizens in an Ethnic Jewish State*. New Haven: Yale University Press.

Sered, Susan. 2000. *What Makes Women Sick? Maternity, Modesty, and Militarism in Israeli Society.* Boston: Brandeis University Press.

Shalev, Carmel and Sigal Gooldin. 2006. "The Uses and Mis-uses of In Vitro Fertilization (IVF) in Israel: Some Sociological and Ethical Considerations," *Nashim: A Journal of Jewish Women's Studies and Gender Issues* 12: 151–176.

Turner, Bryan S. 2001. "The Erosion of Citizenship," *The British Journal of Sociology* 52, no. 2: 189–209.

Yuval-Davis, Nira. 1997. *Gender and Nation*. London: Sage.

Ethnography, Exegesis, and Jewish Ethical Reflection: The New Reproductive Technologies in Israel

Don Seeman

The State of Israel has emerged as a leader in the use and development of new reproductive technologies. It is well-known for example, that Israel boasts more IVF clinics per capita than any other country in the world, and is one of the only nations to make this technology available at public expense to women without regard to their marital status or sexual orientation (Kahn 2000). More surprising perhaps is that Israel, where determinations of personal status and the legality of reproductive technologies are subject to veto by state-authorized religious authorities, specifically legalized donor insemination at least a decade before the militantly secular Republic of France, where the practice had been determined as early as 1880 to be "repugnant to the laws of nature," and was effectively banned until 1973 (Ball 2000: 548). The tendency of scholars who study Israel to assume a self-explanatory rift between religious-conservative and secular-scientific worldviews must obviously be reexamined (cf. Seeman 1999). One of the primary arguments of this chapter is that we need a more nuanced analysis of the ways in which ethical reflection upon new medical technology grows out of culturally grounded interpretive practices.

The French comparison is instructive here because of the way in which an avowedly secular yet deeply metaphysical discourse on the "laws of nature" has helped to inform contemporary decisions about social and public health policy. In France, judgments about the propriety of reproductive technology were made not primarily by recourse to sacred texts but to foundational documents of modern secularism like the 1789 Declaration of the Rights of Man, which encodes a complex web of ideas about the "natural" and the "good." This secularized version of natural law theory did not invoke revelation, but it did invoke ideas about the natural "rights and dignity of man" in order to call into question practices like IVF treatment for post-menopausal women or post-mortem sperm collection (Ball 2000: 553) that seemed to stretch the definition of what could be considered "natural." Policy makers asserted the importance of establishing "natural paternity" as a criterion of human dignity that would necessarily entail a challenge to the notion of anonymous sperm banking (ibid.: 573), for example, upon which several contemporary reproductive technologies rely. Ultimately, French policy makers limited the legal practice of IVF to sterile, heterosexual couples of childbearing years—"natural" parents in other words, whose inability to bear children could be conceived as *extrinsic* to their social position or cultural identity.

Concerns of this type have been relatively peripheral to the Israeli Jewish context, but they echo the concerns of modern Catholic writers, who continue to view most forms of artificial reproductive technology with suspicion or hostility as counter to nature. Ball (2000) adds that the French debate should be contextualized in the light of a strong literary tradition extending back to Rousseau's valorization of nature and the rise of the novel in France as a tool for shaping sentiments about kinship. She also urges policy makers to engage in an explicit consideration of this inherited literary tradition, which is, she believes, inherently "freer than a restrictive legal text," allowing for non-consensus, "so that ethical questions can be explored more fully" (ibid.: 587). The call to engage more fully with the literary traditions that help to shape moral sentiments in different societies is one that I will endorse wholeheartedly in the course of this chapter, though I will also argue that the flip distinction between "literary" and "legal" modes of ethical analysis is quite simply ill-informed.

Bioethical deliberation cannot be severed from the broader hermeneutical concerns that shape other styles of reading and forms of thought, including religious worldviews. This holds true for French debates on the Rights of Man (Ball 2000), feminist reflection on Marge Piercy's fictional accounts of human reproduction (Adams

1993), and the use of abortion as a ubiquitous metaphor of social and moral breakdown in early modernist English language poetry (Hauk 2003). Recently, a Hindu writer (Batthacharyya 2006) has argued that Hindus should follow the example of Christian bioethics to derive a formal set of ethical principles for assisted reproduction from the sacred narrative of the Mahabharata. But Jewish bioethical discourse has drawn primarily from a legacy of *legal* writing that is no less intrinsically flexible than narrative models, and sometimes much more so. My goal in this chapter is simply to outline some of the distinctive hermeneutic strategies that have helped to define Jewish and Israeli approaches to the new reproductive technologies, and to differentiate them from their Christian and Western-secular counterparts. At the same time, I will argue as an anthropologist that our understanding of these textual strategies and traditions ought to be complicated by calling ethnographic attention to the situated character of human experience in real-world settings of possibility and constraint.

Textual practices and reproductive practices

Jews have arguably had one of the longest continuous literary pre-occupations with problems of human reproduction of any group in history. In the Hebrew Bible, notes Thierry Maertens, the womb "is the organ that all along the elect people's history" serves as "the privileged locus of divine benedictions" (LaCocque and Ricoeur 1998: 24). One of the inescapably dominant themes in Genesis is in fact the desperate attempt by both men and women to bring forth children from childlessness by almost any means (Seeman 1998). In Genesis 16, for example, the matriarch Sarah gives her Egyptian servant Hagar to her husband Abraham in what we to-day would probably call a "traditional surrogacy" arrangement to produce the child that had eluded her. "Behold now, the Lord has restrained me from bearing; go in, I pray thee, unto my handmaid; *it may be that I shall be built up through her*" (cf. Gen. 30). Some commentators have resisted reading this story as a surrogacy arrangement for the simple reason that later Jewish *halachah* (religious law) makes no provision for the formal transference of maternal identity from a birth mother to another woman—the birth mother remains the mother for many halachic purposes no matter who may raise the child—but biblical scholars have found ample precedent for true surrogacy involving concubines in the ancient Near East (see Speiser 1964: 20).

This biblical story is driven by the fact that both Sarah and her surrogate ultimately do bear sons, whereupon Sarah's magnanimity collapses into a rivalry that threatens to tear the household of Abraham apart. Yet this rivalry is of more than purely theological interest, as the troubled descendants of Isaac and Ishmael continue to compete even today for reproductive preeminence in the Promised Land they share (Kanaaneh 2002; Kahn 2000). For Jews and Muslims, the importance of the story and its Koranic cognate involves the transference of blessing (who really inherits Abraham's covenant?), but it is worth mentioning that many Protestant writers cite this story today in support of the view that surrogacy is against the divine "reproductive paradigm" (cf. Storey 2000; Meilander 1991; McColley 1991) because of all the strife that it caused in Abraham's household! At least one modern feminist writer has followed suit in arguing that the Sarah-Hagar episode proves that surrogacy makes women "interchangeable" and should be disallowed (Rothman 1991), but this only serves to highlight the very different attitude towards assisted reproduction that might also be fairly derived from this biblical text.

Every one of the matriarchs in Genesis struggles with barrenness, which comes to define the very architecture of biblical narrative. Women's movement across the thresholds of tents comes to signify a literary enactment of the problematic quest for motherhood (Seeman 1998), and contributes to a uniquely biblical idiom of the relationship between gender, fecundity, and national identity. This is very far from the concern with nature and natural reproduction that has characterized many modern responses to assisted reproduction. Sarah's miraculous conception in old age ("Sarah had stopped having the periods of women" [Gen. 18:11]) betrays no hint of the ethical conflict surrounding post-menopausal reproduction that continues to bedevil some modern policy makers (cf. Parks 1999; Ball 2000). Nor is Sarah the last of the biblical women to reproduce in unexpected ways. Jacob's wife Rachel has trouble conceiving and prays bitterly for death if God refuses to give her a child (Gen. 30). She resorts to pharmacological measures through fertility-enhancing "mandrakes" (a kind of plant) and competes with her sister Leah over who can produce the most sons for their common husband through surrogacy involving each of the two women's female servants: "She [Rachel] said [to Jacob], 'Here is my maidservant Bilhah; come in to her and she will give birth upon my knees *so that I also may be built up through her*" (Gen. 30:3).

The fact that servant-surrogacy seems to be an assumed element of the biblical kinship system need not deflect modern thinkers—even religious ones—from raising the whole knot of thorny ethical problems raised by surrogacy in its different settings. The text can be read to raise important and highly relevant contemporary questions about the ways in which surrogacy in some contexts may be said, for example, to put poor women's reproductive capacities at the disposal of rich women along clearly established lines of social and economic power. But we must also acknowledge that this is very far from the text's primary and explicit concern with the possibilities for reproductive success on the part its protagonists, and with the ambiguity and instability in local kin relations that surrogacy can sometimes introduce. Classical midrashic literature is filled with allusions not just to tensions between the families of Rachel and Leah but also to tensions and hierarchies pitting the sons of the wives against the sons of the concubines among Jacob's progeny, without thereby implying that servant-surrogacy was in any way ethically problematic. Though we may sometimes read biblical texts for contemporary edification, this should not come at the expense of imposing foreign or anachronistic modern concerns upon them.

Indeed, what I am arguing here is that if biblical texts sometimes seem to prefigure modern (or post-modern) reproductive dilemmas, this is because such dilemmas are common to many cultural settings and may inhere to some degree in the human condition. They were not created by the specific technological solutions that have been applied or debated in recent decades, and these technologies themselves may have rough analogues in different kinds of cultural and religious practices described in sacred texts. Returning to Genesis, we find that even "post-mortem" fatherhood, decried as unnatural in the French bioethics debate, makes a brief appearance in the rule of the Levirate, which requires a man whose brother has died without progeny to marry the widow and provide "seed" (i.e. sons) for the sake of his dead brother's patrilineal kin-group. The children of this arrangement are accounted the children of the dead man rather than the "donor" in biblical usage, and a brother's refusal to carry out this responsibility is considered a grave lapse in filial piety (Gen. 38). Such arrangements may seem counterintuitive to our narrowly "genetic" and literalistic conceptions of kinship in the modern West, but anthropologists have shown that Western conceptions are themselves informed by culturally salient metaphors of continuity through blood (Schneider 1980). Understanding the different ways in which reproductive and bioethical questions are framed in different settings requires among other things a clear recognition that *social* rather than just biological reproduction is almost always at stake in the way people think about these matters.

The biblical Levirate may be compared with a recent case in which Israeli courts allowed the parents of a soldier killed in Lebanon to harvest his sperm after testifying that he had wanted to become a father and that they, his bereaved parents, had no other way of becoming grandparents. Their will towards continuity through progeny in the face of death remains familiar from biblical times, although it is clear that the kinship system which made the Levirate arrangement possible no longer applies. For one thing, the erstwhile grandparents portray their desire for a son's procreation in deeply personalistic terms, as an individual desire for grandchildren rather than a social or economic need of an extended kin group. Newspaper accounts cite the family's concern with the continuity of their "line," but this has mostly symbolic significance, with none of the concrete social and economic implications of the Levirate, which also includes control over land and women. Although the boy's parents searched for a suitable "surrogate" to bear their son's child, for example, they also made it clear that they would foreswear any claims to custody or formal legal connection with the child, thus obviating the main reason offered for Levirate marriage in biblical texts—the *social* continuity of a property-holding corporate group. Neither the frustration of desire for progeny nor the willingness to explore radical reproductive strategies are in any way new to our own era, though we must exercise care in the kinds of analogies we adduce.

One of the ways to avoid an exaggerated belief in our own era's incommensurability is to insist upon shifting from a discourse of ethical, religious, and reproductive *norms* in the language of academic bioethics, to a discourse of cultural, religious, and reproductive *strategies*, in the manner of anthropologists. Strategies differ, but they are rarely incommensurate inasmuch as human beings pursue similar (though culturally inflected) goals in different settings. Surrogacy is a strategy for replacing the womb of a woman who is recognized as the mother of a child in social terms with the womb of a woman who can bear the child in biological terms. Technologies available to accomplish this goal vary, as do the social institutions that make it possible, but modern technological surrogacy and the servant-surrogacy of the Hebrew Bible are at least comparable, as are the Levirate and today's controversial post-mortem collection and delivery of sperm cells. It should be very clear that this is not an argument for the foundational authority of biblical texts or the assertion of seamless cultural and religious continuity between ancient and modern Israel. On the contrary, by insisting on the importance of speaking through and about classical texts on reproductive strategies I am arguing that these ought at least to be appreciated

as "other countries heard from" (cf. Geertz 1973), that can help us
to expand the scope of our moral imagination. Investigation into
the lives of other societies and their literature provides a necessary
counterpoint to that which is assumed to be natural and necessary
in our own. While advocates and opponents of new reproductive
technologies both seem prepared to believe that this technology
stands ready to unhinge traditional families and kinship structures,
or even to bring about "the end of the body" as we know it (cf.
Emily 1992) my experience as an anthropologist as well as a Juda-
ics scholar has conditioned me to treat such claims with caution.
Reproductive strategies have *always* been diverse, and so have the
textual hermeneutic strategies that some societies have deployed to
make sense of them.

Jews and Christians: Leviticus and Genesis

An American Orthodox rabbi with a reputation for expertise in
matters of reproductive ethics and Jewish law recently surprised his
Christian colleagues at a multi-faith academic roundtable when he
openly resisted their suggestion that the discussion of religion and
reproduction should start with consideration of texts from Genesis. Many Christian and some Jewish writers have, after all, sought
strong support in the opening chapters of Genesis for what has come
to be known as "traditional marriage"—monogamous, heterosexual, and procreative—in the language of the American culture wars.
There is no reason to deny that Jewish Orthodoxy today also holds
up this kind of marriage as an ideal, but the halachic or Jewish legal grounding for claims about permitted and forbidden reproductive practices begins not with Genesis but Leviticus, whose largely
non-narrative focus on rules of consanguinity and rules of purity
constitutes the main corpus of biblical kinship norms that underlie
later Jewish family law. This simple fact is one of the reasons that
Jewish law experts (*poskim*) have tended to be so much more favorably inclined towards artificial reproductive technologies than many
of their Christian counterparts, just as the State of Israel has been
more supportive than many other Western states. The discrepancy
between dominant Jewish and Christian approaches derives not just
from a formal normative dispute, but also from an interpretive sty-
listic one.

The single most famous Christian statement on reproductive technologies was the Catholic Church's 1987 *Donum Vitae*, or "Instruction on Respect for Human Life in Its Origins and on the Dignity

of Procreation." Authoritative for Catholics but widely influential beyond the Catholic Church, *Donum Vitae* prohibited almost all new reproductive technologies with the exception, when necessary, of homologous artificial insemination or IVF using a husband's sperm. It is important to understand the logical analysis, grounded in particular ways of reading scripture, upon which these decisions are based. "In its natural structure," writes then Cardinal Ratzinger (now Pope Benedict), "the conjugal act is a personal action, a simultaneous and immediate cooperation on the part of the husband and wife, which by the very nature of the agents and the proper nature of the act is the mutual expression of the gift which, according to the words of Scripture, brings about union 'in one flesh' (Gen. 2:24)."[1]

This observation, punctuated by a biblical proof text drawn from the story of creation, has very specific consequences for the Catholic church's view of many common reproductive technologies:

> Heterologous artificial fertilization violates the rights of the child; it deprives him of his filial relationship with his parental origins and can hinder the maturing of his personal identity . . . It brings about and manifests a rupture between genetic parenthood, gestational parenthood and responsibility for upbringing. Such damage to the personal relationships within the family has repercussions on civil society: What threatens the unity and stability of the family is a cause of dissension, disorder and injustice in the whole of social life. (cited in Shivanadan and Atkinson 2004: 125)

"Rupture" is the fundamental theme around which this whole Catholic critique is organized: rupture between genetic and gestational parenthood, rupture between the child and its embodied connection to its heritage, and rupture between the body and personhood. "One of the critical questions that lies at the heart of the debate over biotechnological procedures," write Mary Shivanadan and Joseph C. Atkinson (2004: 145) in their spirited defense of Catholic teaching, "is the precise relationship of the human person to the body." They point out that Karol Wojtyla (Pope John Paul II) was influenced by the phenomenology of Edmund Husserl (ibid.: 143), who rejected the Cartesian divide between body and self, and add that Cardinal Ratzinger was even critical of Thomas Aquinas for allegedly deemphasizing the importance of human embodiment (ibid.: 145). Artificial reproductive technologies are inimical in this view because they destroy the necessary unity between embodied relation and social identity that characterizes the "one flesh" reproductive paradigm.

Shivanadan and Atkinson (2004: 126) call this a "foundational anthropology" of human reproduction, formulated in response to the question, "[is there] an inherently intelligent design, deriving from the divine will or can [conception and reproduction] be engineered according to any given set of principles?" In the natural law paradigm they invoke, truths of scripture and of reason are meant to reinforce one another, but the specific truths of scripture are those derived from Genesis. Some Catholic writers, possibly aware of the reproductive complications we have already described with respect to the biblical families of Abraham and Jacob, go even further, circumscribing the authoritative reproductive models of Genesis to just those that can be derived from the first few chapters of the creation story, in which divine norms rather than mere "Israelite custom" are ostensibly described (Shanon and Cahill 1988). Most Jewish readers, by contrast, assume the behavior of the patriarchs and matriarchs to be worthy of emulation until proven otherwise, but one begins to see why sharing the same set of scriptures may be less important to bioethical deliberation than sharing the same set of hermeneutic practices and interpretive strategies. To the extent that Jewish writers ever cite the early chapters of Genesis in discussions of reproductive technology, it is typically with reference to the commandment to "be fruitful and multiply," which establishes a positive obligation for men (but not necessarily women) to procreate, and also establishes minimal criteria (one boy and one girl by most accounts) for its fulfillment. Whether or not a man whose wife undergoes heterologous IVF has actually fulfilled this technical reproductive requirement is an important discussion in its own right (cf. Shapiro 1979), but it is analytically distinct from the concern with "natural" reproduction raised by *Donum Vitae*.

Unlike Jewish writers, Catholic and Protestant writers who use the Bible tend to focus on what can be derived from narrative rather than legal portions of the biblical text. While Shivanadan and Atkinson, for example, do marshal some sociological data from studies of adoption to argue that children who are cut off from their embodied (i.e. genetic) heritage experience a sense of trauma and loss, the real weight of their argument against reproductive technologies is a literary one, derived from a specific, philosophically inflected reading of biblical texts. "In Hebrew thought," they write, citing the biblical scholar Pederson, ". . . the body-person is understood as the specific instantiation of all those who have preceded the body-person in his clan. This helps to explain the critical importance of the *toledoth*—the generations of the Hebrew mind . . . The individual Moabite is not a section of a number of Moabite individuals, but a revelation of Moabithood" (ibid.: 135). The practical implication they wish to draw is that children should ideally be raised by parents to whom they are biologically related, but I want to draw primary attention here to their methodological considerations. Patterns of biblical narrative are first seemingly historicized as "Hebrew-thought" before being held up as normative and universal, without reference to anything that most Jews would recognize as *halachah* or Jewish law.

The reason for this disconnect is that Jewish law tends to derive not from the open-ended narrative analysis favored by many Christian ethical writers, but from a more formal and abstract notion of discrete and bounded legal prohibitions (i.e. "Do not uncover the nakedness of your brother's wife" [Lev. 18:16]), that constitute a negative *limit* for human behavior rather than an simulacra of some positive ethical ideal. This is why the discussion of artificial reproductive technologies for Jewish writers tends to start with Leviticus rather than Genesis, and also why implications for kinship relations tend to loom so much larger than the kinds of abstract concerns evinced by the Catholic Church. Yet this is also one of the reasons that Jewish legal decisors have tended to be so much more permissive than Catholics and some Protestants with respect to artificial reproductive technologies. *Halachah* presents itself as a species of positive law that has been revealed, transmitted and elaborated in legal discourse over an extended period; it is relatively difficult to impose new prohibitions on the basis of subjective literary readings of sacred texts. Although some rabbinic writers have expressed discomfort with particular aspects of new reproductive technologies, they typically require a more definite legal basis to rule them definitively impermissible. What this really means is that it is *precisely the legalistic emphasis on discrete prohibitions that has given Jewish bioethical deliberation so much more flexibility* than that derived from narrative-based "foundational anthropology" approaches.

It has often been stated that natural law is foreign to *halachah*, and while a few writers (notably Mackler 2000 and Novack 1995) have disputed this claim, they have done so in large part by invoking those jurists who occasionally make reference to "nature" in their responses, like the late R. Eliezer Waldenman, an important *posek* (decisor) identified with the *Haredi* or ultra-Orthodox community of Jerusalem, which opposed IVF as "unnatural." Yet closer consideration of R. Waldenman's position makes it at least arguable that what really troubled him with respect to IVF were the complications of kinship categories that he foresaw, including the possibility of unwitting future incest that might arise from anonymous sperm donation. Unlike his American colleague R. Moshe Feinstein who permits IVF, furthermore, R. Waldenman presumes that the social pressure for use of this technology must come from women seeking their own reproductive goals at their husbands' expense, leading him to question whether IVF will lead to marital disharmony when men realize that they are being asked to support children who are not their own (a concern also raised by some Protestant writers—cf. Meilander 1991). The reference to IVF as "unnatural" in this context seems to express a certain visceral resistance to the potential confusion of *halachic* kinship categories and to the notion of introducing another man's "seed" into a married woman's body, but it lacks the articulate and generative force associated with Catholic natural law conceptions.

This chapter's focus on interpretive strategies in Jewish bioethical discourse is meant to qualify the often repeated claim that Israel's extraordinary acceptance of reproductive technologies can be traced primarily to sociological factors like the State's consciousness of a "demographic problem" stemming from high Arab birth rates, or the much vaunted pro-natalism (we might really call it survivalism) of post-Holocaust Jews. It would be hard to deny that these are among the factors that contribute to a broad pro-natalism in Israeli social policy (see especially Prainsack 2006), yet it would also be a mistake to underestimate the underlying religious and cultural dispositions that allow such policies to take root, especially given the strong limiting factor imposed by *halachah* upon family law in Israel. By the same token, it should be emphasized that pointing to the historical pro-natalism of Jewish law is also by itself insufficient to explain the extraordinary openness of rabbinic authorities to new reproductive technologies, which have been largely rejected by the equally pro-natal Catholic Church. We need to resist both sociological and religious reductionism in other words, by focusing on the ways in which ethical decision-making is actually embedded in habits of thought and styles of reading that may amount to cultural reflexes that transcend (without becoming wholly independent of) individual social and religious contexts. Pointing in an unsophisticated way to the traditional Jewish obligation to "be fruitful and multiply" or to the State's desire to increase its Jewish population, without demonstrating how these translate into specific hermeneutic and reproductive practices, may obscure more than it reveals.

I have pushed against the grain of anthropological studies of reproductive technology in this chapter by insisting upon careful attention to texts and their interpretation. Yet we also need to consider in an empirical way how these interpretive strategies are deployed in the shaping of local moral worlds. "Living intimately with strangers" through ethnographic research (cf. Kleinman and Seeman 1998) is probably still the best, and possibly even the only reliable tool we have for consistently evaluating what actually happens on the ground in reproductive contexts, how decisions are made, enacted, and finally understood by those who make them. In the best cases, ethnography gives rise to a kind of analytic storytelling that allows readers to access not just the cultural logic of reproduction which we have been discussing, but also the lived experience of differently placed social actors for whom something very real may be at stake in the decision to reproduce through artificial means. This two-pronged approach, based on knowledge of characteristic interpretive strategies alongside ethnographic accounts of reproduction in the real world, holds at least two benefits for contemporary bioethics discourse. First, it has the power to expand moral horizons by showing how moral problems can be construed in ways that are frequently quite different from those presumed in the academy. Yet it can also qualify those interpretive constructs by measuring them against the positioned perspectives of people within local moral worlds (including women, the poor, and other relatively disadvantaged groups), whose experience may be rendered structurally invisible to dominant local conversations about bioethics.

Reproductive technology and ethnography in Israel: what is at stake and for whom?

In her enlightening discussion of a public controversy surrounding the new reproductive technologies in Germany, Kathrin Braun (2005) has observed that this debate went far beyond the advisability of discrete practices like cloning or eugenics to touch on the very meaning of "ethics" and on the role of experts (including both biomedical experts and professional ethicists) in determining social policy. While Americans tend to imagine that bioethical debates are "structured along a line between conservative techno-skeptics on the one hand, who refer to traditional values and the Christian belief system, and liberal techno-optimists on the other, who promote a secular, individualist, rights-based approach," Braun (ibid.: 43) insists that the German debate cannot be parsed in such a neatly partisan way. "Techno-optimists" in Germany are, she argues, drawn from across the political spectrum, but they are united in their belief that "society is able, in principle, to calculate and control potential risks" created by new technology, and by their frequent portrayal of their opponents as irrational or anti-modern. "Techno-skeptics," by contrast, reject this dichotomy, but tend to argue for cautious consideration of the broad ethical and philosophical or religious implications of changes in reproductive practice. While techno-optimists tend to focus on the balancing of rights and the maximization of choice, techno-pessimists tend to focus on broad moral questions like "How can we realize basic values such as human dignity and solidarity within society?" Techno-skeptics raise concerns about the costs of human hubris, and raise troubling historical analogies like the eugenics program of the Third Reich, as a moral touchstone for what should be permitted or prohibited in contemporary biotechnological practice.

Braun also argues that optimists tend to think new biotechnologies raise mainly technical rather than philosophical dilemmas, and that these can best be managed through risk-benefit analysis performed by experts in the field of medicine or of ethics—what she calls "managerial discourse"—while pessimists tend to favor a "republican" style that prizes the deliberation of non-expert stakeholders among the educated public. Some aspects of this debate have played out in the American debate over issues like embryonic stem cell research, but here the partisan context ("liberals" vs. "neo-conservatives") tends to overshadow other considerations. The former chair of the U.S. President's Commission on Bioethics, Leon Kass, went so far as to accuse many professional bioethicists of reflexively affirming whatever choices are favored by the technological community (Kass 2005), prompting Ruth Macklin (2006) to reply that public intellectuals and journalists associated with the political right who were "until recently unknown to bioethicists" have been usurping the prerogative of experts in the field. This push and pull shows no signs of abating in the polarized American context, but Braun's analytic question has also been cast into sharp relief: What *is* bioethics, and who should be permitted to decide the terms of debate?

Managerial styles of deliberation predominate in Israel even though this is complicated by the fact that recognized "experts" include not just academic ethicists and medical professionals but also state-authorized rabbinic authorities, whose expertise in Jewish law is invoked to determine the ways in which reproductive technologies may be used. The problem with this kind of expert-driven discourse, however, is that it frequently ignores or misconstrues the variety of different stakes and stakeholders that may be affected by their decisions. In Israel, unlike Germany for example, there has been no sustained public debate about the ethics or advisability of aggressive and invasive genetic testing of fetuses with its attendant risk to fetuses and the resultant increase in social pressure to terminate pregnancies for relatively minor medical reasons. Tzipy Ivry's (2004) unprecedented comparative ethnography of reproductive genetic testing in Israel and in Japan shows how different cultural attitudes promote radically different biomedical standards and practices.

In Japan, where fetuses are described as babies almost from conception, prenatal genetic testing is typically held to a minimum, especially where potentially risky procedures like amniocentesis are involved, and the needs or desires of women (described already as "mothers") tend to be strongly mediated by notions of the welfare of the child. In Israel by contrast, fetuses are not commonly represented as babies until much later in pregnancy or even at birth and popular discourse correspondingly emphasizes female autonomy. Intensive genetic testing is at one of the highest rates for any Western country, and Ivry documents the subtle rhetorical pressures brought to bear by many genetic counselors and physicians for abortion. Neither the Japanese nor the Israeli construct should be construed as inherently unethical, but they each clearly involve ethical and social tradeoffs that are cultural rather than technological in origin. Israel has so far avoided the painful German debate over eugenics, despite the natural interest one might expect a generation of post-Holocaust Jews to show in this question, and it is worth considering whether a broader public discussion would necessarily lead to a more measured embrace of these technologies. Ivry shows how doctors and genetic counselors often deploy a frankly military language in describing the importance of invasive tests for the production of sound Israeli babies, which only reinforces the conclusion that bioethical practice may have a determinant local context despite its sometimes obfuscating claims of cultureless, scientific objectivity.

One reason for emphasizing professionalized expert discourse in Israel's fractured political landscape is that this serves as a strategy for avoiding paralyzing public debate around contentious social issues. Sue Kahn's (2000) ethnography of IVF practices in Israel demonstrates how rabbinic attitudes towards kinship and reproduction overlap sufficiently with those of medical experts and demographic policy makers to support the wide use of in vitro technology as long as certain requirements (like the use of non-Jewish sperm donors for married women) are met. Unlike those European countries that limit IVF technology to married women, Israel both permits and undertakes to pay for its use by single women as well as lesbian couples alongside married heterosexual couples. Kahn argues that since no significant disability devolves in Jewish law upon a child born out of wedlock, the use of IVF technology by single and lesbian women remains *functionally* invisible to rabbis who are concerned primarily with the prevention of technical anomalies like *mamzerut* (children born of adulterous or incestuous unions), who are subjected by Jewish law to a set of painful exclusions. Despite most rabbis' insistence on the ideal of heterosexual marriage as a precondition for parenthood in other words, their more immediate technical concern with avoiding kinship disasters like *mamzerut* while helping Jewish women to have children pushes the enforcement of this idea much lower on their list of priorities. Both rabbis and secular activists, moreover, seem to understand that they might lose more than they would gain from a protracted legal and political battle over the enforcement of a cultural value like procreation through marriage; the outcome of the struggle would be uncertain, while meanwhile both potential parties to the dispute can enjoy certain pragmatic benefits by veering away from open conflict.

A decision not to collect statistics on the kinds of individuals who seek state-sponsored IVF treatment is therefore also a pragmatic decision to avoid forcing rabbis into a corner by publicizing their de facto acquiescence in a complicated, un-orthodox social reality. Kahn deftly shows how the confluence of rabbinic and public health models at certain critical junctures (like the desire to make IVF available to Israeli women) albeit for different reasons, allows technology to flourish, and allows individuals to maximize their reproductive agency. What Israeli society loses by this strategy is however the ability to have an informed public debate about the tremendous public resources that go into providing this technology at little or no cost and the ethics of its relatively unrestricted use. Each group of experts—rabbis and public health professionals—have reason to prefer that such conversations are minimized. It took an ethnographer like Kahn to point out the cultural contradictions surrounding this issue.

Ethnographic accounts of reproductive practice almost never correspond exactly to what one would be led to expect from the theological, legal, or academic bioethical accounts that ostensibly describe and judge those practices. Jewish law maintains that Jewish status is conferred through birth from a Jewish woman's womb rather than by genetic considerations, so the Israeli religious establishment insists that gestational surrogates for Jewish women be Jewish women as well. Yet ethnographer Elly Teman (2006, 2004) has shown that neither surrogates nor commissioning mothers in Israel *ever* describe surrogate maternity in this way. Indeed, despite rabbinic assertions to the contrary, both surrogates and commissioning couples expend tremendous rhetorical energy on the dissociation of children from any sense of kinship or ongoing relation with their gestational mothers. She shows, furthermore, how this dissociation is embedded in Israeli clinical and legal practice as being psychologically, culturally, *and* bureaucratically necessary to the success of surrogacy arrangements. Rabbinic conceptions notwithstanding, both surrogates and commissioning parents make a point of describing maternity in genetic terms that allow the surrogate to be portrayed as a mere *pundakit* (host) to a child who is not "really" her own—a child she will therefore willingly part with at birth.

The anonymity of babies born to surrogates is protected in Israel by criminal statute, yet the Rabbinate, which defines maternity by birth-mother, is permitted to keep records for the prevention of possible future incest between surrogacy children and their birth siblings. At the same time, Teman shows that some commissioning parents exercise near total control of the medical care that pregnant surrogates receive, and may even serve as their intermediaries in discussions with doctors about medication. Commissioning mothers frequently attend ultrasounds and other procedures, and are encouraged by surrogates to experience "their" pregnancy as directly as possible through long telephone conversations with the surrogate, talking to the fetus, and otherwise participating in the birth process. Teman found several commissioning mothers who insisted that they experienced morning sickness, food cravings, and labor pains along with surrogates, and there have even been cases in which commissioning mothers were rolled into the delivery room along with surrogates, and then admitted to maternity while the surrogate was sent home. Surrogates are physically and legally separated from infants soon after birth and pressured by medical and other personnel to cut off contact with commissioning parents.

Ostensibly designed to prevent custody disputes and to ensure a quick severing of the presumed emotional bonds between birth mother and child, these bureaucratic practices also emerge in Teman's fine ethnography as a set of techniques for the suppression of cultural anomaly and categorical confusion, which might have been treated as "matter out of place" or ritual impurity (Douglas 1966) in a society that lacked the fine bureaucratic apparatus available to contemporary Israelis (cf. Herzfeld 1992). While some individuals do resist this bureaucratic restructuring of experience however, they do so in ways that might be surprising to readers of academic theoretical literature. Rather than expressing regret or turmoil over the relinquishing of a child they have birthed, or concern over the exploitation ("colonization") of their bodies by commissioning families, for example, those surrogates who expressed conflict did so with respect to the severing of their own relationships *with commissioning parents* that they had come to think of as their own families or "sisters" during pregnancy. Teman is correct to distance herself from critiques of surrogacy grounded in feminist concern with women's agency, given most Israeli surrogates' enthusiastic endorsement of their own choices, but her work raises other kinds of ethical problems that are rarely if ever dealt with in current bioethical discourse, like the grief felt for the loss of sisterly companionship at the end of the surrogate agreement, for which some surrogates were ill-prepared.

Something is invariably at stake for participants in assisted reproduction, but those stakes vary from context to context, from one style of ethical hermeneutic to another, and from one positioned engagement to another—and they can only be detailed empirically. Sometimes, as in the case of IVF and surrogacy in Israel, imperatives experienced in different ways by differently positioned social actors can overlap in ways that create realities which never could have been predicted in the abstract. Orthodox rabbis, state planners, public health experts and advocates for single or lesbian women may all agree, for a time, to support free public access to a reproductive technology such as IVF for different reasons, leading to a useful though potentially unstable political alliance. Surrogacy, similarly, may exist and flourish in the interstices of understanding between commissioning mothers, surrogates themselves, and the medical and rabbinic establishments. Understanding cases such as these requires a willingness to forgo simplistic or unitary explanations of social practice and to grapple with the complicated meanings underlying complex human choices. Like ethnography, deeper appreciation for a classical textual tradition can also contribute to this goal by underscoring the multiplicity of possible readings and ethical alternatives available to a reader.

Consider the reproductive leitmotif that informs the biblical book of Ruth. In this story a childless Moabite woman named Ruth forswears the land and house of her father and embraces poverty in order to follow Naomi, the mother of her dead Israelite husband, back to the land of Israel. Eventually, Ruth marries a kinsman of her dead husband named Boaz and bears him a son—a son who will be counted to her dead husband's patriline. Often read in popular culture as an endearing love story, some feminist readers depict Ruth as a story about solidarity between women, despite the ethnic and family divisions that threaten to tear them apart. Classical rabbinic readings view Ruth's trajectory as a paradigm of disinterested religious conversion to Judaism, and even use her words to her mother-in-law—"Whither thou goest I shall go . . . your people shall be my people and your God my God"—as a site for the derivation of laws about conversion practice (Zohar and Sagi 1994; Seeman 2003). Yet the anthropologist cannot help but read this story also in light of the partilineal politics that suffuse most of the Bible's historical books from Deuteronomy to Second Kings (Seeman 2004). For ancient readers, Ruth's heroism would have consisted primarily in her willingness to bear "seed" for her dead husband even though she was not, as a Moabite widow, required to do so. Her love and commitment to Naomi support this deeper structural goal of the narrative leading to the birth and rise of King David. Ruth's role in the redemption of her husband's hereditary land and seed through marriage to his kinsman are the reproductive themes that drive this whole biblical narrative forward.

We have thus come full circle, from a discussion of the ways in which narrative helps to shape reproductive ethics to some of the ways in which reproductive ethics may help to shape narrative, but the point in each case is similar. Good literature and good ethnography each make us more aware of the moral ambiguities and subtle leitmotifs as well as grand cultural narratives and power structures in which reproductive choices are made. They should be thought of as complimentary prisms upon a reality that is more complex than any single descriptive or literary account can accommodate.

Conclusion: expanding the conversation about bioethics and reproductive technology

"Republican discourse" advocates in places like Germany and the United States continue to try to frame conversations about reproductive technology in terms of "big questions" like what it means to be human or how we might lose a measure of our humanity through misguided technological choices. The "fear of the loss of the human" (Kleinman 1998) is perhaps pervasive in our society precisely because of the disordering effects of innovations like biotechnology. Yet neither republican discourse advocates nor those who prefer a more managerial style have yet undertaken the disciplined and rigorous exploration of both cultural categories and lived experience of those who actually make use of this technology. Expanding the empirical parameters of what is at stake in bioethical discourse would mean attending not just to the question of what is "natural" or cost effective, but also to the possibility of completely different configurations of the problem that emerge when different interpretive paradigms (like those of Jewish or Muslim law for example) are also juxtaposed. The Israeli example should be of great interest to bioethics everywhere because of the unique ways in which a distinctive tradition of discourse and adjudication have been brought to bear in ways that differ considerably from dominant Euro-American models of ethical deliberation. What used to be known as "Western medicine" is now no more at home in the West than it is in Israel, India, or Japan, and each of these contexts shapes the ways in which ostensibly universal technologies like IVF or surrogacy are practiced and understood. When we learn to think of this diversity as a resource for comparative deliberation, it will become clear that what happens in Israel should be of concern to North Americans at least as much as North American paradigms have mattered in recent decades to countries like Israel and Japan.

It should be possible within the overlapping (but not identical) spheres of Israeli and Jewish bioethics to expand many ethical conversations beyond their current limits. We might imagine a reinvigorated bioethical discourse that takes into account not just rabbinic concerns with lineage and kinship categories, or philosophical concerns with free agency and informed consent, but also a broader grappling with the kinds of social and experiential issues raised empirically through ethnographic research—like the implicit expectation of intimacy and gratitude held by many surrogates, and the disappointment or resentment encountered when these are not met. With respect to IVF, this might mean reopening the question of how public resources are apportioned and what social ills may be fostered through unrestricted access even to very useful technologies. Are young ultra-Orthodox women being pressured by their communities to resort to artificial reproductive technologies very early in their marriages because of relative ease of access and the demand for many children? If so, does this pose an ethical concern distinct from those that have been posed in other settings, or demand different kinds of sensitivities from those who seek to address it? Medical anthropology is not yet well-developed in Israeli universities, but as the field grows, we can expect that more of these positioned realities will be made visible to analysis through ethnographic research.

One final example I would like to mention involves the potential of reproductive cloning, which is likely to become more significant as a topic of public debate as technology improves and medical/technical risks and barriers diminish over time. A near consensus in the bioethical community today is that this practice should not be permitted. Thus, the Catholic Church, the World Council of Churches, the Methodist Church, and the United Church of Christ have all adopted formal policies opposed on ethical grounds to the eventuality of human cloning, and the President's Council on Bioethics in the United States issued a nearly unanimous report to support a federal ban on research in this area. The two dissenting members of the Council were both Jewish writers who took the view that while technical objections to human cloning were currently valid, broad philosophical objections to "playing God" or to "meddling in nature" were misplaced. As in other areas of reproductive ethics and new reproductive technologies, these and other writers (Breitowitz 2002; Broyde 1998, 2001, 2005) have taken the view that once technology makes it feasible, cloning could in principle be regulated to avoid the specific prohibitions and kinship problems that are of concern to Jewish law (who, if anyone, are the *halachic* parents of a cloned person?) without necessarily compromising values like the dignity and uniqueness of individuals. This case constitutes one more piece of evidence that the lack of an overriding concern with "nature" or natural law in rabbinic jurisprudence can make *halachah* eminently more flexible than some other forms of ethical deliberation when it comes to new reproductive technologies. One author (Broyde 2004) titled an article for a popular audience on this topic provocatively, "In Judaism, Playing God is Good."

Elsewhere, the same author (Broyde 2005) simply dismisses concerns about the human dignity of clones by noting that Jewish law would recognize a cloned human being *prima facie* as a person subject to the same rights and responsibilities as any other person, so that the question of his or her humanity need never arise. These are not merely speculative concerns either, as the State of Israel is today one of the very few countries that has not outlawed state funded research of human cloning, a situation explored with some alarm by Prainsack (2006). Contemporary rabbis tend to be "techno-optimists" in the terms of Braun's comparison. Yet even the most ardent techno-optimist should be able to acknowledge that problems may arise which technical experts have failed to foresee. And while this alone cannot serve as a basis for the prohibition of potentially life-enhancing new reproductive technologies, wisdom should indicate that any conversation about the advisability of new technologies should include multiple voices and perspectives. For now, Jewish and Israeli perspectives on cloning act as an important moral counterweight to attitudes that are seemingly shaped more strongly by visceral distaste and a vague sense of "nature" than by closely reasoned argument. The freedoms of Leviticus, it turns out, may be more conducive to medical technology and assisted reproduction than the constraints of Genesis. Yet caution is in order. We have learned that no moral system can see around every corner, and that every hermeneutic style fosters characteristic blind spots along with distinctive capacities for moral vision. Ethics cannot be reduced to a purely technical craft so long as moral interpretation and human experience remain decisively open-ended.

Note

1. This passage from *Donum Vitae* is actually a quote from Pope Pius XII's Discourse to the Italian Catholic Union of Midwives, delivered in 1951. I am citing from the appendix to Shannon and Cahill (1988: 166).

References

Adams, Alice. 1993. "Out of the Womb: The Future of the Uterine Metaphor," *Feminist Studies* 19: 269–89.

Ball, Nan T. 2000. "The Reemergence of Enlightenment Ideas in the 1994 French Bioethics Debates." *Duke Law Journal* 50: 545–87.

Bhattacharyya, Swasti. 2006. *Magical Progeny, Modern Technology: A Hindu Bioethics of Assisted Reproductive Technology.* Albany: State University of New York Press.

Braun, Kathrin. 2005. "Not Just for Experts: The Public Debate about Reprogenetics in Germany." *Hastings Center Report* 35 (May-June): 42–49.

Breitowitz, Yitzchok. 2002. "What's So Bad about Human Cloning?" *Kennedy Institute of Ethics Journal* 12, no. 4: 325–41.

Broyde, Michael J. 2005. "Modern Reproductive Technologies and Jewish Law," in *Marriage, Sex and the Family in Judaism*, eds. Michael J. Broyde and Michael Ausubel. New York: Rowman and Littlefield: 295–328.

———. 2004. "In Judaism, Playing God is Good," *Voices Across Boundaries* (Winter 2003–2004).

———. 2001. "Cloning and the Noahide Legal Code," *The Torah U-Madda Journal* 9: 207–11.

———. 1998. "Cloning People: A Jewish View," *Connecticut Law Review* 30: 2503–35.

Douglas, Mary. 1966. *Purity and Danger.* New York: Ark Paperbooks.

Geertz, Clifford. 1973. *The Interpretation of Cultures.* Boston: Basic Books.

Hauk, Christina. 2003. "Abortion and the Individual Talent," *ELH* 70: 233–66.

Herzfeld, Michael. 1992. *The Social Production of Indifference: Exploring the Symbolic Roots of Western Bureaucracy.* Chicago: University of Chicago Press.

Ivry, Tsipy. 2006. "At the Back Stage of Prenatal Care: Japanese Ob-Gyns Negotiating Prenatal Diagnosis," *Medical Anthropology Quarterly* 20: 441–68.

———. 2004. "Pregnant With Meaning: Conceptions of Pregnancy in Japan and Israel" (Ph.D. dissertation, the Hebrew University of Israel).

Kass, Leon. 2005. "Reflections on Public Bioethics: A View from the Trenches," *Kennedy Institute of Ethics Journal* 15: 221–50.

Kannaneh, Rhoda. 2002. *Birthing the Nation: Strategies of Palestinian Women in Israel.* Berkeley: University of California Press.

Kahn, Susan Martha. 2000. *Reproducing Jews: A Cultural Account of Assisted Conception in Israel.* Durham: Duke University Press.

Kleinman, Arthur. 1997. "Everything that Really Matters: Social Suffering, Subjectivity, and the Remaking of Human Experience in a Disordering World," *Harvard Theological Review* 90: 315–36.

Kleinman, Arthur and Don Seeman. 1998. "The Politics of Moral Practice in Psychotherapy and Religious Healing," *Contributions to Indian Sociology* 32, no. 2: 237–50.

LaCocque, André and Paul Ricoeur. 1998. *Thinking Biblically: Exegetical and Hermeneutical Studies*, trans. David Pellauer. Chicago: University of Chicago Press.

Mackler, Aaron L. 2001. "Jewish and Roman Catholic Approaches to Access to Health Care Rationing," *Kennedy Institute of Ethics Journal* 11, no. 4: 317–36.

———. 2003. *Introduction to Jewish and Catholic Bioethics: A Comparative Analysis*. Washington, D.C.: Georgetown University Press.

Macklin, Ruth. 2006. "The New Conservatives in Bioethics: Who are they and what do they seek?" *Hastings Center Report* 36 (January-February): 34–43.

Martin, Emily. 1992. "The End of the Body?" *American Ethnologist* 19: 121–38.

Meilander, Gilbert. 1991. "New Reproductive Technologies: Protestant Modes of Thought," *Creighton Law Review* 25: 1637–46.

McColley, Dawn. 1991. "A Biblical Response to Baby-Making: Surrogacy, Artificial Insemination, *In Vitro* Fertilization and Embryo Transfer," *Journal of Biblical Ethics in Medicine* 5, no. 3: 45–48.

McCormick, Richard A. 1991. "Surrogacy: A Catholic Perspective," *Creighton Law Review* 25: 1617–25.

Novack, David. 1995. "Natural Law, *Halachah* and the Covenant," in *Contemporary Jewish Ethics and Morality*, eds. Elliot Dorf and Louis E. Newman. Oxford: Oxford University Press.

Parks, Jennifer A. 1999. "On the Use of IVF by Post-Menopausal Women," *Hypatia* 14: 77–96.

Prainsack, Barbara. 2006. "Negotiating Life: The Regulation of Human Cloning and Embryonic Stem Cell Research in Israel," *Social Studies of Science* 136: 173–205.

Rothman, Barbara Katz. 1991. "Reproductive Technologies and Surrogacy: A Feminist Perspective," *Creighton Law Review* 25: 1599–1607.

Schneider, David. 1980. *American Kinship: A Cultural Account*. Chicago: University of Chicago Press.

Seeman, Don. 2004. "The Watcher at the Window: Cultural Poetics of a Biblical Motif," *Prooftexts* 24: 1–50.

———. 2003. "Agency, Bureaucracy and Religious Conversion: Ethiopian 'Feleshmura' Immigrants to Israel," in *The Anthropology of Religious Conversion*, eds. Andrew S. Buckser and Steven Glazier. London: Rowman and Littlefield: 29–42.

———. 1999. "Subjectivity, Culture, Life-World: An Appraisal," *Transcultural Psychiatry* 36: 437–45.

———. 1998. "Where is Sarah Your Wife? Cultural Poetics of Gender and Nationhood in the Hebrew Bible," *Harvard Theological Review* 91, no. 2: 103–25.

Shanon, Thomas A. and Lisa Sowle Cahill. 1988. *Religion and Artificial Reproduction: An Inquiry into the Vatican "Instruction on Respect for Human Life in its Origin and on the Dignity of Reproduction."* New York: Crossroad.

Shapiro, David S. 1979. "Be Fruitful and Multiply," in *Jewish Bioethics*, eds. Fred Rosner and J. David Bleich. New York: Sanhedrin Press: 59–79.

Shivanadan, Mary and Joseph C. Atkinson. 2004. "Person as Substantive Relation and Reproductive Technologies: Biblical and Philosophical Foundations," *Logos* 7: 124–56.

Speiser, E.A. 1964. *Genesis: translated with an introduction and notes* (Anchor Bible 1). New York: Doubleday.

Storey, Grayce P. 2000. "Ethical Problems Surrounding Surrogate Motherhood," in *Yale-New Haven Teacher's Institute*, vol. VII (Bioethics). <http://www.yale.edu/ynhti/curriculum/units/2000/7/00.07.05.x.html> (accessed 10 February, 2009).

Teman, Elly. 2006. "The Birth of a Mother: Mythologies of Surrogate Motherhood in Israel" (PhD. thesis, Hebrew University).

———. 2003. "The Medicalization of Nature in the Artificial Body: Surrogate Motherhood in Israel," *Medical Anthropology Quaterly* 17, no. 1: 78–98.

———. 2003a. "Knowing the Surrogate Body in Israel," in *Surrogate Motherhood: International Perspectives*, eds. R. Cook, S.D. Sclater and F. Kaganas. Portland: Hart Press: 261–81.

———. 2001. "Technological Fragmentation and Women's Empowerment: Surrogate Motherhood in Israel," *Women's Studies Quarterly* 29: 11–34.

Zohar, Tzvi and Avi Sagi. 1994. *Conversion and Jewish Identity* [Hebrew]. Jerusalem: Bialik Institute.

Notes on Contributors

Gali Ben-Or is a lawyer working as a senior director in the Legal Advice and Legislation Department in the Ministry of Justice of Israel. She is in charge of legal advice and legislation in genetics, cloning, genetic databases, surrogacy, IVF, posthumous reproduction, forensic databases, administrative courts and judicial reviews. Ben-Or was a member of the Intergovernmental Team on the establishment of the National Council on Bioethics and took part in the legislation processes of the Israeli surrogacy law, the prohibition of cloning law, genetic information law, forensic database law, and more. For several years, she was a member of the Bioethics Advisory Committee of the Israel Academy of Science and Humanities.

Daphna Birenbaum-Carmeli is a medical sociologist in the Department of Nursing at the University of Haifa, Israel. Studying women's health in contexts of advanced medical technologies, her research focuses on procreative medicine. Birenbaum-Carmeli's main field of inquiry is Israel, where she has investigated health policy, medical practice, consumers' perceptions and behavior in matters of fertility treatments and reproductive choice. She is the author of *Tel Aviv North: The Making of the New Israeli Middle Class* (2000, Hebrew University Press) and primary editor of *Assisting Reproduction, Testing Genes: Global Encounters with New Biotechnologies* (2009, Berghahn).

Yoram S. Carmeli is an anthropologist at the Department of Sociology and Anthropology at the University of Haifa. His Ph.D. (UCL) and much of his subsequent research and publications focus on the British circus, its history, economics, and symbolic aspects. The circus serves as a vantage point for the study of modernity as well as post modern phenomena. Carmeli has also studied popular culture and consumption in Israel and has collaborated with Daphna Birenbaum-Carmeli in studies of new reproductive technologies.

Martha Dirnfeld is an expert in gynecology, director of the Reproductive Endocrinology–IVF Division in Carmel Medical Centre, Haifa and is an associate Professor in the Faculty of Medicine, Technion, Israel Institute of Technology, Haifa, Israel.

Yali Hashash is a Ph.D. candidate at the Jewish History department, University of Haifa. Her current research focuses on the social history and political thought of the Sephardi and Mizrahi Jews in Palestine in the 19th century. Her M.A. thesis analyzed Israel's reproductive policy in the years 1962 to 1974, and the interplay between class, gender, and ethnicity in formulating a natality policy that would benefit affluent westernized families in Israel.

Yael Hashiloni-Dolev is a sociologist of reproductive technologies in the College of Tel Aviv-Yaffo, and the author of: *What is a Life (un)Worthy of Living? Reproductive Genetics in Israel and Germany* (2007, Springer-Kluwer). Hashiloni Dolev is currently studying the issues of sex selection, fertility awareness and egg freezing.

Helene Goldberg is an anthropologist affiliated with the Department of Health Development, Guldborgsund, Denmark. Her former research explored issues of masculinity, kinship and sexuality, and her work on male infertility in Israel won several prizes. With Inhorn, Tjørnhøj-Thomsen and Mosegaard she edited the recent volume *Reconceiving the second sex: Men, Masculinity and Reproduction* (2009, Berghahn Books), and with Mosegaard she co-authored the children's book *Slottet med de mange værelser* (2008' Turbineforlaget), which explores the various ways children come into being today. At present, she conducts applied research and develops public health programmes.

Tsipy Ivry is a medical anthropologist working on themes of reproductive technologies in diverse socio-cultural settings. Her major work compares medical, popular, and personal conceptions of pregnancy in Japan and Israel and is based on fieldwork in medical institutions in both countries. She is the author of *EmbodyingCulture: Pregnancy in Japan and Israel* (2010, Rutgers University Press). Currently, Ivry studies the politics of assisted reproductive technologies in communities of observant Jews in Israel.

Susan Martha Kahn is the Associate Director of the Center for Middle Eastern Studies at Harvard University and a Lecturer in the Department of Near Eastern Languages and Literatures. She received her M.A. in Middle Eastern Studies and Ph.D. in Social

Anthropology from Harvard University. Her book, *Reproducing Jews: A Cultural Account of Assisted Conception in Israel* (Duke 2000) won a National Jewish Book Award, as well as the 2001 Eileen Basker Memorial Prize, awarded by the Society of Medical Anthropology. She is currently working on an environmental history of canines in the Levant from ancient times to the present.

Roy Mashiach is a Specialist in ObGyn at the Sheba Medical Center, Ramat Gan, Israel. He is Head of Gynecologic endoscopic training at the Israeli center for medical simulation. Dr. Mashiach has published extensively in the field of gynecological surgery and infertility.

Shlomo Mashiach is an expert in obstetrics and gynecology. His main fields of interest are advanced reproductive technology and gynecological endoscopy. Mashiach was the director of the Department of Obstetrics and Gynecology at the Sheba Medical Center, and a professor at Tel Aviv University School of Medicine. He was president of the Israel Society for Reproductive Research and of the Israel Society of Obstetrics and Gynecology and has been awarded international and Israeli prizes for his work. At present, he heads the IVF Department at Assuta Medical Centre, Tel Aviv.

Barbara Prainsack is Reader at the Centre for Biomedicine & Society at King's College London, UK. Her work examines the ways in which science, politics, and religion constitute each other, and how they affect understandings of personhood and citizenship. Together with Richard Hindmarsh she is the editor of *Genetic Suspects: Global Governance of Forensic DNA Profiling and Databasing* (2010, Cambridge University Press). Barbara is also a member of the Austrian National Bioethics Commission.

Vardit Ravitsky is a bioethicist trained in philosophy at the Sorbonne University in Paris, the University of New Mexico in Albuquerque, and Bar Ilan University in Israel. Previously a post-doctoral fellow at the Department of Clinical Bioethics at the National Institutes of Health (NIH) and faculty at the Center for Bioethics of the University of Pennsylvania, Ravitsky is presently an assistant professor at the Faculty of Medicine of the University of Montreal. Her main research interests are ethical aspects of human genetics and reproduction.

Aviad E. Raz is Professor of Sociology and Anthropology at Ben-Gurion University, Israel, where he is also the Director of the Program in Behavioral Sciences. His recent research focuses on social and bioethical aspects of genetic risk and responsibility. He has recently published a monograph on this issue, entitled *Community Genetics and Genetic Alliances: Eugenics, Carrier Testing, and Networks of Risk* (2010, Routledge). Raz has also conducted research and published extensively in the field of organizational culture and medical organizations.

Larissa Remennick is Professor of Sociology and Chair of the Department of Sociology & Anthropology at Bar-Ilan University, Israel. She was born and educated in Moscow, Russia where she holds a Ph.D. in medical sociology and demography from the Russian Academy of Sciences, 1988, and in the U.K., where she had a post-doctoral fellowship at Oxford University in 1989. She moved to Israel in 1991 and since 1994 has worked at Bar-Ilan. Her research interests include sociology of immigration, ethnicity and multiculturalism, sociology of women's health, and the politics of fertility and reproduction. She has published over 40 articles and book chapters in these areas of research.

Nitzan Rimon-Zarfaty is a Ph.D. candidate at the Department of Sociology and Anthropology, Ben-Gurion University, Israel. Her current research centers on the influence of new medical technologies in the beginning of life (PGD, PND, and in-uterus treatments of fetuses) on perceptions of the unborn/preborn "fetus" and prospective of "parenthood" among Israeli parents.

Don Seeman is Associate Professor in the Department of Religion and the Tam Institute for Jewish Studies at Emory University. He is a medical anthropologist and anthropologist of religion who currently chairs the PhD program in Jewish Religious Cultures, combining textual and ethnographic methods. He is author of *One People, One Blood: Ethiopian-Israelis and the Return to Judaism* (2009, Rutgers University Press) as well as numerous articles in medical and psychological anthropology, ritual theory, and Jewish thought. Seeman currently leads a team of ethnographers who work with public health specialists studying the role of religion in the reproductive agency of poor American women.

Shiri Shkedi has earned a B.Sc. MED in Basic Medical Sciences, and her M.MED Sc. in Genetics and Human Genetics from The Hebrew University, Israel. Since 2003 she has been a practicing genetic counselor in Israel. Ms. Shkedi is a Ph.D. student at The Hebrew University, with the collaboration of The Centre for Biomedicine &

Society (CBS), King's College, London. Her dissertation focuses on the impact of being diagnosed as a carrier of an altered susceptibility gene on notions of "self" and identity.

Gil Siegal (MD, LLB, SJD) is a surgeon and a health law professor at the University of Virginia School of Law, USA, and Kiryat Ono College, Israel, where he directs the Center for Health Law and Bioethics. In addition, Dr. Siegal serves as a member of the National Committee for Genetic Research in Humans, National Comittee for Non-Medical Sex Selection, and is a member of the National Advisory Committee on Genetic Information. His areas of expertise are biotechnology, patients' rights, and comparative medical ethics.

Elly Teman is a research fellow at the Penn Center for Integration of Genetic Healthcare Technologies at the University of Pennsylvania. She holds a PhD in anthropology from the Hebrew University. Dr. Teman's areas of interest are the anthropology of reproduction, medical anthropology and Jewish folklore. Her ethnography of gestational surrogacy, *Birthing a Mother: the Surrogate Body and the Pregnant Self* (2010, University of California Press) explores how Israeli surrogates and intended mothers negotiate their cooperative endeavor.

Abortion 2, 8, 10, 16, 25, 28, 29,
  30, 33, 34, 38, 54, 61, 121, 122,
  154, 156, 158, 159, 166, 157–
  180, 186, 188, 190, 193–194,
  196, 202–221, 227, 241, 273,
  278–281
Adoption 16, 21, 23, 24, 92, 93, 96,
  116, 117, 127–144
Adultery 93, 94, 206, 298
Amniocentesis 2, 26, 53, 54, 181,
  198, 211, 213, 214, 353
Animals 2, 52–53, 56, 229, 232,
  233, 234
Anxiety 28, 108, 175–176, 187,
  190, 192–193, 195
Arabs 4, 12, 177, 231, 268, 271,
  274, 318–338, 350
Artificial Insemination, *See* Dona-
  tion, sperm
Ashkenazi Jews 10–13, 16, 121,
  154, 162, 168, 230, 275, 304
Autonomy
Female 334, 353
Fetal 207
Human 77, 79, 168
Professional 272, 278, 283, 289

Bilateral relatedness 85, 86, 88, 93,
  94, 98
Bioethics 63, 64, 68, 69, 73, 74, 79,
  153, 168, 203, 206, 227, 236,
  238, 240, 245, 259, 264–267,
  282, 285, 288, 316, 341–359

Childlessness 6, 97, 110, 321–335
Christian 3, 8, 9, 140, 141, 260,
  282, 342, 342, 346, 349, 351
Cloning 34, 68, 226–249, 259, 267,
  269, 273, 282–289, 292, 351,
  358–359
Committees
  Abortion committee 8, 122, 154,
    202–222, 280
  Bioethics Advisory Committee of
    the Israel Academy of Sciences
    and Humanities 227, 259, 264
  Committee of Ministers on Legis-
    lation 230
  Committee for Examining Prohibi-
    tions on Abortion (CEPA) 279
  Expert committees 58, 59, 259, 286
  Natality Committee 275–276, 279
  PGD committee 36, 64, 68–72,
    76, 79
  Science and Technology Knes-
    set Committee 27, 64, 65, 76,
    228, 230–245, 282–283, 285,
    286–288
  Stem cells Committee 261
  Supreme Helsinki Committee
    284, 285

Surrogacy Committee 108–115,
    120
Confidentiality, *See* secrecy
Consumers'
    Characteristics 25
    Interests 21
    Attitudes 22, 24, 31
Consumerism 25, 30, 174, 179,
    189, 191, 195, 318–338
Contraception 8, 10, 132, 212,
    273–278, 280, 290, 292

Discrimination
    Disabled 205
    Genetic 158, 167, 236, 239, 242,
        247
    Social 13, 277, 328
Doctors 22, 23, 25, 30, 35, 51–59,
    87, 88–97, 101–103, 109, 175,
    179, 185, 190, 193, 196, 209–
    210, 217, 235, 257, 271–293,
    296–317
Demography politics and ideology
    3,4,6,8,25, 30, 113, 117, 196,
    203, 271, 274–276, 282, 290,
    319, 324, 325, 331, 333, 337,
    350, 353
Descent *see* kinship *and* relatedness
Disability 27, 66, 68, 153, 155, 178,
    184, 186–192, 198, 205, 211,
    217–219, 319
Donation
Sperm 84–99, 113, 117, 142, 297,
    302, 347, 349, 353
Egg 17, 22, 24, 37, 57, 111, 112,
    116, 117, 129, 142, 273, 282,
    292, 293, 302, 304, 332
Dor Yeshorim (DY) 25, 26, 33,
    156–170
Down Syndrom 27, 167, 178, 179,
    215
Egg / ova / oocyte 6, 37, 52, 58, 89,
    94, 99, 100, 101, 123, 248, 255,
    265, 266, 269, 297–316

Embryo
    Embryo transfer 20, 123, 197,
        199, 297, 304, 307–308, 315

Embryo-related policies 66–67,
    114, 123, 228, 233, 240
Embryo testing 61–79, 97, 103,
    154
Human embryonic stem cells
    23, 34, 36, 58, 226, 228, 240,
    255–269, 282–288, 352
Human status 28, 34, 62–63, 197,
    226, 227, 228, 242
Embryopathy 33, 34, 203–222
    Mild or Likely 202–205, 207–219
    England / UK 5, 14, 27, 32, 38,
        56, 64–67, 70–71, 74, 77, 79,
        112, 130, 131, 132, 157, 211,
        217, 218, 237, 259, 260–263
    Eugenics 29, 33, 62, 202–203,
        211–214, 217–219, 274, 281,
        351, 352, 353

Family planning, *See* contraception
Fatherhood 6, 84–103, 114, 123,
    138, 212, 303, 344–346
    Genetic fatherhood 22, 36, 76,
        111
Fetus, *See* embryo

Genetic
    Counsellors 28, 29, 34, 153, 154,
        158, 163, 164, 204–205, 208,
        215, 217–219, 222, 281, 353
    Couplehood 31, 33, 156–157,
        166, 169
    Discrimination 158, 167, 236,
        239, 242, 247
    Information Law (Israel) 154,
        236
    Risk 28, 30, 33, 61, 62, 64,
        66–70, 73–74, 78, 79, 97, 111,
        156–160, 180, 212, 216, 217,
        279
Genetic Testing
    Population screening 154
    Preconception 26, 157–160
    Preimplantation (PGD) 2, 27, 32,
        36, 58, 61–83, 97, 103, 154,
        212, 258
    Premarital 1, 30, 33, 157, 159,
        161, 163, 164, 166

Prenatal Diagnosis 202–208, 211–212, 215, 217–219
Germany 5, 14, 15, 27, 32, 38, 51, 52, 64, 65, 67–72, 76–77, 79, 130, 131, 153, 233, 351, 352, 357

Haredi / orthodox / Ultra-orthodox Jews 9–11, 13, 25, 26, 29–30, 33, 36, 89, 91, 93, 97, 101, 103, 105, 141, 153–173, 182, 195, 227, 231, 311, 346, 349, 354, 356, 358
halachah 6, 28, 86, 102, 111, 115, 123, 155, 156, 170, 222, 230, 238, 248, 259, 304, 313, 342, 346, 349, 350, 359
Health care system / *Kupat Holim* 275, 279, 291
Holocaust 6,7, 23, 24, 195, 230, 350, 353
Homosexual 108, 112, 116, 119, 128, 129
Human embryonic Stem cell research 23, 34, 36, 58, 226, 228, 240, 255–269, 282–288, 352

ICSI (Intra Cytoplasmic Sperm Injection) 1, 17, 20, 24, 58, 87, 91, 94, 100, 102, 116
Immigration / immigrants 8, 31, 54, 55, 139, 140, 141, 163, 275, 280
Ethiopian 140, 275
Former Soviet Union 10, 11, 17, 36, 320–338
Oriental/Mizrahi 12, 121, 275, 277, 304, 306, 363
Incest 111, 206, 279, 349, 353, 355
Infertility 16, 18, 21, 25, 111, 112, 128, 287, 313, 315, 334–336
Male 1, 7, 22, 58, 84, 106
Female 52, 54, 55, 56
In vitro fertilization 1, 2, 17–25, 27, 33–35, 37, 56–57, 61, 68, 73, 74, 87, 90–92, 95, 97, 100, 102, 103, 111, 113, 116–118, 123, 128, 129, 132, 140–142, 177, 198, 199, 255–259, 265, 266,

282, 286, 296–317, 320–323, 326–337, 340, 341, 347–350, 353–354, 356, 358
Islam 122, 260, 264, 267–269
Israeli Medical Association 273, 290

Jewish *halachah, see halachah*

Knesset (Israeli Parliament) 22, 37, 108–110, 114–116, 134, 135, 229–249, 268, 282, 283, 288, 291

Laboratory technicians 296–317

Wrongful birth 209, 213, 218

Marriage 5, 12, 25, 138, 139, 156–160, 166, 321, 345–346, 353–354, 357, 358
Arranged 156, 159
Mamzerut (bastardism) 93, 111, 353, 354
Masculinity / manhood 22, 86, 335
Masturbation 90–92, 185
Match-making (Hebr. *Shiduch*), *See* Arranged marriage
Maternity 6, 99, 117–119, 181, 191, 328, 355
Maternity care 277
Maternity leave 7, 14, 15, 135
Matrilineal 6, 85, 86
Medicalization 35, 101, 107, 160, 204, 271–274, 277–278, 280, 288, 319
Ministry of Health (Israel) 12, 24, 55, 64, 68–69, 73, 97, 102, 103, 109, 179, 202, 209, 210, 234, 236–238, 240, 243–246
Motherhood 6, 21, 22, 75, 86, 99, 107, 108, 110, 113–118, 121, 122, 319, 323–228
Multiple birth 18, 20, 129
Muslim / Islam 3, 8, 9, 54, 93, 111, 121, 143, 231, 260, 264, 267, 268, 269, 325, 328, 332–336, 343, 357

National Health Insurance Law 154, 178

Natural Law 341, 348–350, 359
Nazism 3, 37, 51, 55, 138

Oriental Jews 9, 11, 12, 13, 16,
    121, 275

Palestinians 3, 4, 36, 139, 271, 303,
    304, 310, 311, 325, 330, 333, 337
Parenthood 8, 16, 21, 31, 111, 122,
    277, 278, 354
    Biogenetic– 32, 347
    Responsible parenthood 211, 218
    Right to parenthood 19, 114,
        327–329, 337
Paternity 2, 6, 93, 100, 102, 153, 341
Patrilineal 84–86, 93, 94, 97, 98,
    100, 344
PGD (preimplantation genetic diag-
    nosis) 2, 27, 32, 36, 58, 61–83,
    97, 103, 154, 212, 258
Post mortem sperm aspiration 19,
    141, 341, 344, 345
Poverty 10, 12, 13, 14, 16, 31, 276,
    277, 284, 344, 351, 356
Pre-embryo 61–79, 103, 116
Prenatal (fetal) Diagnosis 202–208,
    211–212, 215, 217–219
Privatization of reproduction / par-
    enting 319, 336, 337
Pronatalism 6–16, 21–24, 33, 34,
    108, 115, 120, 121, 194, 196,
    271, 274, 282, 291

Rabbis 6, 55, 86, 87, 91–93, 99,
    100, 101, 102, 105, 110, 111,
    115, 117, 120, 138, 157, 158,
    159, 170, 198, 222, 229, 230,
    232, 238, 248, 303, 304, 307,
    346, 349, 350, 352–359
Relatedness, *see* kinship
Religious authorities (Jewish) 161,
    259, 340
Risk
    Genetic 28, 30, 33, 61, 62, 64,
        66–70, 73–74, 78, 79, 97, 111,
        156–160, 180, 212, 216, 217,
        279

IVF-related 18, 19, 21–22, 319,
    323
Legal 180
Oocyte-donation related 286,
    292
Pregnancy-related 179, 180,
    279

Secrecy 24, 98, 112, 117
Self-determination 165, 167, 168,
    208
Sex selection 2, 27, 36, 62, 64, 69,
    76, 97, 103, 116
Sperm 1, 2, 19, 24, 32, 57, 58,
    84–106, 111, 113, 116, 123, 142,
    297, 298–316, 331, 335, 341
Sperm donation, *See* donation,
    sperm
Stigma
    Abortion 203, 220
    Disability 27
    Donor insemination 95
    Infertility 86, 313, 327,
        334–336
    Large family 12–13
    Mutation carrier 156–159, 166
Surrogacy 1, 2, 17, 19, 24, 31,
    32, 68, 85, 89, 90, 101, 107–
    127, 177, 342–345, 354–356,
    358

Terrorization of pregnancy 177,
    185, 190–194
The silent scream (American
    pro-life video) 175, 176, 178,
    187

Ultrasonography 2, 26, 33, 56, 58,
    174–201, 208, 214, 217, 306,
    307, 312, 315, 355

Womanhood 75, 122, 323

Zionism 7, 12, 21, 29–30, 35, 36,
    154, 194, 219, 226, 228, 320,
    324, 336, 337
Zondek, Prof. 23, 51–54